CLINICAL AND LABORATORY MANUAL OF IMPLANT OVERDENTURES

CLINICAL AND LABORATORY MANUAL OF IMPLANT OVERDENTURES

Hamid R. Shafie

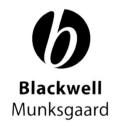

Blackwell
Munksgaard

Dr. Hamid R. Shafie received certification in Advanced Graduate Study of Prosthodontics from the Goldman School of Dental Medicine at Boston University. He founded the Center for Oral Implantology at Johns Hopkins University, where he trained many dentists in various aspects of implant dentistry. Dr. Shafie is president of the American Institute of Implant Dentistry, based in Washington, D.C. He is a faculty member in the Department of Oral and Maxillofacial Surgery at Washington Hospital Center, where he teaches postgraduate courses in oral implantology. He is an adjunct faculty member of the Boston University Center for Implantology.

Editorial Offices:
Blackwell Publishing Professional,
2121 State Avenue, Ames, Iowa 50014-8300, USA
Tel: +1 515 292 0140
9600 Garsington Road, Oxford OX4 2DQ
Tel: 01865 776868

Blackwell Publishing Asia Pty Ltd,
550 Swanston Street, Carlton South,
   Victoria 3053, Australia
Tel: +61 (0)3 9347 0300
Blackwell Wissenschafts Verlag, Kurfürstendamm 57,
   10707 Berlin, Germany
Tel: +49 (0)30 32 79 060

First published 2007 by Blackwell Munksgaard, a Blackwell Publishing Company

Library of Congress Cataloging-in-Publication Data

Clinical and laboratory manual of implant
   overdentures/[edited by] Hamid R. Shafie.
      p. ; cm.
   Includes bibliographical references and index.
   ISBN-13: 978-0-8138-0881-9 (alk. paper)
   ISBN-10: 0-8138-0881-2 (alk. paper)
   1. Implant-supported dentures.   2. Dental
implants.   I. Shafie, Hamid R.
   [DNLM: 1. Denture, Complete.   2. Dental
Prosthesis, Implant-Supported.   3. Denture,
Overlay. WU 530 C641 2006]

RK667.I45C55 2006
617.6′93—dc22

                                        2006036528

Set in India by TechBooks
Printed and bound by COS Printers Pte Ltd

For further information on Blackwell Publishing, visit our website: www.blackwellpublishing.com

Dedication

I am dedicating this book to the memory of my beloved daughter Melody. I wrote most of this book sitting next to her hospital bed during her fight with neuroblastoma cancer. She was a symbol of strength and hope in life.

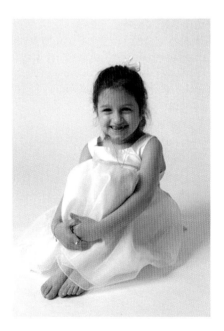

And . . .
To my parents, Mehdi and Minoo, who gave me a love of life,
To my wife Maryam, who gave me a life of love,
To my daughter Ava, who gave joy and meaning to it all.

Acknowledgments

My enormous gratitude to the Blackwell Publishing team for their willingness to go to bat with me: Antonia Seymour, Vice President, Professional Publishing; Dede Andersen, Managing Editor; Don Kehoe, Marketing Manager; Judi Brown, Project Manager/Editor; Martin Nielsen, Business Development Executive; and all of the other supporters at the Blackwell Publishing. They stood by me during the toughest period of my life and they never gave up on me.

My special thanks to Natalie Baratpour, the medical illustrator from Globalgraphic. She spent countless hours working with me to create all of the beautiful artwork for this book.

I would like to extend my special appreciation to my invaluable business manager Amanda Ludwa and my friend Christopher "Chris" Ludwa.

Contents

CONTRIBUTORS, xiii

FOREWORD, xv
Dennis Tarnow

FOREWORD, xvi
Zhimon Jacobson

INTRODUCTION, 1
Hamid Shafie

1 **Patient Preferences and
   Expectations, 3**
   Hamid Shafie

   Implant Overdenture vs. Conventional
      Denture, 3
   Implant Overdenture vs. Fixed
      Implant-Supported Prosthesis, 4
   Indications for Implant Overdenture, 4
   Comparison of Treatment Strategies for
      Implant Overdentures, 4
   The Breda Implant Overdenture Study, 5
   Overdenture Treatment Strategies, 6
   Common Mistakes in Constructing
      Implant-Supported Overdentures, 6
   Successful Implant-Supported
      Overdenture, 6
   References and Additional Reading, 6

2 **Diagnosis and Treatment
   Planning, 11**
   Hamid Shafie

   Diagnostic Workup for Implant
      Overdenture, 11
   Benefits of Diagnostic Mounting, 11
   Radiographic Evaluation, 12
      Panoramic Radiograph, 12
      Occlusal Radiograph, 13
      Computed Tomography
         (CT Scan), 14
   Joint Treatment Planning, 15
   Anatomical Considerations During
      Diagnosis and Treatment Planning
      Process, 15
      Available Bone Quantity, 15
      Classification of Fully Edentulous
         Ridges Based on Bone
         Quantity, 15
      Classification of Edentulous Ridges
         Based on Bone Quality, 17
   References and Additional Reading, 19

3 **Surgical Guide and Diagnostic
   Stent, 24**
   Hamid Shafie, Wolfram Stein, and
   Amir Juzbasic

Classification of Surgical Guides, 26
Gingiva Supported, 26
Bone Supported, 26
Components and the Advantages of the
med3D Technology, 27
Implant 3D Planning Software, 27
Stationary Robot or Positioning
Device X1, 29
Procedural Steps, 29
References and Additional Reading, 29

4 **Principles of Attachment
Selection**, 31
Hamid Shafie

Types of Attachments Based
on Resiliency, 32
Rigid Non-Resilient
Attachments, 32
Restricted Vertical Resilient
Attachments, 32
Hinge Resilient Attachments, 32
Combination Resilient
Attachments, 32
Rotary Resilient Attachments, 32
Universal Resilient Attachments, 32
Attachment Selection Criteria, 32
Different Attachment Assemblies, 33
Factors Influencing the Design and
Resiliency Level of the Attachment
Assembly, 33
Biomechanical Considerations, 33
Distal Extension to the Bar, 33
Load Distribution of Stud vs. Bar
Attachments, 33
Biomechanics of Maxillary
Overdenture, 33
References and Additional Reading,
34

5 **Stud Attachments**, 37
Hamid Shafie and James Ellison

Important Considerations Regarding the
Alignment of Stud Attachments, 37
ERA Attachment, 37
Chair-Side Utilization Procedure, 39
Changing ERA Male Component, 43
VKS-OC rs Stud Attachment, 44
Different Types of Matrices/Clips, 45

Clinical and Laboratory Procedures
for VKS-OC rs Attachment
Embedded in the Acrylic
Denture Base, 45
Clinical and Laboratory Procedures
for VKS-OC rs Attachment Cast
within the Chrome Cobalt
Framework, 49
Home Care, 52
Straumann Retentive Anchor
Abutment, 52
Contraindications for Using
Retentive Anchors, 53
Design Specifications of the
Retentive Anchor and Its
Corresponding Elliptical
Matrix, 53
Adjusting the Retention of the
Female Component, 54
Chair-Side Utilization of the
Retentive Anchor Abutment and
Elliptical Matrix, 55
Clix® Attachment and the Astra Implant,
57
Design Specification of the Clix®
Female Component, 57
Design Specification of the Astra Ball
Abutment, 57
Chair-Side Utilization Procedure, 58
Replacing Clix® Inserts, 59
References and Additional Reading,
60

6 **Bar Attachments**, 63
Hamid Shafie and James Ellison

Bar Materials, 63
Classification of Bar Attachments
Based on Cross-Sectional
Shapes, 63
Classification of Bars Based on the
Nature of Their Resiliency, 64
Factors that Influence the Flexibility of
the Bar, 64
Fundamentals of Bar Arrangement,
64
Vertical Relationship of the Bar to the
Alveolar Ridge, 66
Sagittal Relationship of the Bar to the
Alveolar Ridge, 66

Sagittal Relationship of the Bar to the
    Hinge Axis, 67
Anterior-Posterior Distance
    Rule, 68
Guidelines for Denture Base
    Extension, 68
Hader Bar, 69
    Fabrication Procedures for a
        Castable Hader Bar Attachment
        with Plastic Clips/Riders, 70
    Fabrication Procedures for a
        Castable Hader Bar Attachment
        with Gold Alloy Clips/Riders, 71
    Hader Clip Placement, 71
    Plastic Hader vs. Metal Clips, 72
    Mandibular Implant-Supported
        Overdenture Utilizing Hader
        Bar and Castable ERA
        Attachment, 72
    Troubleshooting for Hader Bar
        Attachment Assembly, 72
Dolder Bar, 72
    Indications, 72
    Contraindications, 73
    Dimensional Specifications, 73
    Fabrication Procedure for a Dolder Bar
        Unit, 75
    Relining an Overdenture with a
        Dolder Bar Unit Attachment
        Assembly, 75
    Fabrication Procedure for a Dolder Bar
        Joint, 75
    Relining an Overdenture with a
        Dolder Bar Joint Attachment
        Assembly, 76
Vario Soft Bar Pattern VSP, 76
    Advantages of Prefabricated
        Titanium Bar, 77
    Advantages of Plastic Castable
        Bar, 77
    Shapes of VSP Bar, 77
    Shapes of VSP Bar's Clips, 77
    Fabrication Procedures of a Rigid
        Fully Implant-Borne
        Overdenture Using a Parallel
        Bar, 78
    Fabrication Procedures of a Hinge
        Resilient Overdenture Using a
        Bredent VSP Bar, 81

Verification of Passive Seat of the
    Bar, 82
Incorporation of the Bar Assembly
    into the Denture, 82
References and Additional
    Reading, 82

7   Spark Erosion, 85
    Hamid Shafie, Eduard Eisenmann,
    and Günter Rübeling
    Sheffield Test, 85
    Most Common Reasons for Ill Fit, 88
    Spark Erosion Process, 88
        Clinical Steps, 89
        Laboratory Steps, 90
        Second Case, 96
    References and Additional Reading, 102

8   Treatment Success with Implant
    Overdenture, 104
    Hamid Shafie
    Implant Survival, 104
    Prosthetic Success, 104
    Patient Related Factors, 105
    Biomechanical Risk Factors for Upper
        Implant Overdenture, 105
    Biomechanical Risk Factors for Lower
        Implant Overdenture, 106
    Shape of the Mandible and Its Effect on
        the Loading of the Supporting
        Implants, 107
    References and Additional Reading, 108

9   Occlusion and Implant-Supported
    Overdenture, 112
    Hamid Shafie and Frank Luaciello
    Different Occlusal Schemes Formed by
        Denture Teeth, 112
    Set-Up Procedure for the Balanced
        Occlusion Utilizing Vita Physiodens
        Teeth, 113
        Setting Up the Premolars, 113
        Setting Up the Molars, 116
    Important Points to Remember During
        the Occlusal Adjustment, 120
        Semi-Anatomic, 120
        Non-Anatomic, 120
        Lingualized, 122

History of Lingualized (Lingual Contact)
    Occlusion, 123
Set-Up Procedure for Lingualized
    Occlusion Utilizing Ivoclar
    Ortholingual Teeth, 123
    1: Position Mandibular Teeth, 124
    2: Position Maxillary Teeth, 125
    3: Eliminate Maxillary Buccal Cusp
        Interferences, 126
    4: Eliminate Anterior Interferences,
        127
    5: Eccentric Balance, 127
Equilibration after Processing, 128
    1: Re-Establish Centric Occlusion
        Contacts, 128
    2: Eliminate Maxillary Buccal Cusp
        and/or Anterior Interferences,
        129
    3: Complete Equilibration by
        Adjusting Only the Incline
        Planes of the Mandibular
        Posterior Teeth, 129
Eccentric Jaw Movements, 129
References and Additional Reading, 130

10   **Surgical Considerations for Implant
     Overdenture, 132**
     Richard Green, George Obeid, Roy
     Eskow, and Hamid Shafie

Presurgical Instructions, 132
    Treatment Room Preparation and
        Utilization Protocol, 133
    Patient, 133
    Instruments, 133
Incisions and Flap Design, 133
    Incision and Flap Design
        Objectives, 133
    Basic Flap Designs, 133
Mandibular Surgery, 134
    1: Crestal Incision, 134
    2: Extended Crestal Incision, 134
    3: Vestibular Incision, 135
Maxillary Surgery, 136
    1: Crestal Incision, 136
    2: Palatal Incision, 136
    3: Buccal Incision, 136
    Tissue Punch Technique, 136
Osteotomy and Implant Placement, 137
Procedural Considerations during the
    Surgery, 137

Suturing Techniques Used for Implant
    Overdenture Surgeries, 138
    1: Simple Interrupted, 138
    2: Continuous (Locking or
        Non-Locking), 138
    3: Horizontal Mattress, 139
    Most Common Suturing Techniques
        for Implant-Supported
        Overdenture Cases, 139
    Suture Material, 139
Post-Surgical Care, 139
    Post-Healing Criteria for Successful
        Integration of the Implant with
        Surrounding Tissues, 140
    Procedural Considerations after
        Surgery, 140
Site Preparation for Overdentures, 140
    Techniques for Site Development,
        140
    Bone Grafting Materials, 140
    Available Resorbable Membranes,
        142
Split-Control System, 144
    Bone-Spreading Sequence, 144
Surgery-Related Problems, 146
References and Additional Reading,
    148

11   **Straumann Implant System, 153**
     Hamid Shafie

Two Sections of Straumann Implants,
    153
    Rough Surface on the Implant Body,
        153
    Polished Collar, 153
Endosseous Diameters, 154
Recommended Attachment Assemblies
    for Straumann Implants, 155
Surgical Steps for Standard Implants
    Ø 4.1mm RN (Regular Neck), 155
    1: Preparation of the Implant Bed, 155
    2: Drilling Sequence for Standard
        Implants Ø 4.1mm RN (Regular
        Neck), 156
    3: Tapping the Implant Site, 156
    4: Implant Insertion, 156
Wound Closure, 159
Healing Period for Straumann Implants
    with SLA Surface, 160

12 Endopore® Dental Implant System, 161
Hamid Shafie

Basic Facts, 161
  External Connection, 162
  Internal Connection, 162
Mechanical Rational for Short
    Endopore® Dental Implants, 162
  Advantages of the Endopore® Dental
    Implant System, 162
  Surgical Steps, 163
  Postsurgical Instructions, 166
  Implant Uncovering Steps, 167
  Prosthetic Steps, 167

13 Overdenture Implants, 168
Hamid Shafie

Classification of Overdenture Implants
    Based on Attachment Design
    Features, 168
Two Basic Purposes for Overdenture
    Implants, 169
  Providing Immediate Stabilization
    for an Overdenture, 169
  Acting as Transitional Implants
    During Initial Healing Phase, 169
Maximus OS Overdenture Implant,
    169
  Unique Features, 170
  Clinical Considerations, 170
  Surgical Steps, 171
  Prosthetic Steps, 178
ERA® Overdenture Implant, 179
  Design Specifications, 180
  Surgical Steps, 180
  Prosthetic Steps, 187
  Changing ERA Male
    Component, 189
References and Additional Reading,
    191

**14 Loading Approaches for Mandibular
Implant Overdentures, 192**
Dittmar May, George Romanos, and
Hamid Shafie

Healing Period before Loading, 192
Three Concepts in Premature Loading,
    192

Early Loading, 192
  Progressive Loading, 192
  Immediate Loading, 192
Critical Factors in Determining Loading
    Strategies, 192
Important Indicating Factors for
    Success of Prematurely Loaded
    Implants, 193
Advantages of Immediate Loading in
    Implant-Supported Overdenture
    Cases, 193
Important Requirements for Treatment
    Protocol, 193
SynCone® Concept, 194
  Advantages of Telescopic Crown
    Techniques, 194
  Patient Selection, 194
  Pre-Surgical Steps, 194
  Surgical Steps, 194
  Prosthetic Steps, 198
  Postoperative Instructions for
    Patient, 201
  Delayed Loading Protocol with
    SynCone® Concept, 202
Troubleshooting, 202
SynCone® Abutments and Framework-
    Reinforced Overdenture, 203
Procedural Sequences, 203
References and Additional Reading, 204

**15 Clinical Applications for the
Measurement of Implant Stability
Using Osstell™ Mentor, 206**
Hamid Shafie and Neil Meredith

Clinical Stages When ISQ Measurement
    Can Be Recorded, 208
Clinical Conditions Affecting the
    Outcome of Immediately
    Loaded Implants, 208

**16 Follow Up and Maintenance of the
Implant Overdenture, 210**
Valerie Sternberg Smith and
Roy Eskow

Characteristics of Ideal Peri-Implant
    Tissues, 210
Consequences for Failure to Achieve
    Cleansable Attachment Design, 210

Home Care Implements, 211
  Toothbrushes, 211
  Flossing Cords, 212
  Denture Brushes, 212
  Antimicrobials, 212
Recommended Routines at Recall
    Visits, 213
  Radiographic Examination, 213
  Removal of Accretions, 213
  Cleaning the Prosthesis, 213
  Evaluation of the Attachment
      Assembly Components, 213
References and Additional Reading, 214

**17   Core Principles of the Successful
        Implant Practice, 216**
Sean Crabtree, Paul Homoly, Andress
Charalabous, Peter Warkentin, and
Kornelius Warkentin

Vision, Team, Systems, Sales,
    Marketing, 216
  Center Point VISION, 216
  Organizational Model/Systems, 217
  People, 218
  Sales, 220
  Marketing, 223

Why Making Implant Overdentures Can
    Make Your Restorative Practice
    Click, 224
  Attracting Older Patients, 224
  Case Acceptance for Complete
      Dentistry, 225
Branding of an Implant Practice, 226
  Identity Ambassadors, 226
  External Marketing
      Objectives, 227
  Marketing Research, 227
  Create a Brand Name for Your
      Practice, 227
  Website, 227
Design Criteria for an Implant
    Practice, 228
  Reception Area, 229
  Waiting Room, 229
  Consultation Room, 230
  Surgical Operatory, 230
  Prosthetic Operatory, 230
  Hygiene and Recall Operatory, 231
  Sterilization Area, 231
  Staff Lounge, 231

INDEX, 233

Contributors

Andreas Charalambous, AIA, BArch
Cornell University
Principal, FORMA Design, Inc.

Sean M. Crabtree, BBA
Chairman/CEO Fortune Management
    of TN, Inc.

Eduard Eisenmann, DMD
Assistant Professor and Clinical Lecturer
Charite-University Medizin Berlin
Campus Benjamin Franklin,
Department of Restorative Dentistry
Berlin, Germany
Private Practice Limited to Implant
    Prosthodotics
Mannheim, Germany

James T. Ellison, CDT, BA, AAS
Director of Education for the ERA Academy

Roy L. Eskow, DDS
Practice Limited to Periodontics, Oral
    Medicine, Implant, and Regenerative
    Surgeries
Bethesda, Maryland

Robert N. Eskow, DMD, MScD
Clinical Professor,
The Ashman Department of Implant Dentistry,
New York University,
College of Dentistry
Private Practice,
Livingston, New Jersey

Richard J. Green, DDS, MScD
Staff Periodontist
VA Hospital,
Baltimore, Maryland
Private Practice Limited to Periodontics,
    Regenerative, and Implant Dentistry
    Bethesda, Maryland

Paul Homoly, DDS, CSP
President
Homoly Communications Institute

Amir Juzbasic, MDT
Director of Laboratory Services
American Institute of Implant Dentistry

Frank Lauciello, DDS
Associate Professor
State University of New York at Buffalo

Dittmar May, DMD
Oral and Maxillofacial Surgeon
Practice Limited to Implant Dentistry
Lunen, Germany

Neil Meredith, BDS., MSc., FDS, RCS, PhD (U.Lond.), PhD (U.Got.)
Visiting Professor
University of Bristol,
England

George Obeid, DDS
Chairman, Department of Oral and
    Maxillofacial Surgery
Washington Hospital Center

George Romanos, DDS, Dr.med.dent., PhD
Clinical Professor of Implant Dentistry
New York University,
New York, USA
Associate Professor of Oral Surgery
    and Implantology
University of Frankfurt, Germany

Günter Rübeling, MDT
Head of Department SAE DENTAL
    VERTRIEB + Development, Bremerhaven
Head of Department Rübeling + Klar
Dental-Labor GmbH,
Berlin, Germany

Wolfram Stein, MSc., PhD
Department of Cranio-Maxillo-Facial Surgery,
University of Heidelberg, Germany
Research Group for Computer Assisted
    Surgery

Valerie Sternberg Smith, RDH, BS
Clinical Instructor,
The Ashman Department of Implant Dentistry,
New York University,
College of Dentistry
Private Practice
Livingston, New Jersay

Kornelius Warkentin
Archetectual Solutions and Human Factor
Specialist
IS2 Teaching Center
Washington, DC

Peter Warkentin
Director of Patient/Doctor Interactive Interior
Design Courses
IS2 Teaching center
Washington, DC

Foreword

With all of the books available today on implants, it is refreshing to see one that is so well documented and thought out. It is a great honor for me to write this Foreword for Dr. Shafie's *Clinical and Laboratory Manual of Implant Overdentures*. With more than 20 million Americans being fully edentulous, there is no better time for this book to be written and utilized. Undergraduate programs across the country are finally realizing that the two implant overdenture is, by far, the recommended treatment of choice over leaving someone fully edentulous. The amount of bone loss that we in dentistry have seen in fully edentulous patients during past generations is frightening to consider. We actually thought and were teaching that this aveolar bone atrophy was "normal"
and continuous after extraction. What we now know is that two implants in the anterior mandible will stop this progressive bone loss and preserve the ridge instead of compressing it slowly as time passes.

Dr. Shafie should be complimented for his outstanding and detailed work. He describes each chapter with diagrams that are easy to follow, along with clinical pictures to document his thoughts. He also has covered the various abutment connections from many of the commercial companies that are being used today by clinicians all over the world. The discussion of occlusion and loading is particularly important for the technician and the clinician to understand. This manual is well organized and easy to follow with its step by step breakdown of each topic and technique. Besides the different implants and abutments that are available, the manual also goes into great detail on the construction of bars and how to best utilize them for different clinical situations. There is even a practice management chapter to help the clinician incorporate this technology into a practice. This clinical laboratory manual should become the gold standard for technicians and clinicians when dealing with overdentures. My deepest congratulations for a job well done to Dr. Shafie and his contributors.

Dennis Tarnow, Professor and Chairman
Department of Implant Dentistry
New York University College of Dentistry

Foreword

Given the increasing number of totally edentulous patients around the world, having the knowledge to plan treatment and place and restore implant-supported overdentures is more important than ever. Totally edentulous patients can become dentally-functional through the placement of dental implants to support complete dentures. It is a great injustice to allow patients, especially those who are financially restricted, to go through their lives without the renovating benefit of implants. The best venue for dentists to learn to treat patients with implants is in dental school as part of the regular curriculum. Dental education around the world has been lacking in training dental students about implantology, especially with regards to implant-supported complete dentures. This inadequacy has forced many dentists to seek training in implantology through short courses sponsored by implant companies. With several hundred implant systems available today, making sense of different options, surgically and prosthetically, is a monumental task. Dentists need accurate information regarding all aspects of implantology, presented scientifically and without commercial bias, and this book has fulfilled those requirements. Dr. Hamid Shafie has authored a very comprehensive and complete book that addresses the most common problems general dentists face in restoring implant-supported dentures. *Clinical and Laboratory Manual of Implant Overdentures* is invaluable as an educational tool and will be effective as a resource for both inexperienced and experienced dentists in treating edentulous patients. As a prosthodontic alumnus of Boston University Goldman School of Dental Medicine, Dr. Shafie has used his vast knowledge and experience to put together a very informative book on how to plan treatment and how to utilize attachments in implant-supported removable dentures. I congratulate Dr. Shafie for his hard work in compiling this information and presenting it in such a logical manner.

Zhimon Jacobson, Professor/Director
Center for Implantology
Boston University Goldman School of Dental Medicine

CLINICAL AND LABORATORY MANUAL OF IMPLANT OVERDENTURES

Introduction

Hamid Shafie

Total edentulism has been noted in 5 percent of adults who are 40 to 44 years old. This percentage gradually increases to almost 42 percent in seniors. However, these percentages are deceptively low because the baby boomer generation outnumbers the current population over 65. We will see a significant increase in the number of fully edentulous patients by the time baby boomers reach ages 65 and above.

The majority of general dentists still fabricate conventional complete, removable dentures for their fully edentulous patients. One of the main complaints of these patients is the instability of the lower denture. Since the conventional denture is fully tissue born and transfers all of the masticatory forces to the residual ridge, patients tend to experience significant and rapid loss of the alveolar ridge. Therefore, even an ideally fabricated, lower, removable, complete denture will be unstable after several months. This problem has helped denture adhesive manufactures build a multimillion-dollar market. Denture adhesive can be a quick solution for instability of removable prostheses but it does not eliminate the etiology; that is, constant bone loss due to direct transmission of masticatory forces to the residual alveolar ridge.

Dental implants have changed the face of prosthetic dentistry. They have shown a great success rate, as recorded in over 35 years of documentation. Dental implants were introduced to the United States in 1984 as an alternative treatment option for fully edentulous patients. Since then, however, most restorative dentists have focused on utilizing them more in the treatment of partially edentulous patients and less in treating fully edentulous patients. Probably one of the main reasons for devoting more attention to fixed partial dentures supported by implants is the significant demand by the sophisticated baby boomer generation. When this section of population reaches retirement age, we will see a significant demand for implant-supported overdentures.

The main benefit that the patient receives from any kind of implant treatment is prevention of further bone loss in areas where tooth or teeth are missing. Implant-supported overdentures not only provide required stability for the patient but also eliminate the etiology of this problem by preventing further bone loss.

All of the money that patients are paying for denture adhesive and fabrication of new conventional, removable dentures in the course of several years can be invested in more successful and predictable treatment options such as implant-supported overdentures.

One of the main reasons why restorative dentists may be reluctant to offer implant-supported overdentures to their patients is the complexity of attachment assemblies. About two hundred different attachments are available, making it difficult to choose the right attachment for a particular patient.

This book encourages the use of implant overdentures for fully edentulous patients and provides the information required to simplify the procedure:

- An easy way of classifying attachments regardless of brand name.

- Guidelines for the indications of each attachment assembly.
- Clinical steps fully illustrated with color pictures and schematic drawings.
- Treatment plan presentations for potential candidates of each type of treatment.
- Internal and external marketing methods related to each treatment modality.

Implant-supported overdentures should be the standard of care for all fully edentulous patients. Conventional, removable, complete dentures should be offered to a patient only if there is a medical or dental contraindication for implant placement or if the patient is not in a financial situation to afford an ideal treatment plan.

1
Patient Preferences and Expectations

Hamid Shafie

Results from some studies show a weak association between a patient's satisfaction with their prosthesis and the clinical qualities of the prosthesis as assessed by dentists. Some reports also show very little correlation between a patient's satisfaction and the clinical evaluation of the denture fit. On the other hand, a strong association does exist between a patient's perceived masticatory efficiency and their satisfaction with the prosthesis.

IMPLANT OVERDENTURE VS. CONVENTIONAL DENTURE

A major problem for edentulous patients has been a lack of satisfaction with their complete dentures. A survey of elderly patients showed that 66 percent were dissatisfied with their complete dentures. The main reasons for this dissatisfaction were discomfort, poor fit and retention, soreness, and pain, especially with mandibular dentures. Patients typically experience significantly less chewing difficulties with implant-supported overdentures than with conventional dentures. An evaluation of the mastication time and the magnitude of masticatory strokes show an almost equal efficiency for implant-supported overdentures and fixed implant-supported prosthesis. The implant procedure is relatively simple, and the treatment time is similar to that for complete dentures.

The data from several randomized studies confirm that implant-supported overdentures provide a better outcome than conventional dentures. Benefits include psychological effects such as satisfaction and oral health-related quality of life, as well as functional benefits such as chewing ability. This improved function could increase the range of foods that an edentulous patient can eat and, as a result, improve their nutrition and general health.

IMPLANT OVERDENTURE VS. FIXED IMPLANT-SUPPORTED PROSTHESIS

Creating a natural aesthetic, enhancing facial appearance, and compensating for lost soft and hard tissue is much easier with implant overdentures than with fixed prosthesis. Most patients can afford one type of implant overdenture since they are less expensive compared to fixed prosthesis. If one or more of the supporting implants fail, it is also easier to modify an existing implant overdenture. A two-piece, precision fit implant overdenture is a good solution when the implants are placed in an unfavorable trajectory and cannot be utilized for a fixed prosthesis. A milled substructure bar helps create an ideal path of insertion and an ideal aesthetic outcome.

Overdenture treatment has less clinical involvement compared to the fixed prosthesis, which is especially important in elderly patients with a medically compromised condition. In addition, this treatment option can be used in patients with compromised available bone. Implant survival rate is comparable to that for fixed implant-supported prosthesis.

INDICATIONS FOR IMPLANT OVERDENTURE

- Compromised bone support for conventional denture
- Poor neuromuscular coordination
- Low tolerance of mucosal tissues for a removable acrylic base
- Parafunctional habits leading to instability of prosthesis
- Active or hyperactive gag reflexes, stimulated by upper removable denture
- Psychological inability to wear a removable prosthesis
- Patient dissatisfaction with complete dentures and desire for more stability and comfort

- Congenital or oral and maxillofacial defects that need oral rehabilitation
- High prosthodontic expectations

COMPARISON OF TREATMENT STRATEGIES FOR IMPLANT OVERDENTURES

The implant overdenture obtains support and retention from an attachment assembly affixed to the implant and to the denture base. Considering the nature of masticatory force distribution, three basic types of implant overdentures are available:

- *Mainly Tissue-Supported Implant Overdenture*: When two prefabricated individual attachments are utilized, the overdenture is mainly tissue-born. The attachments provide retention for the overdenture. With this treatment modality, the denture base should provide maximum tissue coverage, similar to a conventional complete denture. During mastication, the residual ridge receives the majority of the masticatory forces, which means that this type of prosthesis is mainly tissue-born rather than implant-born.
- *Tissue-Implant-Supported Overdenture*: Tissue-implant-supported overdenture is more implant-born compared to the previous type of overdenture. To fabricate this type of overdenture, two implants and a resilient bar attachment assembly should be utilized. The denture base should still provide extended tissue coverage. During mastication, the attachment assembly and supporting implants receive most of the masticatory forces. The remainder of the chewing forces are transferred to the posterior aspect of the overdenture and ultimately absorbed by the supporting tissue.
- *Fully Implant-Supported Overdenture*: An attachment assembly that usually includes four or more implants supports the fully implant-supported overdenture. During

mastication, the attachment assembly transfers all of the masticatory forces to the supporting implants. With this type of overdenture, minimum flange and tissue coverage is required since the prostheses are fully implant-born. A minimum of four implants is required. In a patient with an ovoid or pointed alveolar ridge, three implants can be placed between the two mandibular foramens to form a tripod. In this case, the attachment assembly is not resilient, and the prosthesis is fully implantborn.

Successful fabrication of mainly tissue-supported implant overdentures and/or tissue-implant-supported overdentures still must adhere to the basic principles for fabricating a conventional complete dentures:

- Accurate impression of underlying tissue
- Maximum adaptation between the denture base and the residual ridge
- Proper vertical dimension of occlusion
- Accurate centric relation
- Appropriate denture teeth delection and set up

Any clinical or laboratory error in fabricating the implant overdenture may result in instability of the prosthesis, soreness, and ultimately patient dissatisfaction.

The mainly tissue-supported implant overdenture requires two implants placed between the mandibular foramen. The most common position is the canine area. However, placing the implants in the lateral area (approximately 14–15mm center to center) is another viable option. This option provides the opportunity to place more implants posterior in case the prosthesis must be changed to tissue-implant-supported or fully implant-supported in the future.

Another advantage of placing the implants in the lateral position is that it minimizes the hinge movement of the prosthesis around the axis, which passes through the attachments. If the implants were in the canine position, more hinge movement would occur when the patient tries to cut food with the lower incisors. Placing the implant in the lateral position reduces the anterior-posterior distance from the incisal edges to the hinge axis between the implants. This reduces the lift and movement of the posterior section of the overdenture away from the residual ridge, which ultimately increases stability.

THE BREDA IMPLANT OVERDENTURE STUDY

The Breda Implant Overdenture Study (BIOS) was set up as a randomized, controlled clinical trial to compare three different treatment options for edentulous patients using the Straumann implant system. One hundred and ten edentulous patients with atrophic mandibles and persistent conventional complete denture problems were selected. One-third of the patients received a mainly tissue-supported overdenture supported by two implants and two prefabricated ball attachments (2IBA), one-third received a tissue-implant-supported overdenture on two implants with a single bar (2ISB), and one-third received a fully implant-supported overdenture on four implants with a triple bar (4ITB).

For an overdenture with ball attachments, two Dolla Bona matrixes were used. For group 2ISB, an egg-shaped Dolder Bar with a single matrix was used. For group 4ITB, three egg-shaped Dolder Bars and three corresponding matrixes were used. The investigators reported that treatment of the edentulous mandible with four implants and three bar attachments is significantly more expensive than treatment with two individual attachments. However, multiple bar attachment assemblies require less long-term post-care costs. During the 96-month period of this investigation, the two implants and single bar attachment appeared to be the most effective for edentulous patients when considering patient satisfaction, clinical performance of the prostheses, and cost effectiveness. The study also found that patients who smoke are at a higher risk of complications when treated with mandibular implant overdentures.

OVERDENTURE TREATMENT STRATEGIES

The following factors affect the decision-making process regarding overdenture treatment strategies:

- Soreness and discomfort associated with the denture base and its flanges
- Bone quantity
- Patient's expectation for the treatment outcome
- Expected oral hygiene and patient compliance
- Jaw relationship
- Distance between the upper and lower alveolar ridge
- Expertise of the dentist and the lab technician
- Patient's finances

COMMON MISTAKES IN CONSTRUCTING IMPLANT-SUPPORTED OVERDENTURES

- Poor treatment planning
- Imprecise final impression
- Inaccurate master model as well as working model
- Ill fitting framework
- Poor choice of material and attachment.

SUCCESSFUL IMPLANT-SUPPORTED OVERDENTURE

Following are the basic requirements for a successful implant-supported overdenture:

- Stress-free fit of attachment assembly
- Good oral hygiene
- Biocompatibility of the chosen materials

- High biomechanical strength of chosen materials
- Functional and equilibrated occlusion
- Natural looking aesthetics
- Absence of interferences with normal phonetics

REFERENCES AND ADDITIONAL READING

Adell, R. (1983). Clinical results of osseointegrated implants supporting fixed prosthesis in edentulous jaws. *Journal of Prosthetic Dentistry*, 50, 251–254.

Adell, R., Eriksson, B., Lekholm, U., Branemark, P. I., & Jemt, T. (1990). A long-term follow-up study of osseointegrated implants in the treatment of totally edentulous jaws. *International Journal of Oral & Maxillofacial Implants*, 5, 347–359.

Adell, R., Lekholm, U., Rockler, B., & Branemark, P. I. (1981). A 15-year study of osseointegrated implants in the edentulous jaw. *International Journal of Oral Surgery*, 10, 387–416.

Albrektsson, T., Blomberg, S., Branemark, A., & Carlsson, G. E. (1987). Edentulousness—an oral handicap. Patient reactions to treatment with jawbone-anchored protheses. *Journal of Oral Rehabilitation*, 14, 503–511.

Allen, P. F., & McMillan, A. S. (2002). Food selection and perceptions of chewing ability following provision of implant and conventional prostheses in complete denture wears. *Clinical Oral Implant Research*, 13, 320–326.

Anttila, S. S., Knuuttila, M. L., & Sakki, T. K. (2001). Relationship of depressive symptoms to edentulousness, dental health, and dental health behavior. *Acta Odontologica Scandinavica*, 59, 406–412.

Awad, M. A. & Feine, J. S. (1998). Measuring patient satisfaction with mandibular prostheses. *Community Dentistry and Oral Epidemiology*, 26, 400–405.

Awad, M. A., Locker, D., Korner-Bitensky, N., & Feine J. S. (2000). Measuring the effect of intra-oral implant rehabilitation on the health-related quality of life in a randomized controlled clinical trial. *Journal of Dental Research*, 79, 1659–1663.

Awad, M. A., Lund, J. P., Dufresne, E., & Feine, J. S. (2003). Comparing the efficacy of mandibular implant-retained overdentures and conventional dentures among middle-aged edentulous patients: Satisfaction and functional assessment. *International Journal of Prosthodontics*, 16, 117–122.

Awad, M. A., Lund, L. P., Shapiro, S. H., et al. (2003). Oral health status and treatment satisfaction with mandibular implant overdentures and conventional dentures. A randomized clinical trial in a senior population. *International Journal of Prosthodontics*, 4, 390–396.

Axelsson, G. & Helgadottir, S. (1995). Edentulousness in Iceland in 1990. A national questionnaire survey. *Acta Odontologica Scandinavica*, 53, 279–282.

Axelsson, P., Paulander, J., & Lindhe, J. (1998). Relationship between smoking and dental status in 35-, 50-, 65-, and 75-year-old individuals. *Journal of Clinical Periodontology*, 25, 297–305.

Batenburg, R. H. K., van Oort, R. P., Reintsema, H., Brouwer, T. T., Raghoebar, G. M., & Boering, G. (1998). Mandibular overdentures supported by two Branemark, IMZ, or ITI implants. A prospective comparative preliminary study: One-year results. *Clinical Oral Implants Research*, 9, 374–383.

Berg E. (1984) The influence of some anamnestic, demographic, and clinical variables on patient acceptance of new complete dentures. *Acta Odontologica Scandinavica*, 42, 119–127.

Bergendal, T., & Engquist, B. (1998). Implant-supported overdentures: A longitudinal prospective study. *International Journal of Oral & Maxillofacial Implants*, 13, 253–262.

Bergman, B. & Carlsson, G. E. (1972). Review of 54 complete denture wearers. Patient's opinions 1 year after treatment. *Acta Odontologica Scandinavica*, 30, 399–414.

Boerrigter, E. M., Geertman, M. E., Van Oort, R. P., et al. (1995). Patient satisfaction with implant-retained mandibular overdentures. A comparison with new complete dentures not retained by implants—a multicentre randomized clinical trial. *British Journal of Oral & Maxillofacial Surgery*, 33, 282–288.

Boerrigter, E. M., Stegenga, B., Raghoebar, G. M., & Boering, G. (1995). Patient satisfaction and chewing ability with implant-retained mandibular overdentures: A comparison with new complete dentures with or without preprosthetic surgery. *Journal of Oral and Maxillofacial Surgery*, 53, 1167–1173.

Bosker, H. & van Dijk, L. (1989) The transmandibular implant: a 12-year follow-up study. *Journal of Oral and Maxillofacial Surgery*, 47, 442–450.

Bouma, J., Boerrigter, L. M., Van Oort, R. P., van Sonderen, E., & Boering, G. (1997). Psychosocial effects of implant-retained overdentures. *International Journal of Oral & Maxillofacial Implants*, 12, 515–522.

Bouma, J., Uitenbroek, D., Westert, G., Schaub, R. M., & van de Poel, F. (1987). Pathways to full mouth extraction. *Community Dentistry and Oral Epidemiology*, 15, 301–305.

Bouma, J., van de Poel, F., Schaub, R. M., & Uitenbroek, D. (1986). Differences in total tooth extraction between an urban and a rural area in the Netherlands. *Community Dentistry and Oral Epidemiology*, 14, 181–183.

Brodeur, J. M., Benigeri, M., Naccache, H., Olivier M., & Payette, M. (1996). Trends in the level of edentulism in Quebec between 1980 and 1993 [in French]. *Journal of the Canadian Dental Association* 62, 159–160, 162–166.

Budtz-Jorgensen, E. "Epidemiology: Dental and Prosthetic Status of Older Adults." Chapter 1 in *Prosthodontics for the Elderly: Diagnosis and Treatment*. Chicago: Quintessence Publishing, 1999.

Burns, D. R., Unger, J. W., Elswick, R. K. Jr., & Giglio, J. A. (1995). Prospective clinical evaluation of mandibular implant overdentures: Part I: Retention, stability and tissue response. *The Journal of Prosthetic Dentistry*, 73, 354–363.

Carlsson, G. E., Otterland, A., & Wennstrom, A. (1967). Patient factors in appreciation of complete dentures. *Journal of Prosthetic Dentistry*, 17, 322–328.

Centers for Disease Control and Prevention. (1999). Total tooth loss among persons aged > or = 65 years–Selected states, 1995–1997. *MMWR Morbidity and Mortality Weekly Report*, 48, 206–210.

Cune, M. S. "Overdentures on Dental Implants." (thesis, Utrecht, the Netherlands University of Utrecht, 1993).

Davis, D. M., Rogers, J. O., & Packer, M. E. (1996). The extent of maintenance required by implant-retained mandibular overdentures: A 3-year report. *International Journal of Oral & Maxillofacial Implants*, 11, 767–774.

Dolan, T. A., Gilbert, G. H., Duncan, R. P., & Roerster, U. (2001) Risk indicators of edentulism, partial tooth loss and prosthetic status among black and white middle-aged and older adults. *Community Dentistry and Oral Epidemiology*, 29, 329–340.

Douglass, C. W., Shih, A., & Ostry, L. (2002). Will there be a need for complete dentures in the United States in 2020? *Journal of Prosthetic Dentistry*, 87, 5–8.

Eklund, S. A. & Burt, B. A. (1994). Risk factors for total tooth loss in the United States; Longitudinal analysis of national data. *Journal of Public Health Dentistry*, 54, 5–14.

Enquist, B., Bergedal, T., Kallus, T., & Linden, U. (1988). A retrospective multicenter evaluation of osseointegrated implants supporting overdentures. *International Journal of Oral & Maxillofacial Implants*, 3, 129–134.

Esposito, M., et al. (2001). Quality assessments of randomized controlled trials of oral implants. *International Journal of Oral & Maxillofacial Implants*, 16, 783–792.

Feine, J. S., De Grandmont, P., Boudrias, P., et al. (1994). Within-subject comparisons of implant-supported mandibular prosthesis: Choice of prosthesis. *Journal of Dental Research*, 73, 1105–1111.

Feine, J. S., Maskawai, K., de Grandmont, P., Donohue, W. B., Tanguay, R., & Lund, J. P. (1994). Within-subject comparisons of implant-supported mandibular prostheses: Evaluation of masticatory function. *Journal of Dental Research*, 73, 1646–1656.

Fontijin-Teekamp, F. A., Slafter, A. P., van't Hof, M. A., Geertman, M. A., & Kalk, W. A. (1998). Bite forces with mandibular implant-retained overdentures. *Journal of Dental Research*, 77, 1832–1839.

Garrett, N. R., Kapur, K. K., Hamada, M. O., et al. (1998). A randomized clinical trial comparing the efficacy of mandibular implant-supported overtures and conventional dentures in diabetic patients. Part II. Comparisons of masticatory performance. *Journal of Prosthetic Dentistry*, 79, 632–640.

Geertman, M. E., Boerrigter, E. M, van't Hof, M. A., et al. (1996). Two-center clinical trial of implant-retained mandibular overdentures versus complete dentures—chewing ability. *Community Dentistry and Oral Epidemiology*, 24, 79–84.

Geertman, M. E., Boerrigter, E. M., van't Hof, M. A., et al. (1996). Clinical aspects of a multicenter clinical trial of implant-retained mandibular overdentures in patients with severely resorbed mandibles. *The Journal of Prosthetic Dentistry*, 75, 194–204.

Geertman, M. E., van Waas, M. A., van't Hof, M. A., & Kalk, W. (1996). Denture satisfaction in a comparative study of implant-retained mandibular overdentures: A randomized clinical trial. *International Journal of Oral & Maxillofacial Implants*, 11, 194–200.

Gilbert, G. H., Duncan, R. P., & Kulley, A. M. (1997). Validity of self-reported tooth counts during a telephone screening interview. *Journal of Public Health Dentistry*, 57, 176–180.

Hamasha, A. A., Hand, J. S., & Levy, S. M. (1998). Medical conditions associated with missing teeth and edentulism in the institutionalized elderly. *Special Care in Dentistry*, 18, 123–127.

Health Promotion Survey Canada. (1990). Statistics Canada. Available at: www.statcan.ca/english/sdds/3828.html. Accessed April 30, 2003.

Heydecke, G., Locker, D., Awad, M. A., Lund, J. P., Feine, J. S. (2003). Oral and general health status six months after treatment with mandibular implant overdentures and conventional dentures. A randomized clinical trial in an elderly population. *Community Dentistry and Oral Epidemiology*, 31, 161–168.

Johns, R. B., Jemt, T., Heath, M. R., Hutton, J. E., et al. (1992). A multicenter study of overdentures supported by Branemark implants. *International Journal of Oral & Maxillofacial Implants*, 7, 162–167.

Kapur, K. K. & Garrett, N. R. (1988). Requirements to clinical trials. *Journal of Dental Education*, 52, 760–764.

Kapur, K. K., Garrett, N. R., Hamada, M. O., et al. (1999). Randomized clinical trial comparing the efficacy of mandibular implant-supported overdentures and conventional dentures in diabetic patients. Part III: Comparisons of patient satisfaction. *Journal of Prosthetic Dentistry*, 82, 416–427.

Kent G. (1992). Effects of osseointegrated implants on psychological and social well-being; A literature review. *Journal of Prosthetic Dentistry*, 68, 515–518.

Krall, E. A., Dawson-Hughes, B., Garvey, A. J., & Garcia R. I. (1997). Smoking, smoking cessation, and tooth loss. *Journal of Dental Research*, 76, 1653–1659.

Langer, A., Michman, J., & Seiferd, I. (1961). Factors influencing satisfaction with complete dentures in geriatric patients. *The Journal of Prosthetic Dentistry*, 11, 1019–1031.

Lindquist, L. W., Carlsson, G. E., & Hedegard, B. (1986). Changes in bite force and chewing efficiency after denture treatment in edentulous patients with denture adaptation difficulties. *Journal of Oral Rehabilitation*, 13, 21–29.

Marcus, S. E., Drury, T. F., Brown, L. J., & Zion, G. R. (1996). Tooth retention and tooth loss in the permanent dentition of adults: United States, 1991–1998. *Journal of Dental Research*, 75 (spec no), 684–695.

Marcus, S. E., Kaste, L. M., & Brown, L. J. (1994) Prevalence and demographic correlates of tooth loss among the elderly in the United States. *Special Care in Dentistry* , 14, 123–127.

Mericske-Stern, R. (1990). Clinical evaluation of overdenture restorations supported by osseointegrated titanium implants: A retrospective study. *International Journal of Oral & Maxillofacial Implants*, 5, 375–383.

Naert, I., De Clercq, M., Theuniers, G., & Schepers, E. (1988). Overdentures supported by osseointegrated fixtures for the edentulous mandible: A 2.5-year report. *International Journal of Oral & Maxillofacial Implants*, 3, 191–196.

Osterberg, T., Carlsson, G. E., & Sundh, V. (2000). Trends and prognoses of dental status in the Swedish population: Analysis based on interviews in 1975 to 1997 by Statistics Sweden. *Acta Odontologica Scandinavica*, 58, 177–182.

Osterberg, T., Carlsson, G. E., Sundh, W., & Fyhrlund, A. (1995). Prognosis of and factors associated with dental status in the adult Swedish population. 1975–1989. *Community Dentistry and Oral Epidemiology*, 23, 232–236.

Palmqvist, S., Soderfeldt, B., & Vigild, M. (2001). Influence of dental care systems on dental status. A comparison between two countries with different systems but similar living standards. *Community Dental Health*, 18, 16–19.

Palmqvist, S., Soderfeldt, B., & Arnbjerg, D. (1992). Explanatory models for total edentulousness, presence of removable dentures, and complete dental arches in a Swedish population. *Acta Odontologica Scandinavica*, 50, 133–139.

Pietrokovski, J., Harfin, J., Mastavoy, R., & Levy, F. (1995). Oral findings in elderly nursing home residents in selected countries: Quality of satisfaction with complete dentures. *The Journal of Prosthetic Dentistry*, 73, 132–135.

Population projections for Canada, provinces and territories, 2000–2026 [catalogue no. 91-520-XPB]. Ottawa, Ontario: Statistics Canada, March 13, 2001.

Raghoebar, G. M., Meijer, H. J., Stegenga, B., van't Hof, M. A., van Oort, R. P., & Vissink, A. (2000). Effectiveness of three treatment modalities for the edentulous mandible. A five-year randomized clinical trial. *Clinical Oral Implants Research*, 11, 195–201.

Slade, G. D. & Spencer, A. J. (1994). Development and evaluation of the oral health impact profile. *Community Dental Health*, 11, 3–11.

Slade, G. D., Locker, D., Leake, J. L., Price, S. A., & Chao, I. (1990). Differences in oral health status between institutionalized and non-institutionalized older adults. *Community Dentistry and Oral Epidemiology*, 18, 272–276.

Slade, G. D., Offenbacher, S., Beck, J. D., Heiss, G., & Pankow, J. S. (2000). Acute-phase inflammatory response to periodontal disease in the US population. *Journal of Dental Research*, 70, 49–57.

Slagter, A. P., Olthoff, L. W., Bosman, F., & Steen W. H. (1992). Masticatory ability, denture quality, and oral conditions in edentulous subjects. *Journal of Prosthetic Dentistry*, 68, 299–307.

Steele, J. G., Treasure, E., Pitts, N. B., Morris, J., & Bradnock, G. (2000). Total tooth loss in the United Kingdom in 1998 and implications for the future. *British Dental Journal*, 89, 598–603.

Suominen-Taipale, A. L., Alanen, P., Helenius, H., Nordblad, A., & Uutela, A. (1999). Edentulism among Finnish adults of working age. 1978–1997. *Community Dentistry and Oral Epidemiology*, 27, 353–365.

Takala, L., Utriainen, P., & Alanen, P. (1994). Incidence of edentulousness, reasons for full clearance, and health status of teeth before extractions in rural Finland. *Community Dentistry and Oral Epidemiology*, 22, 254–257.

Thompson, G. W. & Kreisel, P. S. (1998). The impact of the demographics of aging and the edentulous condition on dental care services. *Journal of Prosthetic Dentistry*, 79, 56–59.

Tuominen, R., Rajala, M., & Paunio, I. (1984). The association between edentulousness and the accessibility and availability of dentists. *Community Dental Health*, 1, 201–206.

Unell, L., Soderfeldt, B., Halling, A., & Birkhed, D. (1998). Explanatory models for oral health expressed as number of remaining teeth in an adult population. *Community Dental Health*, 15, 155–161.

van Waas MA. (1990). The influence of clinical variables on patients' satisfaction with complete dentures. *Journal of Prosthetic Dentistry*, 63, 307–310.

Warren, J. J., Watkins, C. A., Cowen, H. J., Hand, J. S., Levy, S. M., & Kuthy, R. A. (2002). Tooth loss in the very old: 13–15-year incidence among elderly Iowans. *Community Dentistry and Oral Epidemiology*, 30, 29–37.

Wayler, A. H. & Chauncey, H. H. (1983). Impact of complete dentures and impaired natural detection of masticatory performance and food choice in healthy aging men. *Journal of Prosthetic Dentistry*, 49, 427–433.

WHO (World Health Organization). Oral Health Country/Area Profile Programme. Available at http://www.whocollab.od.mah.se/countriesalphab.html (accessed April 30, 2003).

Wismeijer, D., Van Waas, M. A. J., Vermeeren, J. I. J. F., Mulder, J., & Kalk, W. (1997). Patient satisfaction with implant-supported mandibular overdentures. A comparison of three treatment strategies on ITI dental implants. *International Journal of Oral & Maxillofacial Surgery*, 26, 263–267.

Wismeijer, D., Van Wass, M. A. J., Vermeeren, J. I. J. F., Mulder, J., & Kalk, W. (1999). Clinical and radiological results of patients treated with three treatment modalities for overdentures on implants of the ITI-dental implant system. *Clinical Oral Implant Research*, 10, 297–306.

Wismeijer, D., Vermeeren, J. I. J. F., & van Waas, M. A. J. (1992). Patient satisfaction with overdentures supported by one-stage TPS implants. *International Journal of Oral & Maxillofacial Implants*, 7, 51–55.

Wismeijer, D., Vermeeren, J. I. J. F., & van Waas, M. A. J. (1995). 6.5 year evaluation of patient satisfaction and prosthetic aftercare in patient treatment using overdentures supported by ITI implants. *International Journal of Oral & Maxillofacial Implants*, 10, 744–749.

World Bank Group. Data and statistics. Available at http://www.worldbank.org/data/quickreference/quickref.html (accessed May 15, 2002).

Zarb, G. A. & Schmitt, A. (1990). The longitudinal clinical effectiveness of osseointegrated dental implants: The Toronto study. Part I: Surgical results. *Journal of Prosthetic Dentistry*, 63, 451–457.

2
Diagnosis and Treatment Planning

Hamid Shafie

Diagnosis and treatment planning are the most important parts of the entire implant therapy, determining whether the treatment will be a success or a failure. Skipping any of the recommended steps of the treatment-planning phase compromises the outcome of the final treatment.

DIAGNOSTIC WORKUP FOR IMPLANT OVERDENTURE

1. Perform a radiographic evaluation by utilizing a panoramic x-ray. Determine the magnification error of that image, and then determine the height of available bone.
2. Evaluate the existing conventional upper and lower denture to determine if satisfactory aesthetic, phonetic, and function have been achieved.
3. If the existing denture is satisfactory, it can be duplicated with clear acrylic and used for diagnostic mounting and fabrication of the surgical guide.

4. Take a bite registration record in centric relation for a diagnostic mounting.
5. Mount the duplicated upper and lower denture on an articulator.
6. Choose the proper length and diameter for the designated implant system.
7. Choose the number and location of the implants based on the desired attachment assembly.

BENEFITS OF DIAGNOSTIC MOUNTING

- Creates a surgical template
- Visualizes the relationship of the denture teeth with anticipated implant positions
- Gives the clinician and lab technician a good idea of the position and final design of the bar
- Creates an index for the position of the final overdenture teeth

In patients with a high smile line, a removable overdenture will more likely fulfill the patient's functional and aesthetic demands better than an implant-supported fixed bridge. If the patient's upper lip support needs to be enhanced, an implant-supported overdenture with a labial flange is the preferred choice of treatment.

If the relationship between the maxilla and mandible is unfavorable, such as class II or class III, or if excessive inter-ridge space is present, implant-supported overdentures are preferred over fixed bridges supported by implants.

RADIOGRAPHIC EVALUATION

Panoramic Radiograph

The panoramic radiograph is the most common image used to evaluate implant overdenture cases. This radiograph produces a single image of the maxilla and mandible with all of the anatomical landmarks in a frontal plane. It is very cost effective and practical, because it can be generated in most dental offices. The clinician can easily identify the gross anatomy of the jaws and opposing landmarks, as well as form an initial assessment of the vertical height of the bone. Any pathology within the maxillary and/or mandibular bone can be detected. The patient is exposed to a relatively low radiation dose compared to a CT scan or conventional tomogram.

However, the panoramic radiograph has several disadvantages such as overlapping images, distortion of the special relationship among anatomical landmarks, and magnification errors. Also, fine anatomical details cannot be seen as they appear on a CT scan. This radiograph usually increases the horizontal dimension by about 30–70 percent and increases the vertical dimension by about 20–30 percent.

The use of a diagnostic template while taking the panoramic x-ray can effectively eliminate the magnification error. The diagnostic template is an acrylic base, which has been fabricated over the study cast.

One or more ball bearings (BBs) should be incorporated into the template using self-cured acrylic. Place the BBs as close as possible to the desired implant sites (Figure 2.3).

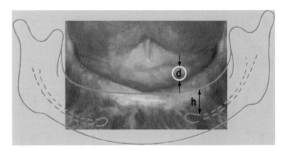

FIGURE 2.1.

DETERMINING MAGNIFICATION ERROR OF PANORAMIC X-RAYS

1. Measure the diameter of the ball bearings before incorporating them into the templates (Figure 2.2).

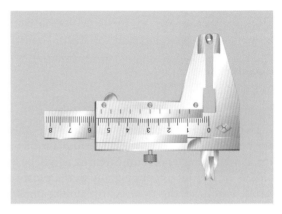

FIGURE 2.2.

2. Incorporate the ball bearings into the acrylic template utilizing self-cured acrylic (Figure 2.3).

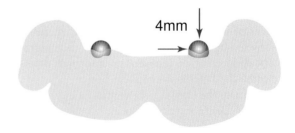

4mm

FIGURE 2.3.

3. Insert the acrylic template in the patient's mouth (Figure 2.1).
4. Take the x-ray image (Figure 2.4).

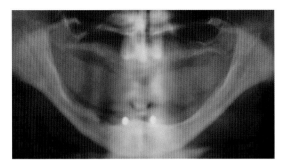

FIGURE 2.4.

5. Measure the diameter of the ball bearings as they appear in the x-ray image.
6. Use the following formula to calculate the actual height of the alveolar process:

d = Actual diameter of the ball bearing
D = Diameter of ball bearing in the panoramic x-ray
H = Height of the bone in the panoramic x-ray
h = Actual height of the bone
Magnification Error: ME = d ÷ D
h = ME × H

PANORAMIC LANDMARKS

- Crest of the ridge
- Opposing landmarks

Note the opposing landmarks in the mandible (Figure 2.5):

- *Anterior*: Inferior border of the symphysis
- *Canine/Premolar Region*: Mental foramina
- *Posterior*: Mandibular nerve canal

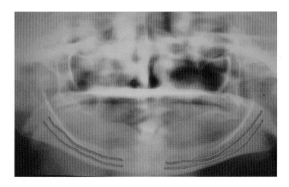

FIGURE 2.5.

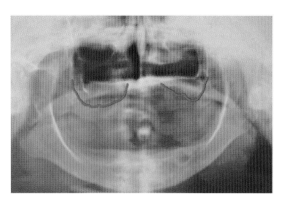

FIGURE 2.6.

Note the opposing landmarks in the maxilla (Figure 2.6):

- *Anterior*: Inferior border of the nasal cavity
- *Canine/Premolar Region*: Lateral walls of the nasal cavity and anterior border of the maxillary sinus
- *Posterior*: Floor of the maxillary sinus

During treatment planning for a mandibular implant overdenture, this radiograph can provide a fair approximation of the position of the most distal supporting implants. The position of the mental nerve, the path of the mandibular nerve canal, and the height of the alveolar ridge have a great influence on the position of most distal implants.

The mandibular nerve canal generally extends 3–4mm anterior to the mental foramen. However, the mandibular nerve may loop forward 6–7mm in some patients. It is recommended that you position the center of the distal implant 7mm mesial to the mental foramen to eliminate any possibility of nerve injury. **Note** that all anatomical variations are patient-specific.

Occlusal Radiograph

An occlusal radiographic image is very helpful in assessing the width of the bone in the mandibular symphysis area. Employ proper techniques such as symmetrical positioning of the central ray and the film.

Make an acrylic base on the lower cast and glue a 5mm diameter ball bearing to the side of the acrylic base in the symphysis area. The patient should wear this acrylic base when the image is taken. Changes in the diameter of the ball bearing in the radiograph will help the clinician determine the magnification error of the radiograph.

Computed Tomography (CT Scan)

Since plain films fail to provide data on bone width and bone density, clinicians started utilizing CT scan technology to enhance their diagnostic and treatment planning abilities (Figure 2.7).

technology results in no magnification error, and all of the images have the exact same dimensions as the patient's anatomical structure being examined. Therefore, this scan permits precise measurement of the bony structure that is relevant to the desirable implant locations in all three planes.

The techniques for producing clinically useful CT image vary, depending upon the equipment employed. However, regardless of the type of equipment, the thickness of each cut must be 1mm or less.

Placing a radioopaque material such as special barium sulfate teeth as a marker in the diagnostic guide identifies the desired site for an implant placement (Figure 2.8). This allows the clinician to see the makers on the CT images and evaluate the underlying bony structure.

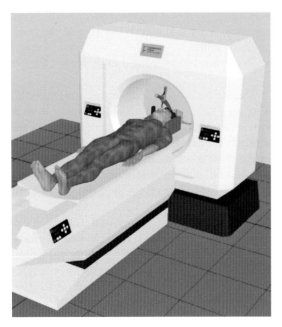

FIGURE 2.7.

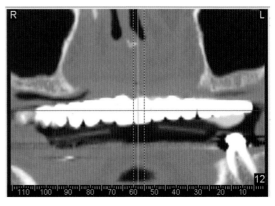

FIGURE 2.8.

CT analysis of the jaws is normally very expensive; the technique is therefore generally used only if additional diagnostic information is necessary due to anatomical complexity or other diagnostic difficulties. The need to assess accurately the position of the inferior alveolar canal, the mental foramen, the contour of the lingual surface of the mandible, and the floor of the sinuses are primary indications for using a CT scan during the treatment planning phase for implant overdenture cases. The advantages of CT scanning when planning for the placement of dental implants must be balanced against the cost and the amount of the radiation exposure incurred with CT scans.

The CT scan creates three-dimensional images of the edentulous arches at 1.00mm intervals from left to right around the entire dental arch in both the mandible and maxilla. The images (cross sections) are sequentially numbered. The clinician has at his or her disposal cross-sectional, panoramic, and occlusal views of the actual osseous topography. This radiographic

JOINT TREATMENT PLANNING

The next phase in the treatment planning process involves an effective conference among the entire implant team, which consists of the restorative dentist, surgeon, and laboratory technician, along with any number of supporting members such as the hygienist and the representative of the implant company.

The crucial factor in building an effective conference is to create a team of people, each of whom knows his or her job and can perform it well. Each member of the team must be committed to listening as well as sharing his or her ideas and observations. Ideally, the treatment planning conference should be done in person. However, it can be conducted via telephone or web conferencing.

The leader of this team will be the restorative dentist. He or she begins the communication with the patient regarding the patient's chief complaint and continues that communication throughout the treatment process and beyond. The secondary leaders in this process are the surgeon and the laboratory technician.

ANATOMICAL CONSIDERATIONS DURING DIAGNOSIS AND TREATMENT PLANNING PROCESS

Available Bone Quantity

Bone quantity is one of the most important factors that dictate the treatment plan. The height, width, length, and shape of the available bone should be assessed.

HEIGHT OF BONE The distance between the crest of the alveolar ridge and opposing anatomical landmarks (e.g., maxilla: floor of the sinuses and the nasal cavity; mandible: the mandibular nerve canal, mental foramina, and inferior border of the symphysis) determines the height of the bone. It is advisable to leave 2mm between the bottom of the implant and border of the opposing landmark. The height of the bone can easily be determined through a panoramic x-ray.

WIDTH OF BONE The distance between the buccal and lingual walls of the alveolar process determines the width of the bone. It is recommended that at least 1mm thickness of the bone should remain on the buccal and lingual aspects of the implants. Very thin buccal and lingual bone plates around the implant will have a compromised blood supply and increase the risk of bone loss. The width of the bone cannot be determined by a panoramic x-ray. However, the occlusal x-ray or the CT scan will provide suitable images for measuring the width of the bone.

SHAPE OF BONE The shape of the alveolar ridge influences the clinician's selection of the shape of the implant body (e.g. choosing a tapered implant vs. parallel sided screw). The shape of the bone influences the trajectory of the implant, which is not always inline with the path of insertion of the overdenture. This problem can cause application of destructive forces to the supporting implants. The shape of the bone can be modified by bone grafting techniques or alveoloplasty.

LENGTH OF BONE The distance from one point of the alveolar ridge to another point in the mesio-distal direction determines the length of the bone. The mesio-distal distance between the supporting implants will be determined based on the design of the attachment assembly.

Misch and Judy described an easy and practical classification for fully edentulous jaws based on the available bone.

Classification of Fully Edentulous Ridges Based on Bone Quantity

GROUP A There is minimum bone loss, which translates to less inter-ridge space. On average, the height of the bone in the anterior mandible is more than 20mm, and the width of

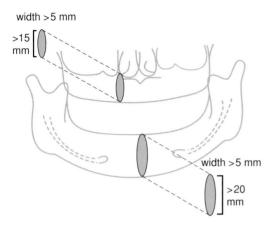

FIGURE 2.9.

the bone is more than 5mm (Figure 2.9). The height of the bone in the anterior maxilla is usually more than 15mm, and most of the time the width of the bone is more than 5mm. Because of small inter-ridge space, patients in this group are not good candidates for a bar attachment assembly. Insufficient room is available to fabricate a cleansable bar and an overdenture with adequate denture base thickness. Patients in this category are good candidates for hybrid prosthesis as well as overdenture supported by stud attachments.

GROUP B   The height and width of the bone is less than group A, which means more interridge space is available. On average, the height of the bone in the anterior mandible is between 15–20mm, and the width is more than 5mm (Figure 2.10). The height of the bone in the an-

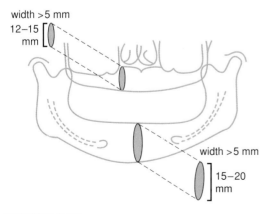

FIGURE 2.10.

terior maxilla is approximately 12–15mm, and the width is more than 5mm. Patients in this group can qualify for any kind of implant overdenture. The bone quantity and inter-ridge space allow the clinician to utilize any type of attachment assembly.

GROUP C   Patients in this group demonstrate severe resorption of the alveolar process. The height of the bone in the anterior mandible is approximately 10–15mm, and the width of the bone in this region is almost 5mm (Figure 2.11). The height of the bone in the anterior maxilla is less than 10mm, and the width of the bone is less than 5mm. This means that patients have expansive inter-ridge space. These patients generally are not good candidates for a stud attachment assembly since the expansive inter-ridge space translates into longer teeth and denture base. This space will increase the chance of lateral dislodgement of the prosthesis if the overdenture is supported by small and short stud attachments. Bar attachments are strongly recommended for this group of patients. However, exceptional situations mandate use of stud attachments for these types of patients. (Refer to Chapter 5, "Stud Attachments.") In some cases, alveolar ridge augmentation, ridge expansion, or sinus lift may be necessary.

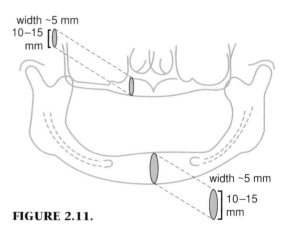

FIGURE 2.11.

GROUP D   Patients in this group demonstrate complete resorption of the alveolar process, as well as part of the basal bone. Generally, the height of the bone in the anterior mandible is

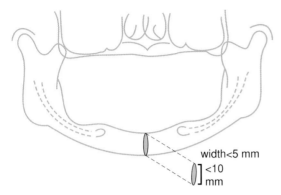

FIGURE 2.12.

less than 10mm, and the width of the bone is less than 5mm (Figure 2.12). The height and width of the bone in the anterior maxilla is severely deficient. Any overdenture treatment for patients in this group requires advanced bone grafting procedures to accommodate implants longer than 10mm length and 4mm in diameter. The other approach to accommodate patients in this group is to utilize shorter implants with expansive surface area instead of subjecting the patient to the bone grafting procedure. The endopore implant has been designed with a porous titanium surface and a tapered body and can be used in most of the group D patients with compromised bone quantity. (Refer to Chapter 12.)

Classification of Edentulous Ridges Based on Bone Quality

A direct correlation exists between the primary stability of the implants and the bone quality. This is a very important factor if the patient has been treatment planned for immediately-loaded overdenture.

Since most of the implant overdenture patients are over 50 years of age, the issue of bone quality plays a roll in the prognosis of the treatment. Most people in this age group, especially women, experience some level of osteoporosis. Generally, in osteoporotic patients, a physiological reduction of the trabecular bone can be observed. The most accurate way to determine the bone quality is by assessing the bone during the surgical steps or when the clinician starts drilling the osteotomy.

Misch described a simple classification for different bone quality osteotomy (Figure 2.13):

- *D1*: Thick, compact bone
- *D2*: Thick, porous, compact bone with a highly trabecular core
- *D3*: Thin, porous, compact bone surrounding a loosely structured cancellous bone
- *D4*: Loose, thin, cancellous bone

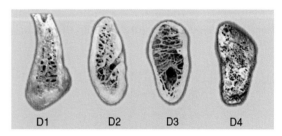

FIGURE 2.13. (Photo courtesy of Dr. Eliane dos Santos Porto Barboza)

D1: THICK, COMPACT BONE This type of bone usually can be found in the symphysis part of the mandible (Figure 2.14).

Advantages
- Provides good primary stability for the implants
- Expansive implant bone interface
- Use of short implants is possible
- Overdenture can be loaded immediately

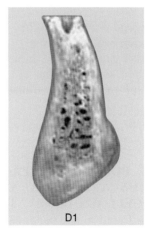

FIGURE 2.14. (Photo courtesy of Dr. Eliane dos Santos Porto Barboza)

Disadvantages
- Reduced blood supply
- Difficult implant bed preparation, which can cause overheating
- Extra step of tapping the bone is required to eliminate the possibility of the pressure necrosis

D2: THICK, POROUS, COMPACT BONE WITH A HIGHLY TRABECULAR CORE

This type of bone can be found in the anterior and posterior portions of the mandible as well as the palatal aspect of the anterior maxilla (Figure 2.15).

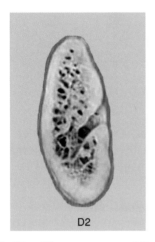

FIGURE 2.15.   (Photo courtesy of Dr. Eliane dos Santos Porto Barboza)

Advantages
- Provides good primary stability
- Easy implant bed preparation
- Overdenture can be loaded immediately
- Good blood supply, which means shorter healing time and faster osseointegration

Disadvantages
- None

D3: THIN, POROUS, COMPACT BONE SURROUNDS A LOOSELY STRUCTURED CANCELLOUS BONE
This type of bone can be found in the facial aspect of the anterior maxilla, posterior maxilla, posterior portion of the mandible, and the remaining bone after the osteoplasty of the D2 bone (Figure 2.16).

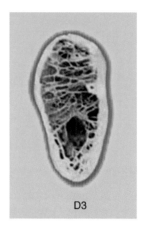

FIGURE 2.16.   (Photo courtesy of Dr. Eliane dos Santos Porto Barboza)

Advantages
- Good blood supply

Disadvantages
- Possibility of unwanted widening of the osteotomy, which can leads to poor primary stability
- Reduced implant bone interface

D4: LOOSE, THIN CANCELLOUS BONE
This type of bone can be found in the posterior maxilla as well as the remaining bone after osteoplasty of the D3 bone (Figure 2.17).

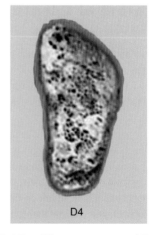

FIGURE 2.17.   (Photo courtesy of Dr. Eliane dos Santos Porto Barboza)

Advantages
- None

Disadvantages
- Poor primary stability
- Reduced implant bone interface

REFERENCES AND ADDITIONAL READING

Abrahams, J. J. & Arjun, K. (1995). Dental implants and dental CT software programs. *Seminars in Ultrasound, CT and MRI* 16(6), 468.

Abrahams, J. J. (1993) The role of diagnostic imaging in dental implantology. *Radiologic Clinics of North America*, 31(1), 163.

Adell, R., Eriksson, B., Lekholm, U., Branemark, P. I., & Jemt, T. (1990). A long-term follow-up study of osseointegrated implants in the treatment of the totally edentulous jaws. *International Journal of Oral & Maxillofacial Implants*, 5, 347–359.

Adell, R., Lekholm, U., Rockler, B., & Branemark, P. I. (1981). A 15-year study of osseointegrated implants in the edentulous jaw. *International Journal of Oral Surgery*, 10, 387–416.

Adell, R. (1983). Clinical results of osseointegrated implants supporting fixed prosthesis in edentulous jaws. *Journal of Prosthetic Dentistry*, 50, 251–254.

Albrektsson, T., Blomberg, S., Branemark, A., & Carlsson, G. E. (1987). Edentulousness—an oral handicap. Patient reactions to treatment with jawbone-anchored prostheses. *Journal of Oral Rehabilitation*, 14, 503–511.

Balshi, T. J., Ekfeldt, A., Stenberg, T., & Vrielinck, L. (1997). Three-year evaluation of Branemark implants connected to angulated abutments. *International Journal of Oral & Maxillofacial Implants*, 12, 52.

Basten, C. H. J. (1995). The use of radioopaque templates for predictable implant placement, *Quintessence International*, 26, 609.

Batenburg, R. H. K., van Oort, R. P., Reintsema, H., Brouwer, T. T., Raghoebar, G. M., & Boering, G. (1998). Mandibular overdentures supported by two Branemark, IMZ, or ITI implants. A prospective comparative preliminary study: One-year results. *Clinical Oral Implants Research*, 9, 374–383.

Benz, O., Mouyen, F., & Razzano, M. "Radiovisiography: concept and applications." Chapter 18 in *Computers in Clinical Dentistry*. Chicago: Quintessence Publishing, 1993.

Bergendal, T. & Engquist, B. (1998). Implant-supported overdentures: A longitudinal prospective study. *International Journal of Oral & Maxillofacial Implants*, 13, 253–262.

Block, M. S. & Kent, J. N. (1995). *Endosseous Implants for Maxillofacial Reconstruction*. Philadelphia: W.B. Saunders Company, 1995.

Borrow, J. W. & Smith, J. P. (1996). Stent marker material for computer tomography-assisted implant planning, *International Journal of Periodontics & Restorative Dentistry*, 16, 61.

Bosker, H. & van Dijk, L. (1989). The transmandibular implant: a 12-year follow-up study. *Journal of Oral and Maxillofacial Surgery* 47, 442–450.

Branemark, P. –I., Zarb, G. A., & Albrektsson, T. *Tissue-Integrated Prostheses: Osseointegration in Clinical Dentistry*. Chicago: Quintessence Publishing, 1985.

Burns, D. R., Unger, J. W., Elswick, R. K. Jr., & Giglio, J. A. (1995). Prospective clinical evaluation of mandibular implant overdentures: Part I: Retention, stability and tissue response. *Journal of Prosthetic Dentistry*, 73, 354–363.

Buser, D., Mericske-Stern, R., Bernard, J. P., et al. (1997). Long-term evaluation of non-submerged ITI implants. Part 1: 8-year life table analysis of a prospective multicenter study with 2,359 implants. *Clinical Oral Implants Research*, 8, 161–172.

Carr, A.B. (1998). Successful long-term treatment outcomes in the field of osseointegrated implants: Prosthodontic determinants. *International Journal of Prosthodontics*, 11(5), 502–512.

Chan, M. F., Narhi, T. O., de Baat, C., & Kalk, W. (1998). Treatment the atrophic edentulous maxilla with implant-supported overdentures. A review of the literature. *International Journal of Prosthodontics*, 11, 207–215.

Cordioli, G., Majzoub, Z., & Castagna, S. (1997). Mandibular overdentures anchored to single implants: A five-year prospective study. *Journal of Prosthetic Dentistry*, 78, 159–165.

Cune, M. S. "Overdentures on Dental Implants." (thesis, Utrecht, the Netherlands University of Utrecht, 1993).

Davis, D. M., Rogers, J. O., & Packer, M. E. (1996). The extent of maintenance required by implant-retained mandibular overdentures: A 3-year report. *International Journal of Oral & Maxillofacial Implants*, 11, 767–774.

Dharmar S. (1997). Locating the mandibular canal in panoramic radiographs, *International Journal of Oral & Maxillofacial Implants*, 12, 113.

Duchmanton, N. A., Austin, B. W., Lechner, S. K., & Klineberg, I. J. (1994). Imaging for predictable maxillary implants. *International Journal of Prosthodontics*, 7, 77.

Dudic, A. & Mericske-Stern, R. (2002). Retention mechanism and prosthetic complications of implant-supported mandibular overdentures: Long-term results. *Clinical Implant Dentistry and Related Research*, 4, 212–219.

Duyck, J., Van Oosterwyck, H., Vander Sloten, J., Cooman, M., Puers, R., & Naert, I. (1999). In vivo forces on implants supporting a mandibular overdenture: influence of attachment system. *Clinical Oral Investigations*, 99, 201–207.

Emmott, L. F. (1999). Digital radiography. *Dentistry Today*, May, 106.

Emmott, L. F. (1999). Digital radiography, how to buy a system in an evolving market. *Dental Economics*, May, 50.

Enquist, B., Bergedal, T., Kallus, T., & Linden, U. (1988). A retrospective multicenter evaluation of osseointegrated implants supporting overdentures. *International Journal of Oral & Maxillofacial Implants*, 3, 129–134.

Esposito, M., et al. (2001). Quality assessments of randomized controlled trials of oral implants. *International Journal of Oral & Maxillofacial Implants*, 16, 783–792.

Farman, A. G., Farag, A. (1993). Teleradiology for dentistry. *Dental Clinics of North America*, 37, 69.

Farman, A. G., Farman, T. T. (1999). Radio VisioGraphy-ui: a sensor to rival direct exposure intra-oral x-ray film. *International Journal of Computerized Dentistry*, 2, 183.

Farman, A. G., Mouyen, F. "Evaluation of the new RadioVisioGraphy: concept and application." Chapter 18 in *Computers in Clinical Dentistry*. Chicago: Quintessence Publishing, 1993.

Feine, J. S., Awad, M. A., & Lund, J. P. (1998). The impact of patient preference on the design and interpretation of clinical trials. *Community Dentistry and Oral Epidemiology*, 26, 70–74.

Feine, J. S., de Grandomont, P., Boudrias, P., et al. (1994). Within subject comparisons of implant-supported mandibular prosthesis: Choice of prosthesis. *Journal of Dental Research*, 73, 1105–1111.

Fontijin-Teekamp, F. A., Slafter, A. P., van't Hof, M. A., Geertman, M. A., & Kalk, W. A. (1998). Bite forces with mandibular implant-retained overdentures. *Journal of Dental Research* 77, 1832–1839.

Fredholm, U., Bolin, A., & Andersson, L. (1993). Pre-implant radiographic assessment of available maxillary bone support. Comparison of tomographic and panoramic technique, *Swedish Dental Journal*, 17, 103.

Frost, H. M. (1999). Changing views about "Osteoporosis" (a 1998 overview). *Osteoporosis International*, 10, 345–352.

Fugazzotto, P. A. (1997). Success and failure rates of osseointegrated implants in function in regenerated bone for 6 to 51 months: a preliminary report, *International Journal of Oral & Maxillofacial Implants*, 12, 17.

Garrett, N. R., Kapur, K. K., Hamada, M. O., et al. (1998). A randomized clinical trial comparing the efficacy of mandibular implant-supported overdentures and conventional dentures in diabetic patients. Part II. Comparisons of masticatory performance. *Journal of Prosthetic Dentistry*, 79, 632–640.

Geertman, M. E., Boerrigter, E. M., van't Hof, M. A., et al. (1996). Clinical aspects of a multicenter clinical trial of implant-retained mandibular overdentures in patients with severely resorbed mandibles. *Journal of Prosthetic Dentistry*, 75, 194–204.

Glantz, P. O. & Nilner, K. (1997). Biomechanical aspects on overdenture treatment. *Journal of Dentistry*, 25(supplement 1), 21–24.

Gotfredsen, K. & Holm, B. (2001). Implant-supported mandibular overdentures retained with ball or bar attachments: A randomized prospective 5-year study. *International Journal of Prosthodontics*, 13, 125–130.

Higginbottom, F. L. & Wilson, T. G. (1997). Three-dimensional templates for placement of root-form dental implants: a technical note., *International Journal of Oral & Maxillofacial Implants*, 12, 52.

I.D.T. Seminar, Atlanta, Georgia, Dec 3–5, 1992.

Jaffin, R. A. & Berman, C.L. (1990) The excessive loss of Branemark fixtures in type IV bone, *Journal of Periodontology*, 61, 300.

Jeffcoat, M., Jeffcoat, R. L., Reddy, M. S., & Berlan, L. (1991). Planning interactive implant treatment with 3-D computed tomography, *Journal of the American Dental Association*, 122, 40.

Johns, R. B., Jemt, T., Heath, M. R., Hutton, J. E., et al. (1992). A multicenter study of overdentures supported by Branemark implants. *International Journal of Oral & Maxillofacial Implants*, 7, 162–167.

Kapur, K. K. & Garrett, N. R. (1988). Requirements for clinical trials. *Journal of Dental Education*, 52, 760–764.

Kiener, P., Oetterli, M., Mericske, E., & Mericske-Stern. (2001). Effectiveness of maxillary overdentures support by implants: Maintenance and prosthetic complications. *International Journal of Prosthodontics* 14, 133–140.

Klein, M., Cranin, A. N., & Sirakian, A. (1993). A computerized tomography (CT) scan appliance for optimal presurgical and preprosthetic planning of the implant patient, *Practical Periodontics & Aesthetic Dentistry*, 5(6), 39.

Klinge, B., Peterson, A., & Maly, P. (1989). Location of the mandibular canal: comparison of macroscopic findings, conventional radiography, and computer tomography, *International Journal of Oral & Maxillofacial Implants*, 4, 327.

Kohavi, D. & Bar-Ziv, J. (1996). A typical incisive nerve: clinical report. *Implant Dentistry*, 5, 281.

Kraut, R. A. (1991). Selecting the precise implant site, *Journal of the American Dental Association*, 122, 50.

Kraut, R. A. (1994). Interactive radiologic diagnosis and case planning for implants, *Dental Implantology Update* 5(7), 49.

Kraut, R. A. "Radiologic planning for dental implants." In *Endosseous Implants for Maxillofacial Reconstruction*. Philadelphia: W.B. Saunders, 1995.

Kraut, R. A. (1993). Effective uses of radiographs for implant placements—panographs, cephalograms, CT scans. Interview in *Dental Implantology Update*, 4(4), 29.

Kraut, R. A. (1992). Utilization of 3D/dental software for precise implant site selection: clinical reports. *Implant Dentistry*, 1(2), 134.

Krennmair, G. & Ulm C. (2001). The symphyseal single tooth implant for anchorage of a mandibular complete denture in geriatric patients: A clinical report. *International Journal of Oral & Maxillofacial Implants*, 12, 589–594.

Kutsch, V. (1999). Digital radiography: how can digital radiography fit into your practice. *Dental Economics*, 12, 56.

Lam, E. W. N., Ruprecht, A., & Yang, J. (1995). Comparison of two-dimensional orthoradially reformatted computed tomography and panoramic radiography for dental implant treatment planning. *Journal of Prosthetic Dentistry*, 74, 42.

Lima-Verde, M. A. R., Morgano, M. (1993). A dual-purpose stent for the implant supported prosthesis. *Journal of Prosthetic Dentistry*, 69, 276.

Maher, W. P. (1991). Topographic, microscopic, radiographic, and computerized morphometric studies of the human adult edentate mandible for oral implantologists. *Clinical Anatomy*, 4, 327.

Makkonen, T. A., Holmberg, S., Niemi, L., Olsson, C., Tammisalo, T., & Peltola, J. (1997). A 5-year prospective clinical study of Astra Tech dental implants supporting fixed bridges or overdentures in the edentulous mandible. *Clinical Oral Implants Research*, 8, 469–475.

Marino, J. E., et al. (1995). Fabrication of an implant radiologic-surgical stent for the partially edentulous patient. *Quintessence International*, 26:111.

McGivney, G. P., et al. (1986). A comparison of computer-assisted tomography and data-gathering modalities in prosthodontics, *International Journal of Oral & Maxillofacial Implants*, 1, 55.

Meijer, H. J. A., Batenburg, H. K., Raghoebar, G. M. (2001). Influence of patient age on the success rate of dental implant supporting an overdenture in an edentulous mandible: A 3-year prospective study. *International Journal of Oral & Maxillofacial Implants*. 16, 522–526.

Menicucci, G., Lorenzetti, M., Pera, P., & Preti, G. (1998). Mandibular implant-retained overdenture: Finite element analysis of two anchorage systems. *International Journal of Oral & Maxillofacial Implants*, 13, 369–376.

Mericske-Stern, R. (1998). Three-dimensional force measurements with mandibular overdentures connected implants by ball-shaped retentive anchors. A clinical study. *International Journal of Oral & Maxillofacial Implants*, 13, 36.

Mericske-Stern, R. (1998). Treatment outcomes with implant-supported overdentures. Clinical considerations. *Journal of Prosthetic Dentistry*, 79, 66–73.

Mericske-Stern, R., Piotti, M., & Sirtes, G. (1996). 3-D in force measurements on mandibular implants supporting overdentures. A comparative study. *Clinical Oral Implants Research*, 7, 387–396.

Mericske-Stern, R., Venetz, E., Fahrlander, F., & Burgin. (2000). In vivo force measurements on maxillary implant supporting a fixed prosthesis or an overdenture pilot study. *Journal of Prosthetic Dentistry*, 84, 535–547.

Mericske-Stern, R. & Zarb, G. A. (1993). Overdentures: An alternative implant methodology for edentulous patients. *International Journal of Prosthodontics*, 6, 203–208.

Mericske-Stern, R. (1990). Clinical evaluation of overdenture restorations supported by osseointegrated titanium implants: A retrospective study. *International Journal of Oral & Maxillofacial Implants*, 5, 375–383.

Naert, I., De Clercq, M., Theuniers, G., & Schepers, E. (1988). Overdentures supported by osseointegrated fixtures for the edentulous mandible: A 2.5-year report. *International Journal of Oral & Maxillofacial Implants*, 3, 191–196.

Naert, I., Gizni, S., & van Steenberghe, D. (1998). Rigidly splinted implants in the resorbed maxilla to retain a hinging overdenture: a series of clinical reports for up to 4 years. *Journal of Prosthetic Dentistry*, 79, 156–164.

Narhi, T. O., Ettinger, R. L., & Lam, E. W. (1997). Radiographic findings, ridge resorption, and subjective complaints of complete denture patients. *International Journal of Prosthodontics*, 10, 183–189.

Oetterli, J., Kiener, P., & Mericske-Stern, R. (2001). A longitudinal study on mandibular implants supporting an overdenture: The influence of retention mechanism and anatomic-prosthetic variables on peri-implant parameters. *International Journal of Prosthodontics*, 14, 536–542.

Payne, A. G. T. & Solmons, Y. F. (2000). The prosthodontic maintenance requirements of mandibular muscosa-implant-supported overdentures: A review of literature. *International Journal of Prosthodontics*, 13, 238–245.

Quirynen, M., et al. (1990). The CT scan standard reconstruction technique for reliable jaw bone volume determination. *International Journal of Oral & Maxillofacial Implants*, 5, 384.

Quirynen, M., Peeters, W., Naert, I., Coucke, W., van Steenberghe, D. (2001). Peri-implant health around screw shaped CP titanium machined implants in partially edentulous patients with or without ongoing periodontitis. *Clinical Oral Implants Research*, 12, 589–594.

Raghoebar, G. M., Meijer, H. J. A., Stegenga, B., van't Hof, M. A., van Oort, R. P., & Vissink A. (2000). Effectiveness of three treatment modalities for the edentulous mandible. *Clinical Oral Implants Research*, 11, 195–201.

Reddy, M. S., Mayfield-Donahoo, T., Vanderven, F. J. J., & Jeffcoat, M. K. (1994). A comparison of the diagnostic advantages of panoramic radiography and computed tomography scanning for placement of root-form dental implants. *Clinical Oral Implants Research*, 5, 229–238.

Scarfe, W. C., Farman, A. G., Brand, J. W., & Kelly, M. S. (1997). Tissue radiation dosages using the RadioVisioGraphy-S with and without niobium filtration. *Australian Dental Journal*, 42, 335.

Scher, E. L. C. (1994). Use of the incisive canal as a recipient site for root form implants: preliminary clinical reports. *Implant Dentistry*, 3, 38.

Shimura, M., et al. (1990). Presurgical evaluation for dental implants using a reformatting program of computed tomography: maxilla/mandible shape pattern analysis (MSPA). *International Journal of Oral & Maxillofacial Implants*, 5, 175.

Smith, J. P. & Borrow, J. W. (1991). Reformatted CT imaging for implant planning. *Oral and Maxillofacial Surgery Clinics of North America*, 3, 805.

Spencer, M. D. (1999). Digital radiography: the value of digital radiography. *Dental Economics*, 12, 54.

Stellino, G., Morgano, S. M., & Imbelloni, A. (1995). A dual-purpose, implant stent made from a provisional fixed partial denture. *Journal of Prosthetic Dentistry*, 74(2), 212.

Tan, K. B. C. (1995). The use of multiplanar reformatted computerized tomography in the surgical-prosthodontic planning of implant placement. *Annals of Academy of Medicine Singapore*, 24, 68.

Tang, L., Lund, J. P., Tache, R., Clokie, C. M., Feine, J. S. (1997). A within-subject comparison of mandibular long-bar and hybrid implant-supported prostheses: Psychometric evaluation and patient preference. *Journal of Dental Research*, 76, 1675–1683.

Todd, A. D., Gher, M. E., Quintero, G., Richardson, A. C. (1993). Interpretation of linear and computer tomograms in the assessment of implant recipient sites. *Journal of Periodontology*, 64, 1243.

Wakoh, M., et al. (1994). Radiation exposures with the RadioVisioGraphy-S and conventional intraoral radiographic films. *Oral Radiology*, (Japan) 10, 33.

Vandre, R. H., Pajac, Farman, T. T., Farman, A. G. (1997). Technical comparison of six digital intraoral x-ray sensors. *Dentomaxillofacial Radiology*, 26, 282.

Verstreken, K. et al. (1996). Computer-assisted planning of oral implant-surgery: a three-dimensional approach. *International Journal of Oral & Maxillofacial Implants*, 11, 806.

Weinberg, L. A. (1993). CT scan as a radiologic data base for optimum implant orientation. *Journal of Prosthetic Dentistry*, 69, 381.

Wismeijer, D., Van Waas, M. A, J., Vermeeren, J. I. J. F., Mulder, J., & Kalk, W. (1999). Clinical and radiological results of patients treatment with three treatment modalities for overdentures on implants of the ITI-dental implant system. *Clinical Oral Implants Research*, 10, 297–306.

Wismeijer, D., Van Waas, M. A. J., Vermeeren, J. I. J. F., Mulder, J., & Kalk W. (1997). Patient satisfaction with implant-supported mandibular overdentures. A comparison of three treatment strategies on ITI-dental implants. *International Journal of Oral and Maxillofacial Surgery*, 26, 263–267.

Wismeijer, D., Vermeeren, J. I. J. F., van Waas, M. A. J. (1995). A 6.5-year evaluation of patient satisfaction and prosthetic aftercare in patient treatment using overdentures supported by ITI-implants. *International Journal of Oral & Maxillofacial Implants*, 10, 744–749.

Wismeijer, D., Vermeeren, J. I. J. F., van Waas, M. A. J. (1992). Patient satisfaction with overdentures supported by one-stage TPS implants. *International Journal of Oral & Maxillofacial Implants*, 7, 51–55.

Zarb, G. A. & Schmitt, A. (1990). The longitudinal clinical effectiveness of osseointegrated dental implants: The Toronto study. Part I: Surgical results. *Journal of Prosthetic Dentistry*, 63, 451–457.

3
Surgical Guide and Diagnostic Stent

Hamid Shafie
Wolfram Stein
Amir Juzbasic

Some clinicians think that the use of a surgical guide for overdenture candidates is unnecessary. Improper implant arrangement in overdenture patients, however, can compromise the design of the attachment assembly and retention of the prosthesis and lead to difficulty in fabrication of the prosthesis and difficulty in maintaining good oral hygiene around the implants and attachment assembly (Figures 3.1 and 3.2).

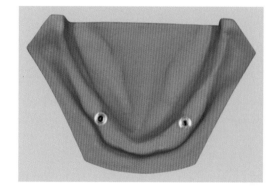

FIGURE 3.2.

Because implant treatment is prosthetic driven, the restorative dentist should make and design the surgical guide, and the guide should dictate the position of the implants based on the planned attachment assembly.

However, when placing two implants and two stud attachments in the anterior mandible, the use of the surgical guide can be replaced by utilizing a paralleling device (Figure 3.3).

If the overdenture design includes a bar attachment assembly, the use of a surgical guide is required, because the length of the bar and its sagittal relationship with the alveolar ridge have a direct effect on the mechanical properties

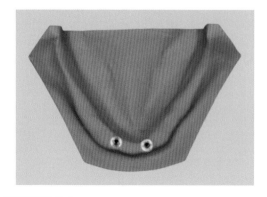

FIGURE 3.1.

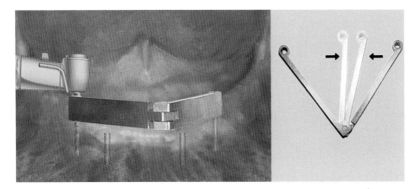

FIGURE 3.3.

of the attachment assembly, as well as the long term prognosis of the treatment.

When the patient's treatment requires a rigid, non-resilient, fixed detachable overdenture (hybrid prosthesis), the use of an accurate surgical guide is necessary. In this situation, the distribution of the implants will determine the anterior posterior distance (AP distance) and ultimately the amount of the distal cantilever.

The surgical guide is made of acrylic and usually is the duplicate of the patient's transitional denture (Figures 3.4 and 3.5).

Avoid duplicating a poorly made existing denture. As a general rule, the transitional denture should meet all of the requirements for setting up an accurate denture.

Mark the location of the implants on the surgical guide and then use a milling machine to drill parallel holes through the acrylic (Figures 3.6, 3.7, and 3.8).

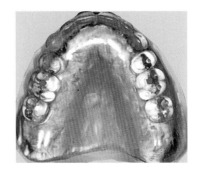

FIGURE 3.6.

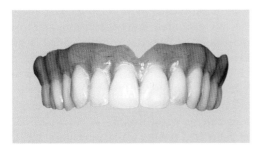

FIGURE 3.4.

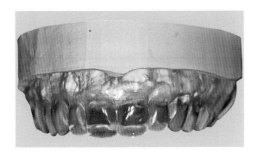

FIGURE 3.5.

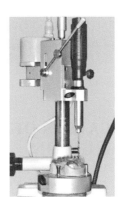

FIGURE 3.7.

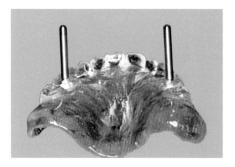

FIGURE 3.8.

A 3mm pilot is recommended for drilling holes in the acrylic, so that when the surgeon starts preparation of the osteotomy with a 2mm pilot drill, the drill does not come in contact with the acrylic. The pilot should go through the holes passively. Otherwise, any contact between the pilot and acrylic would drive acrylic particles into the osteotomy. The ideal situation is to use 2.5mm or 3mm titanium or stainless cylinders and insert them inside of the surgical guide (Figure 3.9). These cylinders allow the surgeon to pass the pilot drill through the metal sleeves instead of the acrylic holes. These cylinders should be installed in the acrylic with proper trajectories.

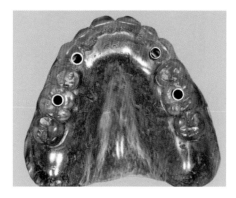

FIGURE 3.9.

CLASSIFICATION OF SURGICAL GUIDES

Surgical guides are classified based on their relationship with the underlying tissues, as described in the following sections.

Gingiva Supported

Typically the surgical guide should be utilized before raising the flap since the elevated flap prevents accurate fitting of the surgical guide. This type of surgical guide is an ideal choice for the biopsy punch (flapless surgery) surgical technique as well as the flap surgery with minimum reflection (Figure 3.10).

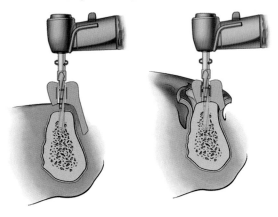

FIGURE 3.10.   **FIGURE 3.11.**

Bone Supported

Since the surgical guide fits directly over the bone, an extended crestal incision and completely elevated flaps are recommended (Figure 3.11). Because of extensive flap reflection the post-operation complications such as pain and swelling are amplified.

More accurate and sophisticated surgical guides can be made based on the anatomical data generated from a CT scan (Figure 3.12).

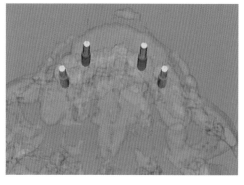

FIGURE 3.12.

Several different technologies are available to fabricate a CT-guided surgical guide. Some of them require that the impressions, casts, and the CT-scan data files be sent to a centralized manufacturing facility. The company med3D has introduced a technology that does not require a centralized manufacturing facility. Any regular dental laboratory is able to fabricate a CT-guided surgical guide.

The med3D implant 3D technology delivers the following advantages:

- Real time 2D and 3D visualization
- Precise transfer of treatment plan data to the surgical guide
- The ability to read the CT data directly from CD ROM (no need for a processing center)

- Parallel kinematics of the positioning device, which provides high precision and stability
- Easy and fast check of calibration for each patient

COMPONENTS AND THE ADVANTAGES OF THE MED3D TECHNOLOGY

Implant 3D Planning Software

3D planning software enables the dentist to analyze the CT scan in DICOM-3-format (Figure 13.3). The DICOM files are saved on a CD-ROM by the radiologist and sent to the dentist.

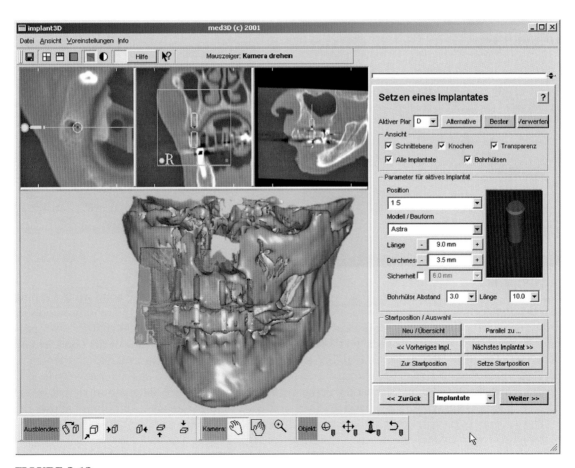

FIGURE 3.13.

During the CT-scanning process, it is recommended that the patient wear a stent with barium-sulfate covered (radioopaque) teeth (Ivoclar) (Figures 3.14 and 3.15). The boundaries of the teeth will be visible in the CT images and provide an extra point of reference to the dentist during the analysis process (Figure 3.16).

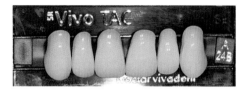

FIGURE 3.14.

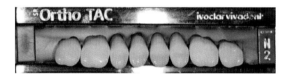

FIGURE 3.15.

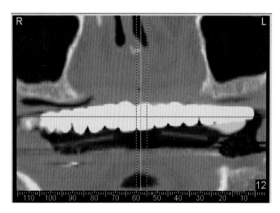

FIGURE 3.16.

The exact geometry and dimensions of the most popular implant systems are incorporated into the med3D's planning software—the Implant 3D. This gives the dentist the ability to develop a treatment plan for the patient based on the actual shape and dimension of the designated implant system (Figures 3.17 and 3.18).

The majority of the CT scan-based treatment planning software enables the dentist to move only the dummy implant over the scan images. However, with med3D software the dentist has

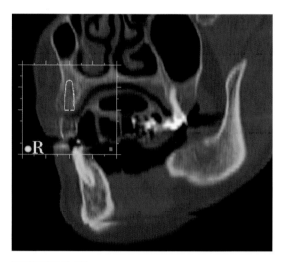

FIGURE 3.17.

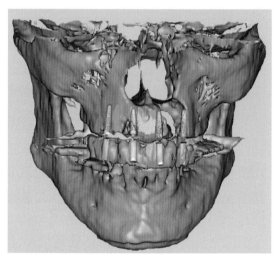

FIGURE 3.18.

the ability to move the jawbone while keeping the implant stationary. The possibility of looking at the data with an "implant centric view" provides an excellent overview of the bone around the implant. The software enables the dentist to move implants freely and interactively in real time through the CT dataset and view it in 2D slices and in 3D images. This ability allows the dentist to explore different treatment alternatives.

After the position, length, diameter, and product type have been chosen for each implant, a drilling plan is generated for the positioning device.

Stationary Robot or Positioning Device X1

The George Schick Dental Company and med3D have developed a positioning device for placing titanium tubes in the acrylic surgical guide. This device transfers the ideal, yet virtual implant positions, from the software planning into the surgical guide.

The device has a highly parallel structure that provides excellent mechanical strength and precision in transferring the data into the surgical guide (Figure 3.19).

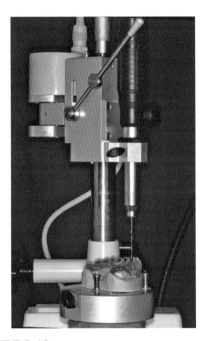

FIGURE 3.19.

PROCEDURAL STEPS

1. Use the software to generate a printout that shows the details of the drilling plan.
2. E-mail or fax this drilling plan to the laboratory that has the positioning device. This plan will describe the position of each implant as well as the appropriate length for all six legs

of the positioning device. The length of each leg is adjustable and will be customized for each patient based on the software-generated data.
3. Start drilling the acrylic surgical guide by using the pre-mounted milling machine attached to the positioning device.
4. Insert a tube holder to keep the titanium tube in place while permanently attaching it to the template using super glue or self-cure acrylic.

Note: For the surgical procedure, only the ready-made surgical guide is needed; neither the software nor the positioning device is required during surgery.

REFERENCES AND ADDITIONAL READING

Barteaux, L., Daelemans, P., & Malevez, C. (2004). A surgical stent for the Branemark Novum bone reduction procedure. *Clinical Implant Dentistry & Related Research*, 6(4), 210–21.

Chiche, G. J., Block, M. S., & Pinault, A. (1989). Implant surgical template for partially edentulous patients. *International Journal of Oral & Maxillofacial Implants*, 4, 289.

Cowan, P. W. (1990). Surgical templates for the placement of osseointegrated implants. *Quintessence International*, 21, 391.

Di Giacomo, G. A., Cury, P. R., de Araujo, N. S., Sendyk W. R., & Sendyk, C. L. (2005). Clinical application of stereolithographic surgical guides for implant placement: preliminary results. *Journal of Periodontology*, Apr, 76(4), 503–7.

Fortin, T., Bosson, J. L., Coudert, J. L., & Isidori, M. (2003). Reliability of preoperative planning of an image-guided system for oral implant placement based on 3-dimensional images: an in vivo study. *International Journal of Oral & Maxillofacial Implants*, Nov–Dec, 18(6), 886–93.

Fortin, T., Champleboux, G., Lormee, J., Coudert, J. L. (2000). Precise dental implant placement in bone using surgical guides in conjunction with medical imaging techniques. *Journal of Oral Implantology*, 26(4), 300–3.

Fortin, T., Coudert, J. L., Champleboux, G., Sautot, P., & Lavallee, S. (1995). Computer-assisted dental implant surgery using computed tomography. *Journal of Image Guided Surgery*, 1(1), 53–8.

Fortin, T., Isidori, M., Blanchet, E., Perriat, M., Bouchet, H., & Coudert, J. L. (2004). An image-guided system-drilled surgical template and trephine guide pin to make treatment of completely edentulous patients easier: a clinical report on immediate loading. *Clinical Implant Dentistry & Related Research*, 6(2), 111–9.

Johnson, C. M., Lewandowski, J. A., & McKinney, J. F. (1988). A surgical template for aligned placement of the osseointegrated implant. *Journal of Prosthetic Dentistry*, 59, 684.

Kitai, N., Yasuda, Y., & Takada, K. (2002). A stent fabricated on a selectively colored stereolithographic model for placement of orthodontic mini-implants. *International Journal of Adult Orthodontics and Orthognathic Surgery*, 17(4), 264–6.

Kopp, K. C., Koslow, A. H., & Abdo, O. S. (2003). Predictable implant placement with a diagnostic/surgical template and advanced radiographic imaging. *Journal of Prosthetic Dentistry*, Jun, 89(6), 611–5.

Morea, C., Dominquez, G. C., Wuo Ado, V., & Toramano, A. (2005). Surgical guide for optimal positioning of mini-implants. *Journal of Clinical Orthodontics*, 39(5), 317–21.

Ng, F. C., Ho, K. H., & Wexler, A. (2005). Computer-assisted navigational surgery enhances safety in dental implantology. Annals of the Academy of Medicine, Singapore. Jun, 34(5), 383–8.

Owings, J. R., Jr. (2003). Virtual imaging guiding implant surgery. *Compendium of Continuing Education in Dentistry*, May, 24(5), 333–6, 338, 340 passim, quiz 344.

Sarment, D. P., Sukovic, P., & Clinthorne, N. (2003). Accuracy of implant placement with a stereolithographic surgical guide. *International Journal of Oral & Maxillofacial Implants*, Jul–Aug, 18(4), 571–7.

Spiekermann, H., Donath, K., Hassell, T., Jovanovic, S., & Richter, J. *Color Atlas of Dental Medicine: Implantology*. Special diagnosis for implant patients (pp. 118–119). New York: Thieme Medical Publishers, Inc, 1995.

Tardieu, P. B., Vrielinck, L., & Escolano, E. (2003). Computer-assisted implant placement. A case report: treatment of the mandible. *International Journal of Oral & Maxillofacial Implants*, Jul–Aug, 18(4), 599–604.

4
Principles of Attachment Selection

Hamid Shafie

One of the most confusing issues for dentists is choosing the appropriate attachment assembly for implant overdenture cases. They usually ask themselves many questions when it comes to selecting the right attachment assembly. First, which attachment should one use? Would a bar or stud attachments be best? Depending on the answers to those questions, more considerations follow. For instance, which bar or stud would be best for this particular case?

Learning about the mechanical properties and the load distribution characteristics of different attachments is the easiest way to determine which one to use. Most available attachments demonstrate different levels of resiliency. Attachment resiliency is associated with the movement between the abutment and the prosthesis in a predetermined direction or directions. The more directions or planes in which the prosthesis can move, the less stress is placed on the implant, in turn transferring more forces to the residual ridge. That being said, the attachment is more resilient.

Various Movements Allowed by Resilient Attachments
- *Vertical Movement*: The prosthesis is allowed to move bodily toward the tissue. This type of movement results in even loading and support from the entire anterior-posterior length of the residual ridge. Typically, movement is stopped by the supporting structure of the residual ridge, meaning as soon as the prosthesis comes into contact with the residual ridge and passes the resiliency of the soft tissue, it stops.
- *Hinge Movement*: Hinge movement is that in which the prosthesis revolves around an axis that has been formed by the most posterior attachments on each side of the arch.
- *Rotation Movement*: Rotation movement allows the prosthesis to rotate around an axis that runs anterior-posteriorly. Anytime masticatory forces are applied to one side of the prosthesis, it rotates around the crest of the ridge, and the opposite side rotates up and across the arch.
- *Translation and Spinning or Fishtailing*: In this type of movement, the prosthesis moves in an anterior-posterior movement, or a bucco-lingual direction, without any

rotation. The prosthesis, in turn, revolves around a vertical axis.

- *Combination of the Above Movements*

TYPES OF ATTACHMENTS BASED ON RESILIENCY

Rigid Non-Resilient Attachments

No movement occurs between the abutment and the implant. When utilizing a rigid non-resilient attachment assembly, the implant receives 100 percent of the chewing forces, providing no relief to the supporting implants.

This type of attachment is recommended when a sufficient number of implants are available. A screw-retained hybrid overdenture is an example of a rigid non-resilient attachment.

Restricted Vertical Resilient Attachments

This type of attachment provides 5–10 percent load relief to the supporting implants, and the prosthesis can move up and down with no lateral, tipping, or rotary movement. In other words, the attachment resists any lateral tipping or rotary movements.

Hinge Resilient Attachments

This type of attachment resists any lateral tipping, rotational, and skidding forces. Hinge resilient attachments provide almost 30–35 percent load relief to the supporting implant. Each time one utilizes an attachment that provides hinge resiliency, the vertical components of the masticatory forces are shared between the attachments and the posterior portions of the residual ridge—the buccal shelf and retro molar pad. A Hader bar or any other kind of round bar can provide hinge resiliency. (Refer to Figures 6.23 through 6.27.)

Combination Resilient Attachments

Attachments of this type allow unrestricted vertical and hinge movements. This attachment uniformly transfers the vertical component of masticatory forces to the entire length of the residual ridge. Anytime we utilize this type of attachment, we increase the tissue support of the prosthesis during mastication. No matter where the masticatory load is applied to the overdenture, the ridge receives the vertical component of the forces. This type of attachment offers 45–55 percent load relief to the supporting implants. The Dolder bar joint (egg shaped) is a combination resilient attachment (Figure 6.30).

Rotary Resilient Attachments

This type of attachment provides vertical hinge and rotation movements. We utilize these attachments so that the prosthesis can move vertically and hinge-wise and rotate around the sagittal plane. Rotary resilient attachments transfer both the vertical and horizontal components of masticatory forces to the residual ridge. Movements of the prosthesis are determined by the location, direction, and magnitude of the forces that have been applied to the prosthesis. Usually this type of attachment provides 75–85 percent load relief to the supporting implants. Some of the stud attachments (prefabricated individual attachments) provide rotary resiliency. (Refer to Chapter 5.)

Universal Resilient Attachments

These attachments provide vertical, hinge, translation, and rotation movements. Basically, you see all types of movement; the attachment provides resistance only to movements away from the tissue. This type of attachment offers 95 percent load relief to the supporting implants. Magnetic attachments are the best example of the universal resilient attachments.

ATTACHMENT SELECTION CRITERIA

- Available bone
- Patient's prosthetic expectations
- Financial ability of the patient to cover treatment costs
- Personal choice and clinical expertise of the dentist
- Experience and technical knowledge of the lab technicians

Patients with advanced resorption of the alveolar ridge are good candidates for bar or telescopic attachment assemblies. These attachments offer a considerable amount of horizontal stability.

Patients with minimum alveolar ridge resorption are good candidates for studs or magnetic attachments assemblies. Magnets provide the least amount of retention compared to the other attachments, and they lose their initial retention capacity very soon. Studs are ideal for patients with a narrow ridge, because in these cases the bar would interfere with the tongue space.

DIFFERENT ATTACHMENT ASSEMBLIES

- Clips and bars
- Studs
- Magnets
- Telescopic copings (rigid or non-rigid)

Rigid telescopic copings transfer most of the masticatory forces to the supporting implants. This increases the risk for implant fatigue and eventual fracture of the implant or its components. Rigid or minimally resilient attachment assemblies transfer the minimum load to the posterior alveolar ridge; therefore, the patient experiences the least alveolar bone resorption.

FACTORS INFLUENCING THE DESIGN AND RESILIENCY LEVEL OF THE ATTACHMENT ASSEMBLY

- Shape of the arch
- Distribution of the implants in the arch
- Length of the implants and degree of implant bone interface
- Distance between the most anterior and the most posterior implants

BIOMECHANICAL CONSIDERATIONS

One hypothesis suggested that the bar connecting the implants should be parallel to the hinge axis; this rule was followed by many clinicians, but no studies have supported this claim. One long-term study (5–15 years) analyzed the influence of placing the bar parallel to the hinge axis on peri-implant parameters, including the clinical attachment level. The outcome of the type of retention, splinted versus unsplinted, was also assessed. No significant correlations were found. (Refer to Chapter 6.)

DISTAL EXTENSION TO THE BAR

Distal extensions provide a high level of stability against lateral forces, particularly in the mandible, and may protect the susceptible denture-bearing tissue from load forces. They should not extend beyond the position of first premolar of the mandibular prosthesis, and they cannot compensate for a short central segment. When distal extensions are used, the splinting effects of implants for better force distribution disappear. In this situation, the force patterns are similar to those that occur with unsplinted implants.

LOAD DISTRIBUTION OF STUD VS. BAR ATTACHMENTS

The in vivo study by Menicucci and colleagues showed that ball anchors are preferred, because they provide better load distribution on the posterior mandibular bone.

Stern and colleagues, through a series of three-dimensional force measurements with two infraforaminal Strauman implants in fully edentulous patients, showed no significant differences among different attachment assemblies and retention mechanisms.

BIOMECHANICS OF MAXILLARY OVERDENTURE

A pilot study by Stern and colleagues compared repeated in-vivo measurements of maxillary implants supporting either a fixed denture or an overdenture with a rigid bar connection. Comparable force magnitudes and patterns were found. This suggests that a rigid bar with a connected overdenture performs in a similar way as a fixed prosthesis under loading condition.

REFERENCES AND ADDITIONAL READING

Academy of Prosthodontics. (1999). *The Glossary of Prosthodontic Terms* (7th edition). *Journal of Prosthetic Dentistry*, 81, 41–110.

Adell, R., Lekholm, U., Rockler, B., et al. (1986). Marginal tissue reactions at osseointegrated titanium fixtures. Part 1. A 3-year longitudinal prospective study. *International Journal of Oral & Maxillofacial Surgery*, 1, 39–52.

Albrektsson T. & Zarb, G. A. (1998). Determinants of correct clinical reporting. *International Journal of Prosthodontics*, 11, 517–521.

Arvidson, K., Bystedt, H., Frykholm, A., et al. (1992). A 3-year clinical study of Astra dental implants in the treatment of edentulous mandibles. *International Journal of Oral & Maxillofacial Implants*, 7, 321–329.

Burns, D. R., Unger, J. W., Elswick, R. K. Jr., & Giglio, J. A. (1995). Prospective clinical evaluation of mandibular implant overdentures: Part II. Patient satisfaction and preference. *Journal of Prosthetic Dentistry*, 73, 364–369.

Carr, A. B. (1998). Successful long-term treatment outcomes in the field of osseointegrated implants: Prosthodontic determinants. *International Journal of Prosthodontics*, 11, 502–512.

Cochran, D. L. (1999). A comparison of endosseous dental implant surfaces. *Journal of Periodontology*, 70, 1523–1539.

Cochran, D. L. (2001). The scientific basis for and clinical experiences with Straumann implants including the ITI Dental Implant System: A consensus report. *Clinical Oral Implants Research*, 11(Supplement 1), 33–58.

Cox, J. F. & Zarb, G. A. (1987). The longitudinal clinical efficacy of osseointegrated dental implants. A 3-year report. *International Journal of Oral & Maxillofacial Implants*, 2, 91–100.

Davis, D. (1990). The role of implants in the treatment of edentulous patients. *International Journal of Prosthodontics*, 3, 42–50.

Davis, D. M. & Packer, M. E. (1999). Mandibular overdentures stabilized by Astra Tech implants with either ball attachments or magnets: 5-year results. *International Journal of Prosthodontics*, 12, 222–229.

de Grandmont, P., Feine, J. S., Tache, R., et al. (1994). Within-subject comparisons of implant-supported mandibular prostheses: Psychometric evaluation. *Journal of Dental Research*, 73, 1096–1104.

Engquist, B., Bergendall, T., Kallus, T., & Linden, U. (1988). A retrospective multicenter evaluation of osseointegrated implants supporting overdentures. *International Journal of Oral & Maxillofacial Implants*, 3, 129–134.

Ericsson, I., Randow, K., Nilner, K., & Peterson, A. (2000). Early functional loading of Branemark implants. 5-year clinical follow-up study. *Clinical Implant Dentistry and Related Research*, 2, 70–77.

Espositio, M., Coulthard, P., Worthington, H. V., Jokstad, A. (2000). Quality assessment of randomized controlled trials of oral implants. *International Journal of Oral & Maxillofacial Implants*, 16, 783–792.

Fourmousis, I. & Bragger, U. (1999). "Radiographic interpretation of peri-implant structures." In *Proceedings of the 3rd European Workshop on Periodontology-Implant Dentistry*, ed. Lang, N. P., Karring, T., & Lindhe, J. Chicago: Quintessence Publishing, 228–241.

Friberg, B., Sennerby, L., Linden, B., Grondahl, U. K., & Lekholm, U. (1999). Stability measurements of one-stage Branemark implants during healing in mandibles. A clinical resonance frequency analysis study. *International Journal of Oral & Maxillofacial Surgery*, 28, 266–272.

Glantz, P. O., & Nilner, K. (1997). Biomechanical aspects on overdenture treatment, *Journal of Dental Research*, 25(supplement I), 21–32.

Gotfredsen, K., Holm, B. (2000). Implant-supported mandibular overdentures retained with ball or bar attachments: A randomized prospective 5-year study. *International Journal of Prosthodontics*, 13, 125–130.

Heckmann, S. M., Winter, W., Meyer, M., Weber, H., & Wichmann, M. G. (2001). Overdenture attachment selection and the loading of implant and denture-bearing area. Part 2: A methodical study of implant and denture-bearing area. Part 2: A methodical study using five types of attachment. *Clinical Oral Implants Research*, 12, 640–647.

Heckmann, S., Farmand, M., & Wahl, G. (1993). Erste Erfahrungen mit Resilienzteleskopen bei der prothetischen Versorgung enossaler Implantate. *Zeitschrif Zahnartzl Implantol*, 188–193.

Helkimo, M. (1979). Epidemiological surveys of dysfunction of the masticatory system. In *Temporomandibular Joint Function and Dysfunction*, ed.

Zarb, G. A. & Carlsson, G. E. Munksgaard, Copenhagen: 175–192.

Hooghe, M. & Naert, I. (1997). Implant-supported overdentures: The Leuven experience. *Journal of Dentistry*, 25, 25–35.

Jemt, T., Chai, J., Harnett, J., et al. (1996). A 5-year prospective multicenter follow-up report on overdentures supported by osseointegrated implants. *International Journal of Oral & Maxillofacial Implants*, 11, 291–298.

Lekholm, U. & Zarb, G. A. (1985). Patient selection and preparation. In *Tissue Integrated Prostheses: Osseointegration in Clinical Dentistry*, ed. Branemark, P. I., Zarb, G. A., & Albrektsson, T. Chicago: Quintessence Publishing, 199–210.

Meijer, H. J. A., Kuper, J. H., Starmans, F. J. M., & Bosman, F. (1992). Stress distribution around dental implants: Influence of superstructure, length of implants, height of mandible. *Journal of Prosthetic Dentistry*, 68, 96–101.

Menicucci, G., Lorenzetti, M., Pera, P., & Preti, G. (1998). Mandibular implant-retained overdenture: Finite element analysis of two anchorage systems. *International Journal of Oral & Maxillofacial Implants*, 13, 369–376.

Mericske-Stern, R. (1988). Three-dimensional force measurements with mandibular overdentures connecting implants by ball-shaped retentive anchors. A clinical study. *International Journal of Oral & Maxillofacial Implants*, 13, 36–45.

Mericske-Stern, R. (1990). Clinical evaluation of overdenture restorations supported by osseointegrated titanium implants: A retrospective study. *International Journal of Oral & Maxillofacial Implants*, 5, 375–383.

Mericske-Stern, R. (1998). Treatment outcomes with implant-supported overdentures: Clinical considerations. *Journal of Prosthetic Dentistry*, 79, 66–73.

Mericske-Stern, R. (2003) Implant overdentures: The standard of care for edentulous patients. UK: Quintessence, 83–97.

Mericske-Stern, R., Piotti, M., & Sirtes, G. (1996). 3-D force measurements on mandibular implants supporting overdentures. A comparative study. *Clinical Oral Implant Research*, 7, 387–396.

Mericske-Stern, R., Venetz, E., & Fahrlander, F. (2000). In vivo force measurements on maxillary implants supporting a fixed prosthesis or an overdenture. Pilot study. *The Journal of Prosthetic Dentistry*, 84, 535–547.

Naert, I., De Clerq, M., Theuniers, G., & Schepers, E. (1988). Overdentures supported by osseointegrated fixtures for the edentulous mandible: A 2.5 year report. *International Journal of Oral & Maxillofacial Implants*, 3, 191–196.

Naert, I., Gizani, S., Vuylskeke, M., & van Steenberghe, D. (1999). A 5-year prospective randomized clinical trial on the influence of splinted and unsplinted oral implants retaining a mandibular overdenture: Prosthetic aspects and patient satisfaction. *Journal of Oral Rehabilitation*, 26, 195–202.

Naert, I., Gizani, S., Vuylsteke, M., & van Steenberghe, D. (1997). A randomized clinical trial on the influence of splinted and unsplinted oral implants in the mandibular overdenture therapy: A 3-year report. *Clinical Oral Investigations*, 1, 81–88.

Naert, I., Gizani, S., Vuylsteke, M., & van Steenberghe, D. (1998). A 5-year randomized clinical trial on the influence of splinted and unsplited oral implants in the mandibular overdenture therapy. Part 1: Peri-implant outcome. *Clinical Oral Implants Research*, 9, 170–177.

Naert, I., Hooghe, M., Quirynen, M., & van Steenberghe D. (1997). The reliability of implant-retained hinging overdentures for the fully edentulous mandible. An up to 9-year longitudinal study. *Clinical Oral Investigations*, 1, 119–124.

Naert, I., Quirynen, M., Hooghe, M., & van Steenberghe D. (1994). A comparative prospective study of splinted and unsplinted Branemark implants in mandibular overdenture therapy: A preliminary report. *Journal of Prosthetic Dentistry*, 72, 144–151.

Naert, I., Quirynen, M., van Steenberghe, D., Duchateau L., & Darius, P. (1990). A comparative study between Branemark and IMZ implants supporting overdentures: Prosthetic considerations. In *Tissue Integration in Oral Orthopaedic and Maxillofacial Reconstruction*, ed. Laney, W. R. & Tolman, D. E. Chicago: Quintessence Publishing, 179–193.

Oetterli, M., Kiener, P., & Mericske-Stern, R. (2001). A longitudinal study on mandibular implants supporting an overdenture: The influence of retention mechanism and anatomic-prosthetic variables on peri-implant parameters. *The International Journal of Prosthodontics*, 14, 536–542.

Payne, A. G. T., Solomons Y. F., Lownie, J. F. (1999). Standardization of radiographs for mandibular implant-supported overdentures: Review and innovation. *Clinical Oral Implants Research*, 10, 307–319.

Payne, A. G. T., Solomons, Y. F., Lownie, J. F., & Tawse-Smith, A. (2001). Inter-abutment and peri-abutment mucosal enlargement with mandibular implant overdentures. *Clinical Oral Implants Research*, 13, 179–187.

Payne, A. G. T., Tawse-Smith, A., Duncan, W. J., Kumara, R., (2002). Conventional and early loading of unsplinted ITI implants supporting mandibular ovedentures: Two-year results of a prospective randomized clinical trial. *Clinical Oral Implants Research*, 13, 603–609.

Payne, A. G. T., Tawse-Smith, A., Duncan, W., & Kumara, R. (2002). Early loading of unsplinted ITI implants supporting mandibular overdentures: Two-year results of a randomized controlled trial. *Clinical Oral Implants Research*, 13, 603–609.

Payne, A. G. T., Tawse-Smith, A., Kumara, R., Thomson, W. M. (2001). One-year prospective evaluation of the early loading of unsplinted conical Branemark fixtures with mandibular overdentures: A preliminary report. *Clinical Implant Dentistry and Related Research*, 3, 9–18.

Petropoulous, V., Smith, W., & Kousvelati, E. (1997). Comparison of retention and release periods for implant overdentures attachments. *International Journal of Oral & Maxillofacial Implants*, 12, 176–185.

Quirynen, M., Naert, I., van Steenberghe, D., & Nys L. (1992). A study of 589 consecutive implants supporting complete fixed prostheses. Part 1: Periodontal aspects. *Journal of Prosthetic Dentistry*, 68, 655–663.

Quirynen, M., Naert, I., van Steenberghe, D., et al. (1990). Periodontal aspects of Branemark and IMZ implants supporting overdentures: A comparative study. In *Tissue Integration in Oral Orthopaedic and Maxillofacial Reconstruction*, ed. Laney, W. R. & Tolman, D. E. Chicago: Quintessence Publishing, 80–92.

Quirynen, M., van Steenberghe, D., Jacobs, R., et al. (1991). The reliability of pocket probing around screw-type implants. *Clinical Oral Implants Research*, 2, 186–192.

Schmitt, A. & Zarb, G. A. (1998). The notion of implant-supported overdentures. *Journal of Prosthetic Dentistry*, 79, 60–65.

Spiekermann H. Implantology. In *Color Atlas of Dental Medicine*, ed. Rateitschak, K. H. & Wolf, H. F. New York: Thieme Medical Publishers, 1995.

Sul, Y. T., Johansson, C. B., Jeong, Y., Wennerberg, A., & Albrektsson, T. (2002). Resonance frequency and removal torque analysis of implants with turned and anodized surface oxides. *Clinical Oral Implants Research*, 13, 252–259.

Szmukler-Moncler, S., Piattelli, A., Favero, G. A., & Dubruille, J. II. (2000). Considerations prelim

inary to the application of early and immediate loading protocols in dental implantology. *Clinical Oral Implants Research*, 11, 12–25.

Tawse-Smith, A., Duncan, W., Payne, A. G. T., Thomson, W. M., & Wennstrom, J. L. (2002). Effectiveness of electric toothbrushes in peri-implant maintenance of mandibular implant overdentures. *Journal of Clinical Periodontology*, 29, 275–280.

Tawse-Smith, A., Payne, A. G. T, Kumara, R., & Thomson, W. M. (2002). Early loading on unsplinted implants supporting mandibular overdentures using a one-stage operative procedure with two different implant systems: A 2-year report. *Clinical Implant Dentistry and Related Research*, 4, 33–42.

Tawse-Smith, A., Payne, A. G. T., Kumara, R., Thomson, W. M. (2001). A one-stage operative procedure using 2 different implant systems: A prospective study on implant overdentures in the edentulous mandible. *Clinical Implant Dentistry and Related Research*, 3, 185–193.

van Kampen, F. M. C, van der Bilt, A., Cune, M. S., & Bosman, F. (2002). The influence of various attachment types in mandibular implant-retained overdentures on maximum bite force and EMG. *Journal of Dental Research*, 81, 170–173.

van Steenberghe, D., Quirynen, M., Calberson, L., & Demanet M. (1987). Prospective evaluation of the fate of 697 consecutive intra-oral fixtures ad modum Branemark in the rehabilitation of edentulism. *Journal of Head and Neck Pathology*, 6, 52–58.

Versteegh, P. A., van Beek, G. J., Slagter, A. P., & Ottervanger, J. P. (1995). Clinical evaluation of mandibular overdentures supported by osseointegrated implants. *International Journal of Oral & Maxillofacial Implants*, 10, 595–603.

Watson, G., Payne, A. G. T., Purton, D. G., & Thomson, W.G. (2002). Mandibular implant overdentures: Comparative evaluation of the prosthodontic maintenance during the first year of service using three different systems. *International Journal of Prosthodontics*, 15, 259–266.

Wismeijer, D., van Waas, M. A. J., Mulder, J., Vermeeren, J. I. J. F., & Kalk, W. (1999). Clinical and radiological results of patients treated with three treatment modalities for overdentures on implants of the ITI Dental Implant System. *Clinical Oral Implants Research*, 10, 297–306.

Zarb, G. A. (1982). Oral motor patterns and their relation to oral prostheses. *Journal of Prosthetic Dentistry*, 47, 472–478.

Zarb, G. A. (1983). The edentulous milieu. *Journal of Prosthetic Dentistry*, 49, 825–831.

5
Stud Attachments

Hamid Shafie
James Ellison

Stud attachments have been available on the market for several decades. They are very straightforward to use and provide reasonable retention and stability for implant overdentures.

IMPORTANT CONSIDERATIONS REGARDING THE ALIGNMENT OF STUD ATTACHMENTS

- *Relationship of the Stud Attachments with Each Other*: Having all of the stud attachments parallel to each other is important. Some universal joint (ball and socket) attachments may be as much as 5–7 degrees out of parallel with each other and still function properly.
- *Relationship of the Stud Attachments with the Path of Insertion*: The attachments should not interfere with the path of insertion of the overdenture.

- *Height of the Stud Attachments*: Achieving an ideal alignment is much more difficult with taller attachments than with shorter ones.

ERA ATTACHMENT

The ERA attachment is a resilient stud attachment that provides hinge and vertical resiliency (Figure 5.1). The fixed component of this attachment is made of titanium alloy with the female

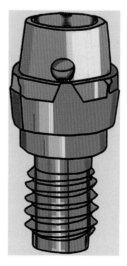

FIGURE 5.1.

37

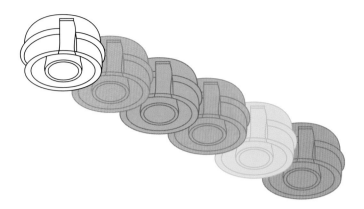

FIGURE 5.2.

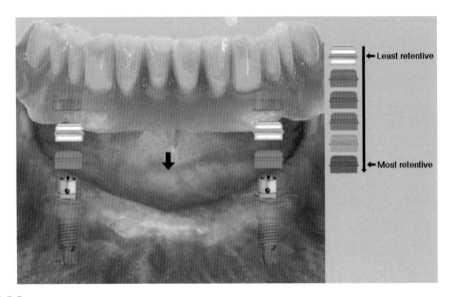

FIGURE 5.3.

attachment portion coated with titanium nitride to decrease attachment wear. The female component comes with different gingival cuff heights: 2mm, 3mm, and 5mm. The nylon male component is captured in the denture acrylic. Six color-coded males correspond to six levels of retention. In order from the least to the most retentive, they are white, orange, blue, gray, yellow, and red (Figures 5.2 and 5.3).

An optional metal housing supports these nylon male components, and the metal housing is preloaded with a black male. The black male is slightly taller (0.4mm) than the final males. Unlike other resilient attachments that have a separate spacer that fits between the male and female during processing, the ERA has a spacer built into the black male. Therefore, when the black male is processed into the denture, removed using two special tools, and replaced with one of the final males, there is 0.4mm of empty space between the male and female. This procedure creates true vertical resiliency and allows a hinging function. Overall height of the male attachment is 3.0mm, and the width of the male is 4.3mm. A new microhead version has a height of only 2.0mm and a width of 3.4mm.

The male attachment (Figures 5.4 and 5.5) accommodates four different implant trajectories: a one-piece with a trajectory of zero degrees, a two-piece with a trajectory of five degrees, a two-piece with a trajectory of 11 degrees, and a two-piece with a trajectory of 17 degrees. The male attachment is available for several implant systems.

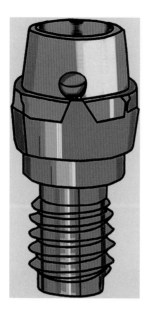

FIGURE 5.4.

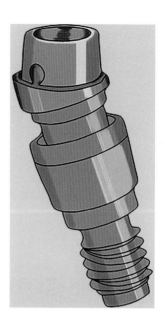

FIGURE 5.5.

The one-piece, zero degree female component screws directly into the implant. The two-piece angled female component has a polished titanium abutment base and a titanium-nitride-coated female component. The abutment base is screwed into the implant, and the angled female component is cemented into the abutment base using a strong resin or resin ionomer cement.

Chair-Side Utilization Procedure

1. Choose the proper ERA abutment according to the implant system that has been used for the patient.
2. Measure the thickness of the soft tissue and choose an abutment with the proper cuff height. When the abutment is completely tightened into the implant, the lateral drain holes should be at or above the tissue surface.
3. The ERA abutments should be parallel in the mouth. The trajectory of the supporting implants and their relationship to each other will determine if you have to chose the zero-degree straight one-piece abutments or the two-piece, 5-degree, 11-degree, or

17-degree angled abutment female attachment. Two methods are available for determining the angulations between the trajectory of the supporting implants that help the clinician to determine the proper angulations for the ERA abutment:

- *Using ERA Plastic Handle Gauges*: Snap one handle onto a zero-degree, one-piece female and screw the abutment fully into the implant using only finger pressure (Figures 5.6, 5.7, 5.8, 5.9, and 5.10).

  Repeat this step for all of the supporting implants. Next, look at the trajectory of each implant. If at least one implant is positioned in the correct path of insertion for the overdenture, use that implant as a guide to make other abutments parallel to that implant or within a maximum of five degrees out of parallel (Figure 5.11). If none of the implants are positioned in the correct path of insertion, make a pick-up impression and a master cast. Then use a surveyor to determine the discrepancy among the trajectory of the supporting implants.
- *Using an ERA Angle Correction Gauge Kit*: There are four different alignment

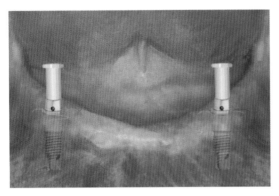

FIGURE 5.6

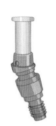 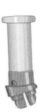 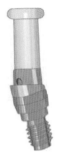

FIGURE 5.7   **FIGURE 5.8**   **FIGURE 5.9**

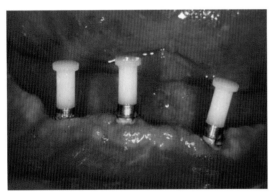

FIGURE 5.10

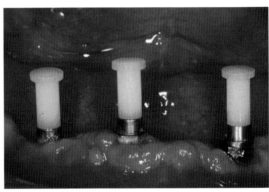

FIGURE 5.11

metal gauges (0, 5, 11, and 17 degrees) that can be use to determine the discrepancy between the trajectory of the supporting implants. The gauges are made of polished titanium. These gauges can be inserted into the screw access holes of most implant systems. These gauges have no thread pattern, just a smooth pin that slides into the screw access hole of the implant. After insertion of the gauge into the implant, manually rotate the gauge until it reaches an ideal trajectory that is aligned with the path of insertion of the overdenture. Choose the proper angled female abutment for each implant by checking the laser mark on each gauge.

4. After choosing the proper female abutments, use an ERA abutment driver and a 20Ncm torque wrench to tighten any zero-degree abutments as well as the base of the two-piece angled female abutment. When using angled ERA abutments, mark the proper relationship of the two pieces with a permanent marker after tightening the bottom piece with a 20Ncm torque wrench (Figure 5.12).

To handle the top piece (the gold titanium nitride part), snap a plastic handle into the selected angled female. The retention of the angled female in the base has been designed only for a hold light enough to retain it during alignment orientation. Use a strong cement (Fuji Plus, GC, or ERA Lock Cement)

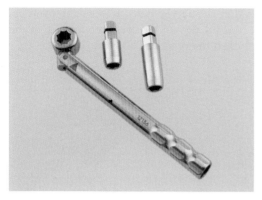

FIGURE 5.12.

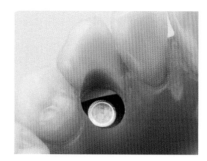

FIGURE 5.15.

to bond the two pieces together based on the permanent marks.

5. Use a large laboratory round carbide bur to cut a hole in the denture base exactly above each ERA abutment (Figure 5.13). Continue the hole toward the lingual flange and create a window (Figure 5.14). This hole should be large enough to insert a pre-loaded metal housing over the female abutment with no contact between the metal housing and the denture base (Figure 5.15).

6. Snap a black male, which is pre-loaded in a metal housing, onto each female abutment (Figure 5.16). Block out any remaining exposed surfaces of the abutments or any potential undercuts with small pieces of rubber dam, soft wax, or block-out resin (Figure 5.17).

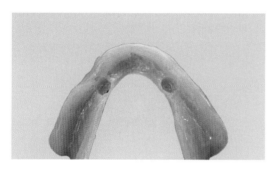

FIGURE 5.13.

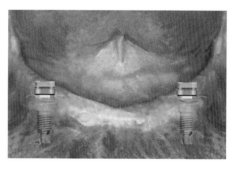

FIGURE 5.16.

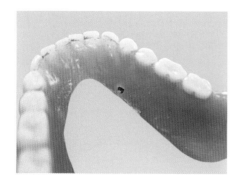

FIGURE 5.14.

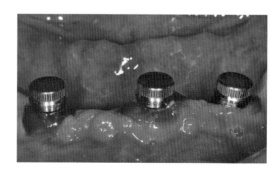

FIGURE 5.17.

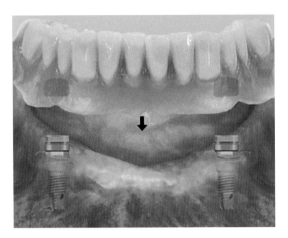

FIGURE 5.18.

9. After the acrylic is set, remove the overdenture, fill any void with acrylic, and finish and polish the prosthesis (Figure 5.20).

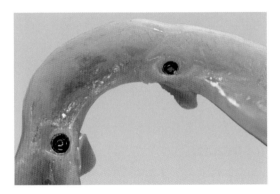

FIGURE 5.20.

7. Insert the denture and verify that there is no contact between each attachment and the denture base (Figure 5.18). If interference exists, trim the denture base.

8. Apply self-cure acrylic around and above each metal housing, as well as inside each hole in the denture base (Figure 5.19). Ensure that the external retention ridge on the outside of the metal housing is completely covered with acrylic. Insert the denture into the patient's mouth over the attachment and guide the patient into maximum intercuspation, but do not allow the patient to close firmly. Allowing the patient to close firmly could cause an improper position of the males to the females.

10. Replace each black male nylon attachment with a white final male (Figures 5.21 and 5.22). Since the final male is 0.4mm shorter than the black male, it creates vertical resiliency for the prosthesis. If the patient desires additional retention, replace the white male with an orange male. Use the blue, gray, yellow, or red male components as necessary.

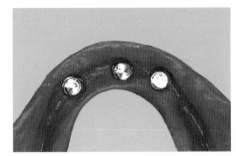

FIGURE 5.21.

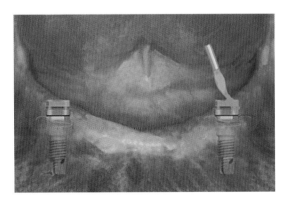

FIGURE 5.19.

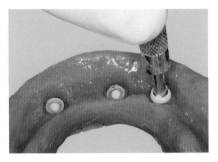

FIGURE 5.22.

11. Verify the occlusion and perform any necessary occlusal adjustments (Figure 5.23).

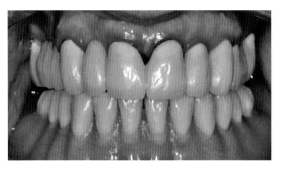

FIGURE 5.23.

Changing ERA Male Component

Note: A dentist's tool kit (core cutter and seating tool) is necessary for replacement of ERA males.

1. Use a core cutter bur and a slow speed hand piece to core the nylon male out of the metal housing (Figures 5.24 and 5.25). This step should be done at a low RPM. Use a short cutting cycle and an in-and-out motion. Push in for about one second at a time. Check to see if the core is removed. The core remains in the core cutter and can be ejected by sliding a thin blade along the cutter's side slot.

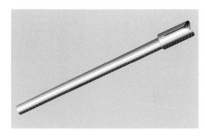

FIGURE 5.24.

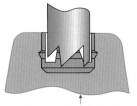

Cross section of denture base

FIGURE 5.25.

2. Use a C scaler and collapse the remaining ring into the open space created by removal of the core, then lift it out (Figure 5.26).

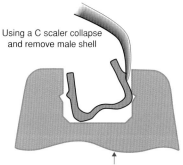

Using a C scaler collapse and remove male shell

Cross section of denture base

FIGURE 5.26.

3. Seat a new male component on the seating tool (Figure 5.27). Push the new male firmly into the metal housing until the male snaps securely into place (Figure 5.28).

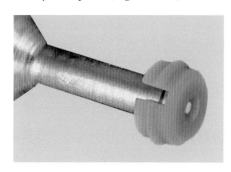

FIGURE 5.27.

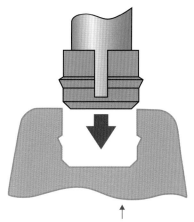

Cross section of denture base

FIGURE 5.28.

VKS-OC RS STUD ATTACHMENT

The Vario Ball-Snap-OC rs stud attachment abutment is designed for implant overdentures that are partly implant born and partly tissue born (Figures 5.29, 5.30, 5.31, 5.32, 5.33, 5.34, and 5.35).

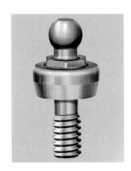

FIGURE 5.29.

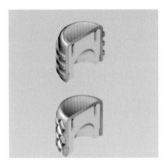

FIGURE 5.30.

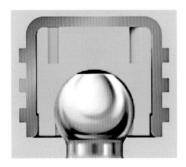

FIGURE 5.31.

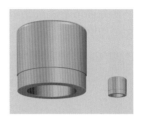

FIGURE 5.32.

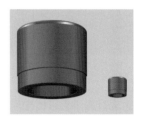

FIGURE 5.33.

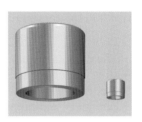

FIGURE 5.34.

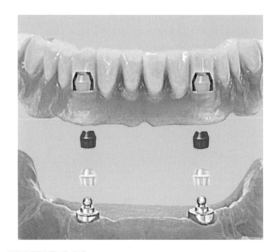

FIGURE 5.35.

This stud attachment is available for the following implants:

- Branemark 3.75 mm, 4.0 mm, 5.0 mm
- 3i external hex 4.0 mm, 5.0 mm, 6.0 mm

The VKS-OC rs stud attachment is available in the following three cuff heights:

- 2mm
- 4mm
- 6mm

Note: As a general rule, the cuff height of the attachment should be approximately 1mm taller than the thickness of the gum.

The male part (ball) of this attachment assembly will be screwed into the implant, and the female matrices will be secured inside the acrylic denture base.

Different Types of Matrices/Clips

Rigid:

- *Green*: Low retention (Figure 5.36)

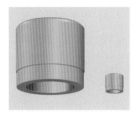

FIGURE 5.36.

- *Yellow*: Medium retention (Figure 5.37)

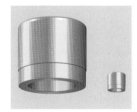

FIGURE 5.37.

- *Red*: Strong retention (Figure 5.38)

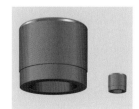

FIGURE 5.38.

This attachment system can be utilized in either of the following two ways:

- Embedded in the acrylic denture base (Figure 5.39)
- Cast within the chrome cobalt framework (Figure 5.40)

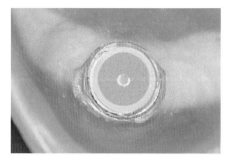

FIGURE 5.39.

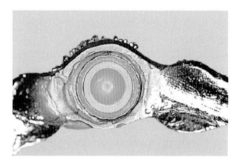

FIGURE 5.40.

Clinical and Laboratory Procedures for VKS-OC rs Attachment Embedded in the Acrylic Denture Base

CLINICAL STEPS

1. After uncovering the implants four weeks later, the patient should be seen for attachment selection. Consider the following factors when choosing a VKS-OC rs stud abutment:
   - Brand of the implant
   - Diameter of the implant
   - Thickness of the gingiva

   Remove the healing abutments, measure the thickness of the gingiva, and determine the cuff height of the stud abutments.

2. Replace the healing abutments with the designated stud abutment (Figure 5.41) and use a 30Ncm torque driver (part # 460 0001 0) to tighten all of the abutments.

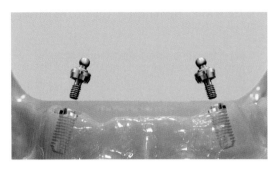

FIGURE 5.41.

3. Place a transfer impression matrix over the stud abutments (Figure 5.42). There should be a slight snap. Then take a pick-up impression with a rigid impression material. After the impression is removed from the patient's mouth, the transfer impression matrices remain in the impression material (Figure 5.43). Retention grooves in the transfer matrices ensure stabilization of the matrices in the impression material.

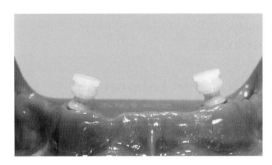

FIGURE 5.42.

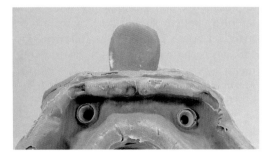

FIGURE 5.43.

LABORATORY STEPS

1. Insert the laboratory analogues inside the transfer impression matrices and pure the impression with a very low expansion or zero expansion stone (Figures 5.44 and 5.45).

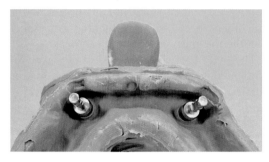

FIGURE 5.44.

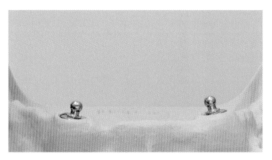

FIGURE 5.45.

2. After fabricating the master cast, snap the axis guide pins (part # 460 0010 2) on the laboratory stud abutments (Figures 5.46 and 5.47) and then use the angle-measuring device to determine the discrepancy between the trajectories of the stud abutments (Figures 5.48 and 5.49). The VKS-OC system can accommodate a maximum 15-degree discrepancy between the trajectory of the

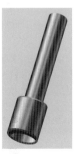

FIGURE 5.46.

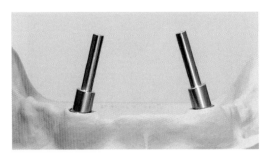

FIGURE 5.47.

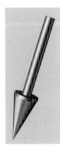

FIGURE 5.48.

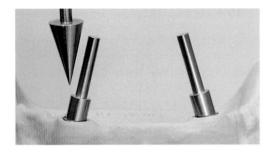

FIGURE 5.49.

stud abutment and the insertion path of the overdenture.

3. Use the matrix-inserting instrument (part # 360 0116 1) and insert a yellow matrix into the matrix metal housing (Figure 5.50).

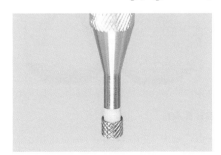

FIGURE 5.50.

4. Snap the matrices over the laboratory stud abutments and change their position manually until they are parallel with each other and follow the overdenture's path of insertion (Figures 5.51 and 5.52). For increased accuracy, use a paralleling mandrel (part # 360 0116 0) and surveyor (Figure 5.53). Repositioning of the matrices over the laboratory stud abutments to offset the discrepancy in the trajectory of the abutments will leave a gap and undercut between the matrix and the laboratory stud abutment, which should be blocked out with plaster

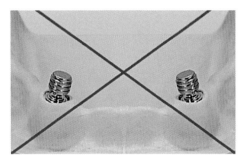

FIGURE 5.51.

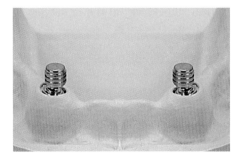

FIGURE 5.52.

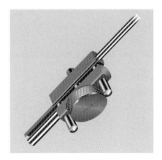

FIGURE 5.53.

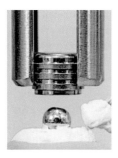

FIGURE 5.54.

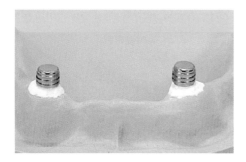

FIGURE 5.55.

(Figure 5.54). The plaster should completely secure the position and orientation of the matrices. Block out all the undercuts under the matrices (Figure 5.55).

5. Make an acrylic base over the master cast. The matrices should be completely embedded into this acrylic base (Figure 5.56).

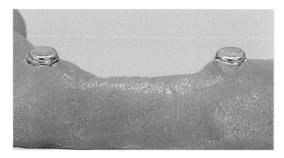

FIGURE 5.56.

6. Make the bite registration wax rim on the record base.
7. After registration of the jaw relationship, set up the teeth based on the lingualized occlusal scheme (Figures 5.57 and 5.58).

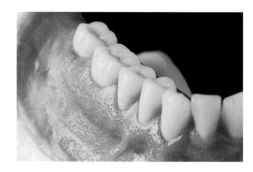

FIGURE 5.57.

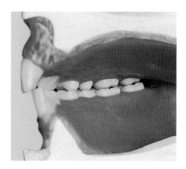

FIGURE 5.58.

8. After trying the denture teeth and verifying the centric relation position, remove the matrices and their metal housing from the acrylic base. Insert the matrices back on the master cast over the laboratory stud abutments.
9. Process the denture utilizing a flasking technique or any other desirable denture processing technique (Figure 5.59). After completion of the processing step, the metal housing will be completely secured in the acrylic base (Figure 5.60).

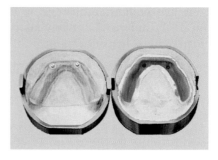

FIGURE 5.59.

10. Finish and polish the overdenture. The plastic matrices can be removed with the matrix pliers (part # 310 0000 6).

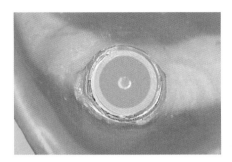

FIGURE 5.60.

Clinical and Laboratory Procedures for VKS-OC rs Attachment Cast within the Chrome Cobalt Framework

CLINICAL STEPS

1. After uncovering the implants four weeks later, the patient should be seen for attachment selection. Consider the following factors when choosing a VKS-OC rs stud abutment:
   - Brand of the implant
   - Diameter of the implant
   - Thickness of the gingiva
   Remove the healing abutments and measure the thickness of the gingiva, and determine the cuff height of the stud abutments.
2. Replace the healing abutments with the designated stud abutments and use a 30Ncm torque driver (part # 460 0001 0) to tighten all the abutments.
3. Place the transfer impression matrix over the stud abutments. There should be a slight snap. Then take a pick-up impression with a rigid impression material. After the impression is removed from the patient's mouth, the transfer impression matrices remain in the impression material. Retention grooves in the transfer matrices ensure stabilization of the matrices/clips in the impression material.

LABORATORY STEPS

1. Insert laboratory analogues inside the transfer impression matrices and pure the impression with a very low expansion or zero expansion stone.

2. After fabricating the master cast, snap the axis guide pins (part # 460 0010 2) on the laboratory stud abutments and then use the angle-measuring device to determine the discrepancy between the trajectories of the stud abutments. A VKS-OC system can accommodate a maximum 15-degree discrepancy between the trajectory of the stud abutment and the insertion path of the overdenture.
3. Snap duplicating matrices (part # 440 0110 8) on the laboratory stud abutments and change their position manually until they are parallel with each other and follow the overdenture's path of insertion (Figures 5.61 and 5.62). For increased accuracy, use a paralleling mandrel (part # 360 0116 0) and surveyor (Figure 5.63). Repositioning of the matrices over the laboratory stud abutments to offset the discrepancy in the trajectory of the abutments will leave a gap and undercut between the matrix and the laboratory stud abutment, which should be blocked out with plaster (Figure 5.64). The plaster

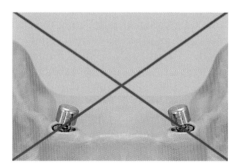

FIGURE 5.61.

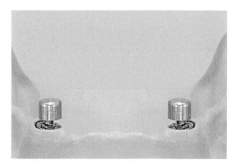

FIGURE 5.62.

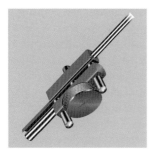

FIGURE 5.63.

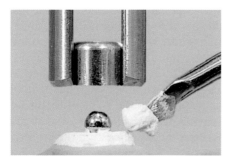

FIGURE 5.64.

should completely secure the position and orientation of the matrices. Block out all the undercuts under the matrices.

4. Start the process of fabricating the chrome cobalt framework as usual. First block out the master cast and then duplicate the master cast to create the refractory cast (Figures 5.65 and 5.66). The duplicating matrices guarantee the correct sizing of the recipient housings in the final chrome cobalt framework.

5. Start waxing the framework pattern (Figures 5.67, 5.68, and 5.69). In order to wax the chrome cobalt framework pattern over the matrix housings, special wax matrix

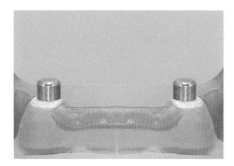

FIGURE 5.65.

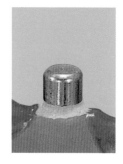

FIGURE 5.66.

copings are available. The special copings ensure the correct thickness of the chrome cobalt framework in the area of the recipient housings.

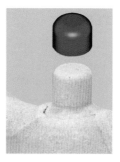

FIGURE 5.67.

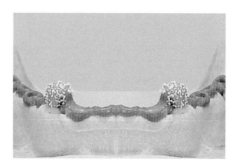

FIGURE 5.68.

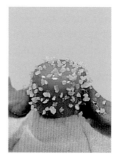

FIGURE 5.69.

6. Cast the framework wax pattern with the usual techniques (Figure 5.70). Finish and polish the chrome cobalt framework using the usual techniques and materials.

   Note: The recipient housing in the framework should not be finished with carbide burs. Clean the recipient site only with a sandblasting process.

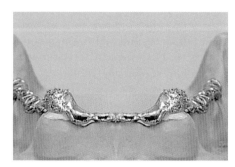

FIGURE 5.70.

7. Press the yellow plastic matrices into the special glueable metal housing (part # 440 0020 2) (Figure 5.71). Medium retention matrices (yellow) are recommended for these laboratory steps.

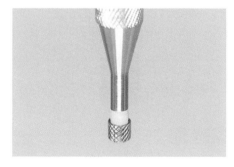

FIGURE 5.71.

8. Snap the matrices with their metal housing on the laboratory stud abutments on the original master cast (Figure 5.72). The plaster block-outs, which were built up by parallel placement of the duplicating matrices, ensure the parallel position of the special metal housing before gluing.

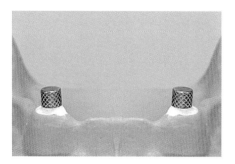

FIGURE 5.72.

9. Make sure that the inside of the recipient housing in the chrome cobalt framework is completely clean and then fill it with DTK Adhesive (Part # 540 0010 6) (Figures 5.73 and 5.74).

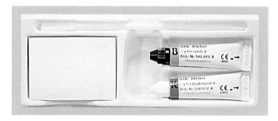

FIGURE 5.73.

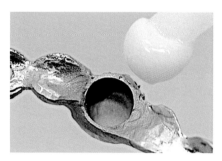

FIGURE 5.74.

   Note: Any residue from the sandblasting process will affect the adhesion strength of the DTK Adhesive.

10. Insert the chrome cobalt framework over the metal housings, which are snapped on the laboratory stud abutments in the master cast (Figure 5.75). Press the framework firmly over the housings to make sure that the excess glue comes out of the recipient sites.

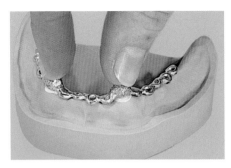

FIGURE 5.75.

11. Make the bite registration wax rim on the record base.
12. After registration of the jaw relationship, set up the teeth based on lingualized occlusal scheme.
13. After trying the denture teeth and verifying the centric relation position, process the denture with the usual techniques (Figure 5.76). Finish and polish the denture (Figure 5.77).

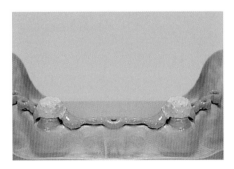

FIGURE 5.76.

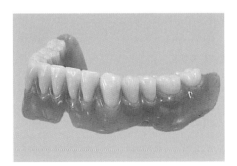

FIGURE 5.77.

14. The yellow matrices can be replaced with any other matrices.

Home Care

The overdenture must be cleaned at least once a day. Cleaning should be carried out using toothpaste and a toothbrush. Cleaning tabs have been proven to be less suitable.

STRAUMANN RETENTIVE ANCHOR ABUTMENT

The Straumann retentive anchor abutment provides rotary and limited vertical resiliency (Figures 5.78, 5.79, and 5.80). The mobile connector shortens the lever arm of the tilting forces applied on the supporting implants. Anytime this type of attachment is utilized, it is important that the implants are placed perpendicular to the plane of occlusion and parallel with each other. This process ensures the axial loading of the implants. This attachment works best when the acrylic base of the overdenture has

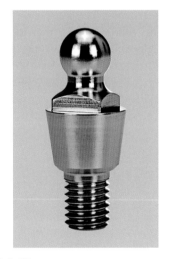

FIGURE 5.78.

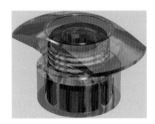

FIGURE 5.79.

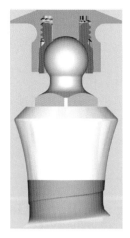

FIGURE 5.80.

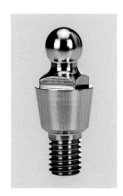

FIGURE 5.81.

maximum adaptation with the supporting tissue and the bilateral balanced occlusal scheme is utilized.

Contraindications for Using Retentive Anchors

- Combined tooth-implant-borne prosthesis
- Use of more than two implants per jaw
- In combination with other attachments that provide a different kind of resiliency
- In cases where the implants have been positioned divergent from each other, which prevents formation of an axis of rotation
- Unfavorable alveolar ridge morphology
- When other implant sizes besides Ø4.1mm, RN (Regular Neck) implants are used

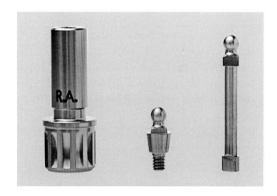

FIGURE 5.82.

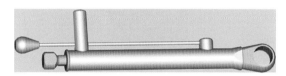

FIGURE 5.83.

Design Specifications of the Retentive Anchor and Its Corresponding Elliptical Matrix

- The Straumann retentive anchor abutment has a square neck to accommodate the driver (Figures 5.81 and 5.82).
- The retentive anchor should be inserted and tightened into the implant with a force of 35Ncm (Figures 5.83 and 5.84).

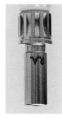

FIGURE 5.84.

- The height of the retentive anchor is 3.4mm, measured from the top of the ball to the bottom of the square neck (Figure 5.85).

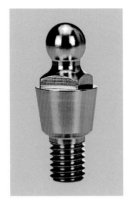

FIGURE 5.85.

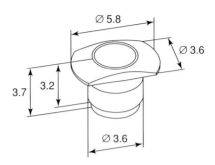

FIGURE 5.87.

- Its corresponding female housing, the elliptical matrix, consists of a titanium housing (pure titanium grade 4) with a gold lamella retentive insert (Au 68.6 percent, Ag 11.8 percent, Cu 10.6 percent, Pd 4.0 percent, Pt 2.5 percent, Zn 2.5 percent, Ir > 1 percent). The insert is screwed into the titanium housing (Figure 5.86).

Adjusting the Retention of the Female Component

A specially designed screwdriver must be used for activating, deactivating, and replacing the lamella retentive insert (Figure 5.88).

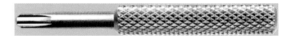

FIGURE 5.88.

The screwdriver should be pushed at a correct angle into the lamella retentive insert as far as it will go. Turning the insert clockwise increases the retention; turning it counterclockwise reduces the retention (Figure 5.89).

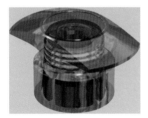

FIGURE 5.86.

- The height of the elliptical matrix is 3.7mm and its width is 5.8mm.

  Note: When insufficient bucco-lingual space is available, the wings of the matrix can be modified to accommodate the tight space. However, a minimum diameter of 3.6mm must be maintained in order to ensure the retention of the matrix in the resin.

One advantage of this attachment assembly compared to other stud attachments is that the level of retention can be adjusted from 200g (0.44lb) to 1400g (3.08lb) without changing any components (Figure 5.87).

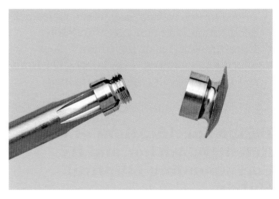

FIGURE 5.89.

The initial retention force (matrix as supplied) is approximately 200g (0.44lb), the minimum that can be set. The maximum retention force is approximately 1400g (Figure 5.90).

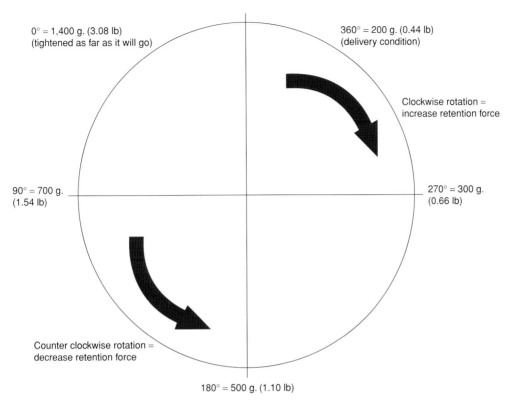

0° = 1,400 g. (3.08 lb)
(tightened as far as it will go)

360° = 200 g. (0.44 lb)
(delivery condition)

Clockwise rotation =
increase retention force

90° = 700 g.
(1.54 lb)

270° = 300 g.
(0.66 lb)

Counter clockwise rotation =
decrease retention force

180° = 500 g. (1.10 lb)

FIGURE 5.90.

Note: The lamella retention insert must not project out of the housing. If the lamella retention insert is no longer providing the acceptable amount of retention, replace it with a new one. There is no need to remove the titanium housing from the denture (Figure 5.90).

Note: Slight deviations from these average values are possible due to unavoidable manufacturing tolerances of the lamella retention insert and the retentive anchor. If signs of wear are evident on the retentive anchor, the retention force may no longer apply, and the retentive anchor abutment must be replaced.

Chair-Side Utilization of the Retentive Anchor Abutment and Elliptical Matrix

1. Insert the retentive anchor abutments into the implants and apply 35Ncm torque to each abutment (Figures 5.91, 5.92, 5.93, and 5.94).

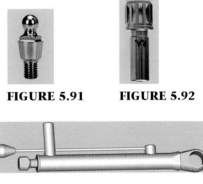

FIGURE 5.91   **FIGURE 5.92**

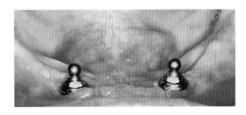

FIGURE 5.93.

FIGURE 5.94.

2. Use a large laboratory round carbide bur to cut a hole in the denture base exactly

above each retentive anchor abutment (Figure 5.95). Continue the hole toward the lingual flange and create a window. This hole should be large enough so there is no contact between the matrix and the denture base after inserting the elliptical matrix over the retentive anchor.

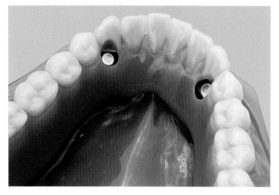

FIGURE 5.95.

3. Place the elliptical matrices over the retentive anchors (Figures 5.96, 5.97, and 5.98).

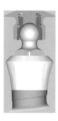

FIGURE 5.96.

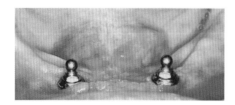

FIGURE 5.97.

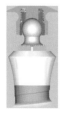

FIGURE 5.98.

Note: The matrices should be parallel with each other and to the path of insertion.

4. Place a small piece of rubber dam over the matrices to block out the undercut created between the lower edge of the matrix and the retentive anchor abutment (Figure 5.99). This dam prevents the acrylic from flowing into the internal aspect of the elliptical matrix, which could lock the denture in the patient's mouth.

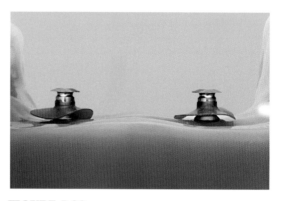

FIGURE 5.99.

5. Insert the denture and verify that there is no contact between each matrix and the denture base. If interference exists, trim the denture base.
6. Apply self-curing acrylic around and above each matrix, as well as inside each hole in the denture base (Figure 5.100). Ensure that the external retention wings on the outside of the matrix are completely covered with acrylic. Insert the denture into the patient's mouth

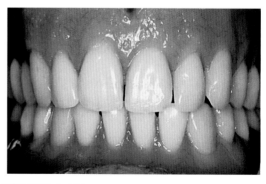

FIGURE 5.100.

over the attachment assembly and guide the patient into maximum inter-cuspation, but do not allow the patient to close firmly. Allowing the patient to close firmly could cause an improper position of the male components to the female components (Figure 5.100).

7. After the acrylic is set, remove the overdenture, fill any void with acrylic, and finish and polish the prosthesis (Figure 5.101).

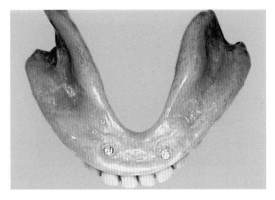

FIGURE 5.101.

8. Verify the occlusion and perform any necessary occlusal adjustments.

CLIX® ATTACHMENT AND THE ASTRA IMPLANT

The Clix® attachment assembly provides hinge and rotational resiliency. The range of movements with this attachment is 10 degrees. It is designed to virtually eliminate wear on the ball component of the attachment assembly. This attachment needs minimum maintenance. Changing the resilient insert is done quickly.

Design Specification of the Clix® Female Component

CLIX® INSERTS

- White (minimum retention)
- Yellow (moderate retention)
- Red (high retention)

Refer to Figure 5.102.

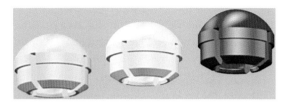

FIGURE 5.102.

METAL HOUSING

- Height 2.6mm
- Diameter 4.0mm
- Titanax (Ti-Al-V)

Refer to Figure 5.103.

FIGURE 5.103.

Design Specification of the Astra Ball Abutment (Figure 5.104)

DIAMETER OF BALL

- 2.25mm

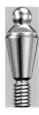

FIGURE 5.104.

ABUTMENT'S GINGIVAL CUFF HEIGHTS

- 0.0mm
- 1.5mm
- 3.00mm
- 4.5mm
- 6.0mm

Chair-Side Utilization Procedure

1. Measure the thickness of the tissue using the depth gauge set, Uni (Figures 5.105 and 5.106).

   Note: The tapered neck of the ball abutment should always stay above the gingival margin (Figures 5.105 and 5.106)

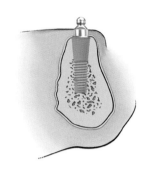

FIGURE 5.107.

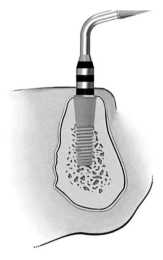

FIGURE 5.105.

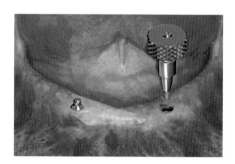

FIGURE 5.108.

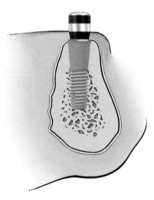

FIGURE 5.106.

2. Choose the appropriate ball abutment and seat the abutment using the ball wrench and the torque driver (Figures 5.107 and 5.108). Tighten the abutment to 20Ncm.

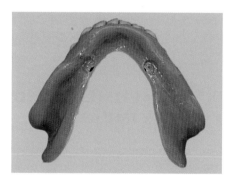

FIGURE 5.109.

3. Use a large laboratory round carbide bur to cut a hole in the denture base exactly above each ball abutment. Continue the hole toward the lingual flange and create a window. This hole should be large enough so you can insert a pre-loaded Clix® metal housing over the ball abutment with no contact between the metal housing and the denture base (Figure 5.109).

FIGURE 5.110.

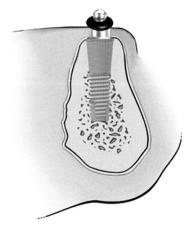

FIGURE 5.111.

4. Place the O-ring spacers over the ball abutments (Figures 5.110 and 5.111).
5. Load the metal housing with the desirable Clix® insert. Snap the female Clix® on each ball abutment (Figures 5.112, 5.113, and 5.114).
6. Block out the undercuts around each attachment assembly with a small piece of the rubber dam or a silicone material.

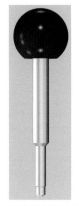
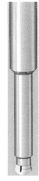

    FIGURE 5.112   **FIGURE 5.113**

FIGURE 5.114.

7. Insert the denture and verify that there is no contact between each female component and the denture base. If interference exists, trim the denture base.
8. Apply self-cure acrylic around and above each metal housing as well as inside each hole in the denture base. Ensure that the external retention ridge on the outside of the metal housing is completely covered with acrylic. Insert the denture into the patient's mouth over the attachment assembly and guide the patient into maximum intercuspation, but do not allow the patient to close firmly. Allowing the patient to close firmly could cause an improper position of the males to the females.
9. After the acrylic is set, remove the overdenture, fill any void with acrylic, and finish and polish the prosthesis.

Replacing Clix® Inserts

1. Remove the old Clix® insert by using a round bur or a hot instrument. Do not damage the retentive metal ledge of the housing (Figure 5.115).

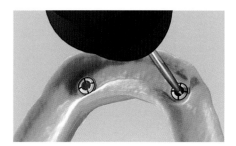

FIGURE 5.115.

2. Snap a new Clix® insert on the insertion tool (Figures 5.116, 5.117, and 5.118). Choose the new insert based on the amount of the desirable retention.

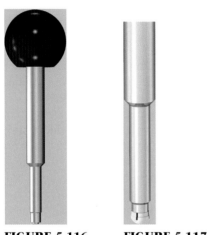

FIGURE 5.116   **FIGURE 5.117**

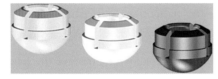

FIGURE 5.118.

3. Press the new Clix® insert into the metal housing (Figure 5.119).

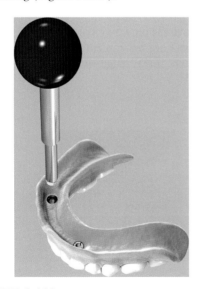

FIGURE 5.119.

Note: With this attachment system removing the metal housing from the denture base is unnecessary.

4. Insert the overdenture in the patient's mouth and verify that the required retention is obtained.

REFERENCES AND ADDITIONAL READING

Academy of Prosthodontics. (1999). *The Glossary of Prosthodontic Terms* (7th edition). *Journal of Prosthetic Dentistry*, 81, 41–110.

Albrektsson, T. & Zarb, G.A. (1998). Determinants of correct clinical reporting. *International Journal of Prosthodontics*, 11, 517–521.

Awad, M. A., Locker, D., Korner-Batinsky, N., & Feine, J. S. (2000). Measuring the effect of implant rehabilitation on health related quality of life in a randomized controlled clinical trial. *Journal of Dental Research*, 79, 1659–1664.

Awad, M. A., Lund, J. P., Dufrense, E., & Feine, J. S. (2003). Comparing the efficacy of mandibular implant-retained overdentures and conventional dentures among middle-aged patients: Satisfaction and functional assessment. *International Journal of Prosthodontics*, 16, 117–122.

Batenburg, R. H. K., Meijer, H. J. A., Raghoebar, G. M., Vissink, A. (1998). Treatment concept for mandibular overdentures supported by endosseous implants: A literature review. *International Journal of Oral & Maxillofacial Implants*, 13, 539–545.

Buser, D., Merickse-Stern, R., Dual, K., Lang, N. P. (1999). Clinical experience with one-stage, non-submerged dental implants. *Advances in Dental Research*, 13, 153–161.

Buser, D., von Arx, T., ten Bruggenkate, C., & Weingart, D. (2000). Basic surgical principles with ITI implants. *Clinical Oral Implants Research*, 1(supplement 1), 59–68.

Carr, A. B. (1998). Successful long-term treatment outcomes in the field of osseointegrated implants: Prosthodontic determinants. *International Journal of Prosthodontics*, 11, 502–512.

Cochran, D. L. (1999). A comparison of endosseous dental implant surfaces. *Journal of Periodontology*, 70, 1523–1539.

Cochran, D. L. (2001). The scientific basis for and clinical experiences with Straumann implants including the ITI Dental Implant System: A consensus report. *Clinical Oral Implants Research*, 11(supplement 1), 33–58.

Ericsson, I., Randow, K., Nilner, K., & Peterson, A. (2000). Early functional loading of Branemark implants. 5-year clinical follow-up study. *Clinical Implant Dentistry and Related Research*, 2, 70–77.

Espositio, M., Coulthard, P., Worthington, H. V., & Jokstad A. (2000). Quality assessment of randomized controlled trials of oral implants. *International Journal of Oral & Maxillofacial Implants*, 16, 783–792.

Fourmousis, I. & Bragger, U. (1999). "Radiographic interpretation of peri-implant structures." In *Proceedings of the 3rd European Workshop on Periodontology-Implant Dentistry*, ed. Lang, N. P., Karring, T., & Lindhe, J. Chicago: Quintessence Publishing, 228–241.

Friberg, B., Sennerby, L., Linden, B., Grondahl, U.K., & Lekholm, U. (1999). Stability measurements of one-stage Branemark implants during healing in mandibles. A clinical resonance frequency analysis study. *International Journal of Oral Maxillofacial Surgery*, 28, 266–272.

Jemt, T., Chai, J., Harnett, J., et al. (1996). A 5-year prospective multicenter follow-up report on overdentures supported by osseointegrated implants. *International Journal of Oral & Maxillofacial Implants*, 11, 291–298.

Lekholm, U. & Zarb, G. A. (1985). "Patient selection and preparation." In *Tissue-integrated Prostheses: Osseointegration in Clinical Dentistry*, ed. Branemark, P. L., Zarb, G. A., & Albrektsson, T. Chicago: Quintessence Publishing, 199–210.

Mericske-Stern, R. & Zarb, G. A. (1993). Overdentures: An alternative implant methodology for edentulous patients. *International Journal of Prosthodontics*, 6, 203–208.

Mericske-Stern, R. (1998). Three-dimensional force measurements with mandibular overdentures connected to implants by ball-shaped retentive anchors. A clinical study. *International Journal of Oral & Maxillofacial Implants*, 13, 36–43.

Mericske-Stern, R. (1998). Treatment outcomes with implant-supported overdentures: Clinical considerations. *Journal of Prosthetic Dentistry*, 79, 66–73.

Mericske-Stern, R., Piotti, M., & Sirtes, G. (1996). 3-D in vivo force measurements on mandibular implants supporting overdentures. A comparative study. *Clinical Oral Implants Research*, 7, 387–396.

Naert, I., Gizani, S., Vuylskeke, M., & van Steenberghe D. (1999). A 5-year prospective randomized clinical trial on the influence of splinted and unsplinted oral implants retaining a mandibular overdenture: Prosthetic aspects and patient satisfaction. *Journal of Oral Rehabilitation*, 26, 195–202.

Payne, A. G. T., Solomons, Y. F., & Lownie, J. F. (1999). Standardization of radiographs for mandibular implant-supported overdentures: Review and innovation. *Clinical Oral Implants Research*, 10, 307–319.

Payne, A. G. T., Solomons, Y. F., Lownie, J. F., & Tawse-Smith, A. (2001). Inter-abutment and peri-abutment mucosal enlargement with mandibular implant overdentures. *Clinical Oral Implants Research*, 13, 179–187.

Payne, A. G. T., Tawse-Smith, A., Duncan, W. J., Kumara, R., (2002). Conventional and early loading of unsplinted ITI implants supporting mandibular ovedentures: Two-year results of a prospective randomized clinical trial. *Clinical Oral Implants Research*, 13, 603–609.

Payne, A. G. T., Tawse-Smith, A., Kumara, R., Thomson, W. M. (2001). One-year prospective evaluation of the early loading of unsplinted conical Branemark fixtures with mandibular overdentures: A preliminary report. *Clinical Implant Dentistry and Related Research*, 3, 9–18.

Sadowsky, S. J. (2001). Mandibular implant-retained overdentures: A literature review. *Journal of Prosthetic Dentistry*, 86, 468–473.

Schmitt, A. & Zarb, G. A. (1998). The notion of implant-supported overdentures. *Journal of Prosthetic Dentistry*, 79, 60–65.

Sul, Y. T., Johansson, C. B., Jeong, Y., Wennerberg, A., & Albrektsson, T. (2002). Resonance frequency and removal torque analysis of implants with turned and anodized surface oxides. *Clinical Oral Implants Research*, 13, 252–259.

Szmukler-Moncler, S., Piattelli, A., Favero, G. A., Dubruille, J. H. (2000). Considerations preliminary to the application of early and immediate loading protocols in dental implantology. *Clinical Oral Implants Research*, 11, 12–25.

Tawse-Smith, A., Duncan, W., Payne, A. G. T., Thomson, W. M., & Wennstrom, J. L. (2002). Effectiveness of electric toothbrushes in peri-implant maintenance of mandibular implant overdentures. *Journal of Clinical Periodontology*, 29, 275–280.

Tawse-Smith, A., Payne, A. G. T., Kumara, R., & Thomson, W. M. (2001). A one-stage operative procedure using 2 different implant systems: A prospective study on implant overdentures in the edentulous mandible. *Clinical Implant Dentistry and Related Research*, 3, 185–193.

Tawse-Smith, A., Payne, A. G. T., Kumara, R., & Thomson W. M. (2002). Early loading of un-splinted implants supporting mandibular overden-tures using a one-stage operative procedure with two different implant systems: A 2-year report. *Clinical Implant Dentistry and Related Research*, 4, 33–42.

Watson, G., Payne, A. G. T., Purton, D. G., & Thom-son, W. G. (2002). Mandibular implant overden-tures: Comparative evaluation of the prosthodon-tic maintenance during the first year of service using three different systems. *International Journal of Prosthodontics*, 15, 259–266.

Wismeijer, D., van Waas, M. A., Vermeeren, J. I., Mulder, J., & Kalk, W. (1997). Patient satisfac-tion with implant-supported mandibular overden-tures. A comparison of three treatment strate-gies with ITI dental implants. *International Journal of Oral & Maxillofacial Implants*, 26, 263–267.

Wismeijer, D., van Waas, M. A. J., Mulder, J., Ver-meeren, J. I. J. F., & Kalk W. (1999). Clinical and radiological results of patients treated with three treatment modalities for overdentures on implants of the ITI Dental Implant System. *Clinical Oral Implants Research*, 10, 297–306.

Zarb, G. A. (1983). The edentulous milieu. *Journal of Prosthetic Dentistry*, 49, 825–831.

6
Bar Attachments

Hamid Shafie
James Ellison

BAR MATERIALS

Bar attachments can be prefabricated type IV gold like the original 1.6mm Dolder Bar. Prefabricated type IV gold bars should be soldered to the abutments with a low fusing solder. The other types of bars come in castable pre-milled plastic patterns. These bars are available in 0, 2, and 4 degrees for telescopic milled restorations. The bar castings should only be made with hard alloys. A minimum Vickers hardness of 200 and at least 95,000psi ultimate tensile strength is required. Non-precious alloys are contraindicated for implant reconstruction.

Examples of Castable Bars
- Round bar
- Plastic Dolder Bar
- I bar
- EDS bar
- Hader Bar

Bar clips or riders are available in different materials and configurations. The metal clips/ riders are fully adjustable. Plastic Hader/EDS clips are non-adjustable, but they can easily be replaced at chair side. Use of a metal housing with Hader/EDS plastic clips is strongly recommended.

Classification of Bar Attachments Based on Cross-Sectional Shapes

- Round (Figure 6.1)

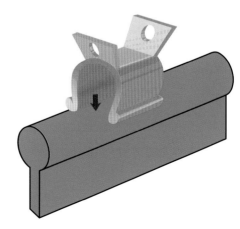

FIGURE 6.1.

63

- Egg shaped (Figures 6.2 and 6.3)

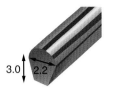

FIGURE 6.2.

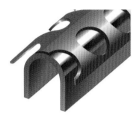

FIGURE 6.3.

- Parallel sided "U" shape (Figure 6.4)

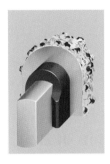

FIGURE 6.4.

Classification of Bars Based on the Nature of Their Resiliency

- Bar joints (resilient) provide vertical and/or hinge resiliency (Figure 6.5)

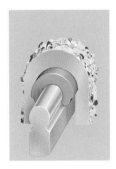

FIGURE 6.5.

- Bar units (non-resilient) (Figure 6.6)

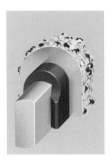

FIGURE 6.6.

Factors that Influence the Flexibility of the Bar

- Length of the bar between the two implants
- Number of implants that support the bar
- Height of the bar
- Physical properties of the alloy
- Magnitude of the masticatory loads

FUNDAMENTALS OF BAR ARRANGEMENT

As a general rule if a single bar is being utilized, the ideal length should be 20–22mm to accommodate two clips/riders. This means the center of the implants should be 24–26mm apart if standard diameter 4mm implants are being used (Figure 6.7 and 6.8).

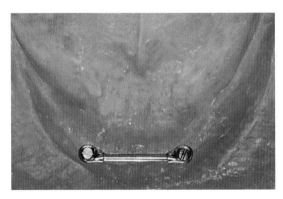

FIGURE 6.7.

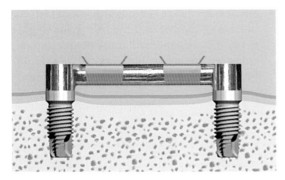

FIGURE 6.8.

If the two implants are too close, the short bar cannot provide enough retention and stability for the overdenture (Figure 6.9).

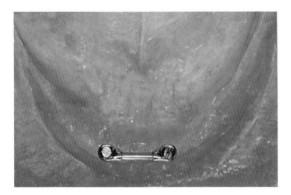

FIGURE 6.9.

This distance, however, depends on following conditions:

- Size and curvature of the mandibular arch
- Type of attachment assembly

If the implants are placed too far distally, a straight-line bar will interfere with the tongue space and create problems in fabricating the prosthesis, also it will be at risk of bending (Figure 6.10 and 6.11).

If the bar has been positioned diagonally, it will not allow friction free anterior hinge movement of the prosthesis. This condition creates excessive torsional loading on the supporting implants (Figure 6.12).

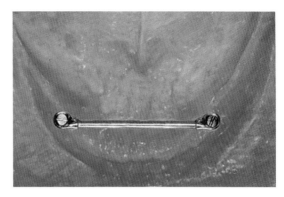

FIGURE 6.10.

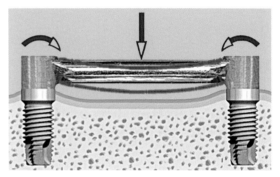

FIGURE 6.11.

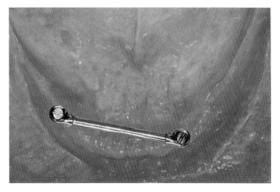

FIGURE 6.12.

As a general rule the bar should be perpendicular to the line that bisects the angle formed by the two posterior mandibular arch segments (Figure 6.13).

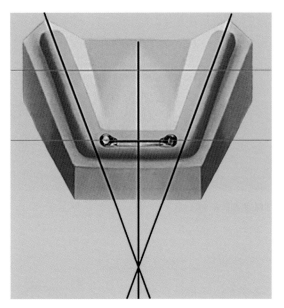

FIGURE 6.13.

Vertical Relationship of the Bar to the Alveolar Ridge

- *Wide Gap:* There is 2mm or more between the bottom of the bar and the soft tissue (Figure 6.14). This distance allows easy passage of saliva and food particles as well as cleaning tools. Hygiene maintenance in this situation is very easy.

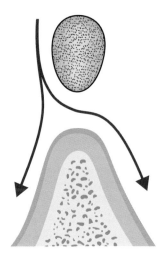

FIGURE 6.14.

- *Small Gap:* There is 1mm or less between the bottom of the bar and the soft tissue (Figure 6.15). This distance will cause plaque and calculus accumulation and it would be very difficult to perform oral hygiene maintenance.

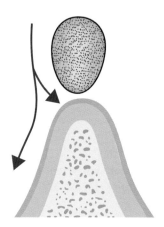

FIGURE 6.15.

- *Compression of the Mucosa by the Bar:* This causes hyperplasia of the gum (Figure 6.16). It is impossible to clean underneath the bar. The bar should be replaced or modified to solve this problem.

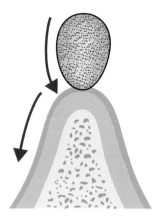

FIGURE 6.16.

Sagittal Relationship of the Bar to the Alveolar Ridge

The bar should be positioned directly above the crest of the ridge (Figure 6.17). This position makes it easy to clean the bar and fabricate the prosthesis above the bar.

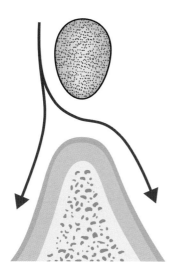

FIGURE 6.17.

If the bar is positioned lingual to the crest of the ridge, it will interfere with tongue space and its function and the patient's speech (Figure 6.18). This problem is a common situation in patients with a narrow and pointed alveolar ridge. One way to prevent this situation is to re-locate the bar further anteriorly. Another solution is to use individual attachments.

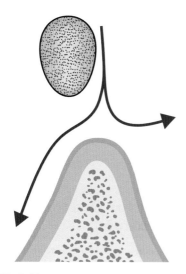

FIGURE 6.18.

If the bar is positioned labial to the crest of the ridge, it will interfere with lip support (Figure 6.19). Both of these scenarios will make fabrication of the prosthesis very difficult.

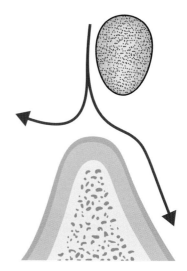

FIGURE 6.19.

Sagittal Relationship of the Bar to the Hinge Axis

It would be ideal if the anterior bar in the edentulous mandible were parallel to the hinge axis. However, this relationship is another reference for better positioning of the bar and this orientation can't be achieved in every case. This rule has been followed by many clinicians, but no studies have supported this claim. The long term study (5–15 years) by Oetterli, Kiener and Mericske-Stern analyzed the influence of placing the bar parallel to the hinge axis on peri-implant parameters, including the clinical attachment level. The outcome as far as the type of retention, splinted versus unsplinted, was also assessed. No significant correlations were found.

Sometimes the anatomical shape of the alveolar ridge will not allow the surgeon to position the implants with the bar parallel to the hinge axis (Figure 6.20 and 6.21). In this situation, the lab technician and restorative doctor can modify the bar design to achieve this goal.

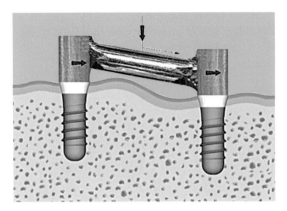

FIGURE 6.20.

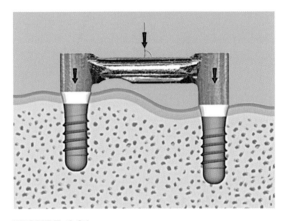

FIGURE 6.21.

Anterior-Posterior Distance Rule

The anterior-posterior distance rule is good for determining the distal cantilever extension of the bar or distal extension of the hybrid (fixed detachable) prosthesis from the most posterior implants.

- Draw a line through the center of the most posterior implants on each side of the arch (Figure 6.22).
- Draw another line through the center of the most anterior implants on each side of the arch.
- The distance between these two lines is the Anterior–Posterior spread (A–P distance).

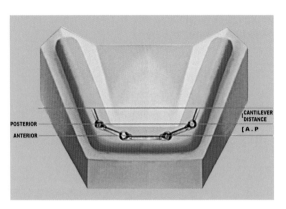

FIGURE 6.22.

- Generally, the distal cantilever should not exceed more than half of the Anterior–Posterior distance.

If the patient has a small mandible, with limited room for four implants, putting the distal implants as far back as possible to the mental nerve can enhance the A–P distance. In addition, the anterior implants should be brought forward as far as possible. These steps will improve the A–P distance to ensure that the basic biomechanical rules are not violated. The maximum cantilever in these cases is generally 8–12mm.

If the patient has a square arch, the implants will be in a straight line in the anterior segment of the mandible. In this situation, any cantilever design must be avoided since the A–P distance will be non-existent or significantly reduced. Resilient bar assemblies are suggested for these patients. The prosthesis should be implant and tissue born so that the buccal shelf and retromolar pad will receive a share of the occlusal load.

To minimize the compressive load on the bar, the denture base can be relieved in the area over the distal extensions.

Guidelines for Denture Base Extension

- *Mainly Tissue Supported Implant Overdenture:* The borders of the overdenture in the anterior area should not extend to the end of the sulcus. There should be minimum extension in the anterior region but maximum extension in stress bearing areas such as buccal shelves. The denture base should extend distally onto the retromolar pads and lingually onto the mylohyoid ridge.

- *Tissue-Implant-Supported Overdenture:* The borders of the overdenture are significantly shorter than conventional dentures; however, they can't be eliminated since this type of prosthesis is still partly tissue supported.
- *Fully Implant-Supported Overdenture:* Since the prosthesis is completely implant born, flanges can be eliminated.

HADER BAR

In 1973, Helmut Hader, master technician and dental manufacturer, developed a unique attachment system that even today is mainly known in the USA as Hader Bar and Hader Vertical. The Hader Bar is a semi-precision bar attachment that provides hinge movement as long as a single Hader Bar has been utilized in an attachment assembly design. The function of this bar is based on the mechanical snap retention concept (Figures 6.23 and 6.24).

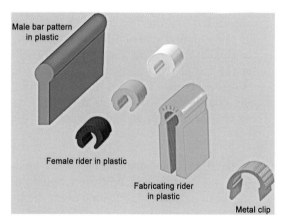

FIGURE 6.23.

Three color-coded clips/riders are available with three retentive strengths. In order from the least to most retentive, they are white, yellow, and red. Use of a metal housing with the Hader

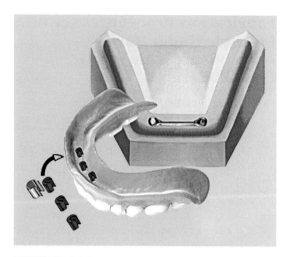

FIGURE 6.24.

plastic clips/riders is strongly recommended. In addition to plastic clips/riders, the option of adjustable gold alloy clips/riders is available (Figures 6.25 and 6.26).

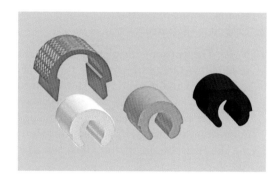

FIGURE 6.25.

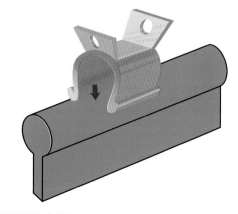

FIGURE 6.26.

Fabrication Procedures for a Castable Hader Bar Attachment with Plastic Clips/Riders

1. Choose matching pick-up impression copings based on the implant type and diameter.
2. Make a full arch pick-up impression utilizing a rigid impression material such as polyether.
3. Fabricate the master cast with soft tissue model.
4. Choose matching gold base non-hex plastic UCLA abutments.
5. Adjust the length of the plastic bar based on the distance between the UCLA abutments and the shape of the alveolar ridge.
6. Connect the plastic bar to the UCLA abutments with wax.
7. Sprue the bar and UCLA abutments. The sprues should always be placed on the connecting points of the bar.
8. Complete the casting steps.

   Note: The burnout for plastic components requires two stages. First, raise the temperature slowly to 600°F (316°C) and hold for 30 minutes. This assures a clean and complete burnout of the plastic piece. Second, complete the burnout procedure by following the instructions of the alloy manufacturer.

9. Finish and polish the casting.

   Note: Do not grind the round bar with stones, burs, or rubber wheels. Grinding reduces the bar diameter and alters the fit and retention of the clips/riders. Finish and polish with polishing compound or with Tripoli and rouge.

10. Try the bar in the mouth by using the Sheffield test. (Refer to Chapter 7.)

    Note: If a removable die model was used for fabricating the bar, or if the bar has to be cut and soldered, then a new impression should be made picking up the bar and retainers. A new, solid master model is fabricated from this impression.

11. Insert the polished bar on the solid master cast. Snap plastic clips/riders on the bar. Insert as many clips/riders on the bar as space allows, which will provide space for additional clips/riders to be inserted to increase retention if necessary. Block out the undercuts of the bar and over the abutments. Do not block out the retentive undercuts of the clips/riders.

    Note: Recommended block-out materials are Rubber Sep. Sterngold order #812045 and Litebloc UV–Bredent order #52000980.

12. In order to fabricate a duplicate cast for denture processing, make an impression of the master cast with the undercuts blocked out on the screwed bar and clips/riders that are snapped on the bar.

13. Insert laboratory clips/riders into the impression in exactly the same position as the imprints of the actual clips/riders and pour the impression. The laboratory clips/riders will be held in the proper position in the duplicate cast by the extensions of the riders in the stone.

    Note: Do not try to shorten the extension of the laboratory riders/clips and place them on the bar. Shortening the extension will cause improper fit of the laboratory clips/riders on the bar, which will create larger retention spaces in the denture base. In this situation, the final clips/riders will not be completely stable in the denture base. When the patient removes the overdenture, the clips/riders will tend to be pulled out of the denture base and remain on the bar.

    Note: If metal housings are used, slide them onto the laboratory clips/riders from the side of the clip after fabrication of the duplicate cast. Do not snap the metal housings on the laboratory riders/clips from the occlusal direction, which could deform the housings and cause the final riders/clips to pull out of the denture.

14. Try the denture teeth setup in the mouth. Send the teeth back to the lab for processing.

15. Insert the prosthesis on the duplicate cast and process it with the technique of choice.
16. Deflask the prosthesis. Remove all of the stone and then remove the laboratory clips/riders with pliers or a hemostat. Finish and polish the denture.
17. Insert actual clips/riders in their position in the denture base by using a special seating tool, which has been supplied in the attachment kit. Press the clips/riders into the prepared receptacles in the acrylic denture base or into the metal housings, which are already positioned in the denture base. There should be a snap when the clips/riders are pushed into position. The clips/riders are easily seated and can be easily replaced. The special shape of the receptacle in the acrylic denture base or metal housing provides secure retention of the clips/riders, while providing leeway space in the labiolingual direction to allow the clips/riders some flex during insertion or removal of the prosthesis.

Fabrication Procedures for a Castable Hader Bar Attachment with Gold Alloy Clips/Riders

1. Choose the desirable gauge of the castable bar and matching gold alloy clips/riders.
2. Wax the gold base non-hex UCLA abutments and the bar.
3. Cast the whole assembly with a hard alloy to eliminate premature wear. Finish and polish the bar assembly.

Note: Palladium copper alloys are recommended for fabrication of the bar. This alloy has sufficient surface hardness as well as very high yield strength. These physical properties increase the clinical wear resistance of the bar. Following are some examples:

- Columbus (Sterngold)
- Argelite 76 SF+ (Argen)
- Pegasus ceramic alloy
- Sterngold 100 crown and bridge alloy
- Argenco 60 M crown and bridge alloy (Argen)

4. Insert the bar over the analogs in the master cast. Block out all of the undercuts and make an impression of the master cast and the bar to create a duplicate cast for denture processing.
5. Adapt the supplied spacer sheet over the stone representation of the bar. Snap the metal clips/riders onto the spacer and the stone representation of the bar (Figure 6.27).

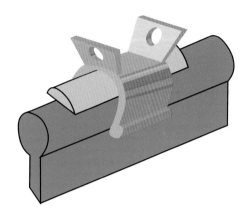

FIGURE 6.27.

6. Block out all of the undercuts on the duplicate cast. Be sure that the block-out material has covered half of the cylindrical portion of the clips/riders. This coverage provides a free space between the acrylic denture base and each side of the clip/rider, allowing the clinician to adjust the amount of retention provided by each clip/rider. This free space lets the patient easily insert and remove the overdenture.
7. Complete the denture teeth setup, waxing, processing, finishing, and polishing of the prosthesis. Be careful when finishing the acrylic around the clips/riders to avoid any contact between the burs and the clips/riders.

Note: The metal clips/riders can be picked up with self-curing resin in the denture base.

Hader Clip Placement

Hader clips can wear out prematurely due to improper bar design and overloading. The denture base should sufficiently contact the top of the bar and avoid concentrating force on the clip(s).

To achieve this contact, the denture base should be relined precisely. Hader clips can be replaced chair side.

Chair-Side Replacement of Hader Clip

1. Remove the worn clip with a hand instrument. The clip usually comes out very cleanly and in one piece.
2. Place a new Hader clip on the insertion tool.
3. Place the clip into the undercut area of the recipient site and gently roll until it snaps into place.

Caution: Do not push straight down into the recipient site, because the insertion of the clip has a rotational path.

The clips should hold their properties for at least six to nine months if they are well designed.

Plastic Hader vs. Metal Clips

ADVANTAGES OF METAL CLIPS

- Metal clips have more wear resistance compared to plastic clips.
- The bar dimensions can be smaller with metal clips.

DISADVANTAGES OF METAL CLIPS

- To replace a metal clip, it has to be cut off of the denture base with a bur.
- Metal clips do not come out as cleanly as plastic clips.
- Metal clips require chair-side pickup with self-cure acrylic.

Mandibular Implant-Supported Overdenture Utilizing Hader Bar and Castable ERA Attachment

This design is very popular when four implants have been placed with a good A–P distance. This attachment assembly includes a Hader Bar between two anterior implants and two ERA attachments off the distal of the attachment assembly. ERA attachments should be positioned lingually in relationship to the crest of the ridge (Figure 6.28).

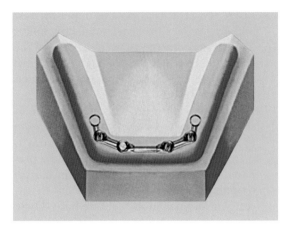

FIGURE 6.28.

Troubleshooting for Hader Bar Attachment Assembly

Refer to Table 6.1 for guidance in troubleshooting the Hader Bar Attachment Assembly.

DOLDER BAR

The Dolder Bar is a prefabricated precision bar attachment. This bar was developed by Dr. Eugen Dolder in Switzerland. It comes in two forms:

- *Rigid:* U-shaped with parallel walls. The rigid type is also called a *bar unit*.
- *Resilient:* Egg-shaped and provides vertical and hinge resiliency. The resilient Dolder Bar is also called a *bar joint*.

The Dolder Bar and its sleeve are made of gold alloy (Elitor). The Dolder Bar is an adjustable bar, so the clinician can control the amount of retention provided by the bar. The Dolder Bar should be soldered to the abutments, and the sleeve should be secured in the denture base with self-cure acrylic.

Indications

- Overdenture patients with adequate or relatively large inter-ridge space

TABLE 6.1. Troubleshooting for Hader Bar Attachment Assembly

Problem	Possible Reason	Solution
Failure in achieving a one-piece casting of the bar and abutments.	Plastic bar pattern was not connected well to the abutments with wax, or the connection broke loose during investing.	Use adequate wax to connect plastic bar to abutments. Invest carefully without excessive vibration.
Failure of the plastic riders to stay in the receptacle in the acrylic denture base.	The laboratory clips/riders were placed over the bar prior to taking the impression rather than the actual retentive clips/riders, which causes the gingival extension of the laboratory clips/riders to expand and cause an oversized receptacle to be processed in the resin.	Position the actual clips/riders, not the laboratory clips/riders, on the cast bar prior to taking the impression for the duplicate processing cast.
Insufficient retention of the plastic clips/riders on the bar.	a) The round bar was reduced in diameter due to overfinishing and polishing. b) The plastic clips/riders are worn.	a) Do not use stones or rubber wheels on the round bar when finishing; polish only. b) Replace plastic clips/riders, or use gold alloy clips/riders that have retention adjustment capability.
The prosthesis is difficult to insert and remove.	a) The plastic retention clips/riders have been processed into the resin incorrectly. The denture acrylic base is preventing the flanges of the clips/riders from flexing. b) The prosthesis was designed to engage a severe labial undercut. This causes the prosthesis to be positioned labially at time of insertion, thus the plastic clips/riders are not properly aligned to snap onto the bar.	a) Use rebasing procedure to replace clips/riders. b) Remove the labial flange area which engages the severe undercut from the prosthesis.

- When minimum resiliency and maximum retention from a removable overdenture is expected, the Dolder Bar is the bar attachment of choice.

Contraindications

- Patients with minimum inter-ridge space

- Patients with poor compliance in maintenance and oral hygiene
- Patients with financial limitations

Dimensional Specifications

The Dolder Bar is available in two sizes: large and small. Refer to Table 6.2 (Figures 6.29 and 6.30).

TABLE 6.2. Dimensional Specifications

Type	Height	Width	Lengths	Combined height of the bar and sleeve	Outside width of sleeve wings
Small Bar Unit	2.3mm	1.6mm	3, 5cm	2.8mm	3.5mm
Large Bar Unit	3.00mm	2.2mm	3, 5cm	3.5mm	4.5mm
Small Bar Joint	2.3mm	1.6mm	3, 5cm	3.5mm	3.5mm
Large Bar Joint	3.00mm	2.2mm	3, 5cm	4.5mm	4.5mm

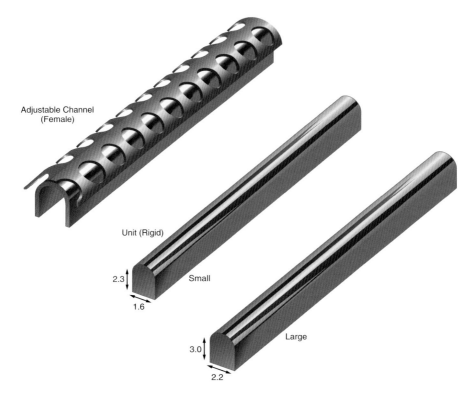

FIGURE 6.29.

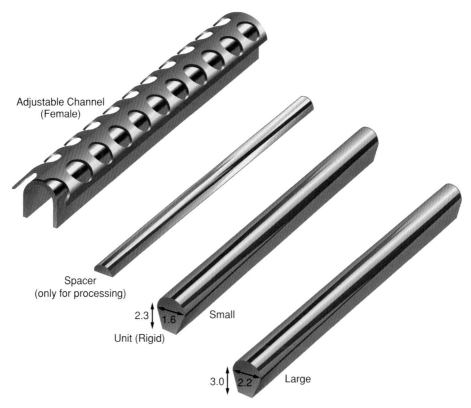

FIGURE 6.30.

74

Fabrication Procedure for a Dolder Bar Unit

1. Choose matching pick-up impression copings based on the implant type and diameter.
2. Make a full arch pick-up impression utilizing a rigid impression material such as polyether.
3. Fabricate the master cast with soft tissue model.
4. Choose gold cylinders or abutments that are compatible with the implant system that has been used. The lab technician should be able to solder or weld the bar to those gold abutments.
5. Cut the bar to the desirable length. Stabilize and secure the bar between the two gold abutments and then solder or weld it to those abutments.
6. After soldering, finish each end of the bar to a rounded contour and then insert the finished bar over the implant analogs.
7. Verify the accuracy and passive fit of the bar by performing the Sheffield test. This test should be repeated in the patient's mouth as well.
8. Adjust the length of the sleeve according to the length of the bar. Snap the sleeve on the bar and then start setting the teeth, which will give the lab technician a good idea about space management and how to contour the teeth.
9. Try the bar and denture teeth in the patient's mouth. Repeat the Sheffield test in the patient's mouth.
10. After trying the denture teeth setup, remove the sleeve from the acrylic base. Insert the bar on the master cast and snap the sleeve on the bar.
11. Block out the space between the bottom of the bar and the soft tissue model, as well as over the abutments and the screw access holes. Rubber-sep, Litebloc UV, or plaster can be used for block out. The block-out material should cover both sides of the sleeve to approximately half its height and along its entire length.
12. Finish any necessary adjustments to the denture teeth and complete the final wax up. Process the dentures as usual.

13. Deflask, finish, and polish the overdenture. Remove the block-out material and adjust the retention of the sleeve as desired.

Relining an Overdenture with a Dolder Bar Unit Attachment Assembly

Fill the sleeve with petroleum jelly, and take the final impression. Place the processing jig in the sleeve in the impression and pour the model. Reline the prosthesis with the usual technique.

Note: Dolder Bar matrix must cover the entire length of the bar. This will maximize the absorption of the horizontal forces.

Fabrication Procedure for a Dolder Bar Joint

1. Choose matching pick-up impression copings based on the implant type and diameter.
2. Make a full arch pick-up impression utilizing a rigid impression material such as polyether.
3. Fabricate the master cast with soft tissue model.
4. Choose gold cylinders or abutments that are compatible with the implant system that has been used. The lab technician should be able to solder or weld the bar to the gold abutments.
5. Cut the bar to the desired length. Stabilize and secure the bar between the two gold abutments and then solder or weld it to those abutments. Since this type of Dolder Bar provides vertical and hinge resiliency, the bar should be positioned parallel to the occlusal plane and at a right angle to the mid-sagittal plane.
6. After soldering, finish each end of the bar to a rounded contour and then insert the finished bar over the implant analogs.
7. Verify the accuracy and passive fit of the bar by performing the Sheffield test. (Refer to Chapter 7.) This test should be repeated in the patient's mouth as well.
8. Adjust the length of the sleeve according to the length of the bar. Snap the sleeve on the bar and then start setting the teeth, which will give the lab technician a good

idea about space management and how to contour the teeth.

9. Try the bar and denture teeth in the patient's mouth. Repeat the Sheffield test in the patient's mouth.

10. After trying the denture teeth setup, remove the sleeve from the acrylic base. Insert the bar back on the master cast and then cut the proper length of spacer wire and place it between the bar and the sleeve. Seat the sleeve on the spacer and rotate it until it makes contact with the anterior section of the bar. This position provides a positive stop to prevent any undesirable posterior lift of the prosthesis.

11. Block out the space between the bottom of the bar and the soft tissue model, as well as over the abutments and the screw access holes. Rubber-sep, Litebloc UV, or plaster can be used for block out. The block-out material should cover both sides of the sleeve to approximately half its height and along its entire length.

12. Finish any necessary adjustment to the denture teeth and complete the final wax up. Process the dentures as usual.

13. Deflask, finish, and polish the overdenture. Remove the block-out material and spacer wire and adjust the retention of the sleeve as desired.

Relining an Overdenture with a Dolder Bar Joint Attachment Assembly

Use sticky wax to secure the spacer wire in the sleeve, and fill the sleeve with petroleum jelly. Take the final impression. Place the processing jig into the sleeve in the impression and pour the model. Reline the prosthesis with the usual technique and remove the spacer wire before delivery.

Note: Always insert the spacer between the matrix and the Dolder Bar joint before incorporating the matrix into the denture base. This ensures the vertical resiliency of the overdenture.

Note: Dolder Bar matrix must cover the entire length of the bar. This maximizes the absorption of the horizontal forces.

VARIO SOFT BAR PATTERN VSP

The Vario Soft Bar Pattern VSP is manufactured by Bredent. This bar is available in two kinds of castable plastic patterns as well as solid grade 5 titanium. The gingival portion of the castable pattern and titanium bars are rounded to make it easy for the patient to maintain good oral hygiene. The bar patterns have been made of a non-distorting, fully burnable thermoplastic material that guarantees optimum precision in castings. This material will not leave any residue after the burn-out process. This plastic material is also very rigid, so it is very easy to trim with an acrylic bur (Figures 6.31, 6.32, and 6.33).

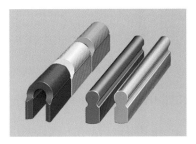

FIGURE 6.31.

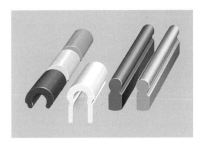

FIGURE 6.32.

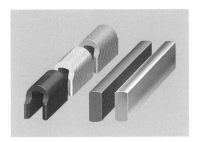

FIGURE 6.33.

Advantages of Prefabricated Titanium Bar

- Saves considerable laboratory steps, time, and material for dental technician
- More cost effective
- More accurate relationship between the bar and clips
- Eliminates all inaccuracies related to the casting process
- Guarantees high biocompatibility

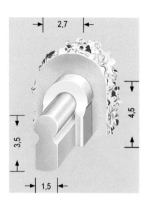

FIGURE 6.35.

Advantages of Plastic Castable Bar

- Provides more opportunities for the lab technician to create functional and aesthetic reconstruction even in the most difficult cases.
- Can be cast with different alloys
- Can be combined with castable stud attachment systems

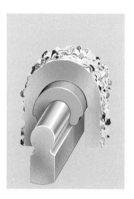

FIGURE 6.36.

Shapes of VSP Bar

- *Rectangular Shape:* It has parallel sides and provides complete rigidity (Figure 6.34).

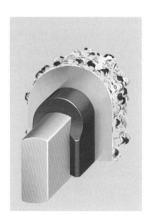

FIGURE 6.34.

- *I Shape:* Depending on what kind of matrix/clip has been used, it provides either complete rigidity or hinge resiliency (Figures 6.35 and 6.36).

Shapes of VSP Bar's Clips

- *Parallel-Sided Matrices/Clips for Rectangular Bar:* These matrices/clips provide complete rigidity through friction only (Figure 6.37).

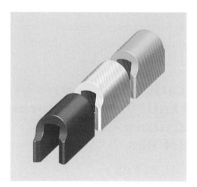

FIGURE 6.37.

- *Snap-on Matrices/Clips with Parallel-Sided Extension:* These matrices/clips fit on the I bar and provide complete rigidity through friction and a snap-on connection with the bar (Figure 6.38).

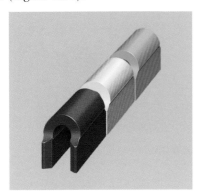

FIGURE 6.38.

- *Snap-on Matrices/Clips with No Extension:* These matrices/clips fit on the I bar and provide hinge resiliency (Figure 6.39).

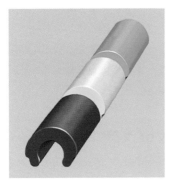

FIGURE 6.39.

Matrix/Clip Retention Levels
- *Green:* Low retention 4Ncm
- *Yellow:* Medium retention 6Ncm
- *Red:* High retention 8Ncm

Fabrication Procedures of a Rigid Fully Implant-Borne Overdenture Using a Parallel Bar

CLINICAL STEPS

1. Make an impression of the supporting implant by using transfer copings and a rigid impression material.

2. After the bar assembly is finished and polished, perform the Sheffield test in the patient's mouth to verify the passive fit of the bar assembly. (Refer to Chapter 7.)
3. Register the centric relation as well as the vertical dimension of the occlusion.
4. Try the denture teeth before denture processing and verify the centric relation, vertical dimension, aesthetic, and phonetic.
5. On the day of delivery of the final prosthesis, perform an occlusal adjustment and, preferably, perform a clinical remount.

LABORATORY STEPS

1. Screw the corresponding lab analogs into the transfer copings and pure the impression with a minimum expansion stone (Bredent "Thixo Rock").
2. Choose gold abutments if utilizing a castable bar pattern, but if utilizing a titanium bar, choose the appropriate titanium abutments.
3. Place the titanium bar between the implant abutments using the paralleling mandrel (item # 430 0623 0). If multiple bars are used, make sure that all of the bars are parallel to each other. Cut the bar to the desired length and then laser-weld it to the titanium abutments. For this step, follow the entire laser-welding instructions recommended by the welding unit manufacture. Do not grind or mill the bar to reduce the thickness. If required, polish the friction surfaces of the bar slightly to a higher luster; do not use coarse or abrasive polishing paste (Figure 6.40).

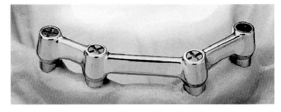

FIGURE 6.40.

If using a castable bar pattern, measure the distance between the gold abutments and cut the plastic bars to the designated length. If using a multiple bar design, repeat the same step for each bar. After cutting the bar, it should be fitted between the implant abutments by utilizing the paralleling mandrel (part # 430 0623 0) (Figure 6.41).

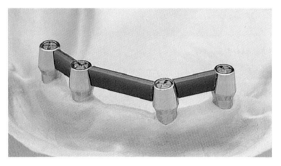

FIGURE 6.41.

4. Cast the plastic bars, finish, and polish them. Do not grind or mill the bar to reduce the thickness. If required, polish the friction surfaces of the bar slightly to a higher luster; do not use coarse or abrasive polishing paste or rouge.
5. Mount the finished bar on the paralleling mandrel and position it between the two gold abutments (Figure 6.42). Secure its position with pattern resin (Bredcnt PiKuPlast HP36 order # 540 0022 0) and solder the bar to the gold abutments (Figure 6.43). If multiple bars are in the attachment assembly design, repeat the same step for each bar (Figure 6.44).

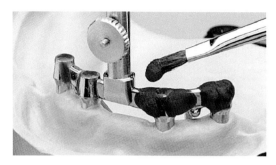

FIGURE 6.43.

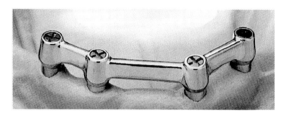

FIGURE 6.44.

6. Start the duplication process to create the refractory cast. First snap on a yellow matrix/clip over the bar assembly. Using the yellow matrix/clip provides the optimum conditions for changing the level of retention. Next, block out all of the undercuts and make a refractory cast (Brevest Rapid 1) using the usual duplicating technique (Figures 6.45 and 6.46).

Note: No spacer wax should be applied around the matrix.

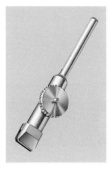

FIGURE 6.42.

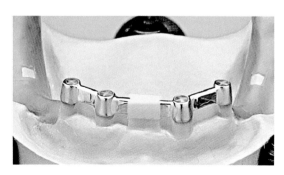

FIGURE 6.45.

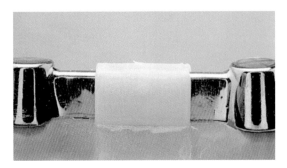

FIGURE 6.46.

7. In the refractory cast, the matrix/clip is also duplicated, which will create space for the recipient housing in the chrome cobalt (Brealloy F 400) framework (Figure 6.47).

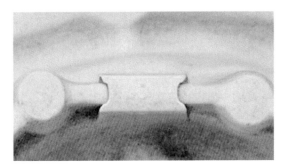

FIGURE 6.47.

8. Duplication of the bar and the matrix in the refractory cast should be covered with wax and plastic beads. The remaining sections of the framework should be waxed as required and planned (Figure 6.48).

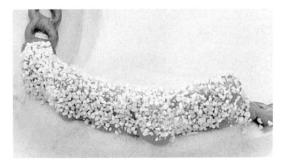

FIGURE 6.48.

9. Cast the metal housing and then finish and polish it (Figure 6.49).

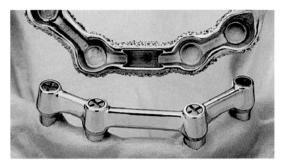

FIGURE 6.49.

Note: Do not grind the inside of the matrix recipient site in the metal housing with a carbide bur. Do not electro-polish the metal housing from the inside. Simply finish it with sandblasting (aluminum oxide 110 micron).

10. Before inserting the final and designated matrix/clip into its recipient site in the chrome cobalt metal housing, check the housing for high spots.

11. Choose the matrix with the desirable degree of retention and press-fit it inside the chrome cobalt recipient site utilizing an insertion tool (part # 430 0622 0) (Figures 6.50, 6.51, 6.52, and 6.53).

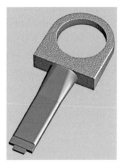

FIGURE 6.50.

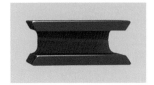

FIGURE 6.51.

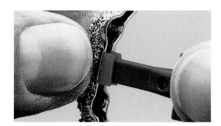

FIGURE 6.52.

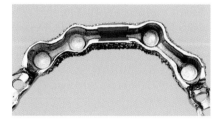

FIGURE 6.53.

12. Make the wax rim for the jaw relationship record.
13. After registration of the centric relation and vertical dimension on the occlusion, set up the denture teeth in the lingualized occlusion.
14. After verification of the teeth and centric relation, process the denture as usual.
15. Finish and polish the denture (Figure 6.54).

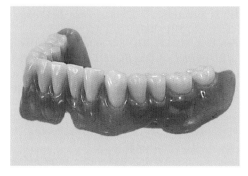

FIGURE 6.54.

Fabrication Procedures of a Hinge Resilient Overdenture Using a Bredent VSP Bar

CLINICAL STEPS All of the clinical steps are similar to the rigid bar.

LABORATORY STEPS All of the laboratory steps are very similar to the rigid bar except the following steps:

- After the bar is soldered and welded, but prior to the duplicating step to produce the refractory cast, the implant abutments and vertical extension of the bar should be covered with block-out wax. The thickness of the wax should be 0.3mm. This thickness will allow hinge movement of the overdenture.

   Note: Make sure the rounded part of the bar (top portion) is not covered with wax.

- Insert the duplicating matrix over the bar. Block out under the side of the bar as well as any other undercut area on the bar (Figure 6.55).

   Note: Make sure the hinge resilient matrix/clip has fit exactly on the bar and is not covered by block-out wax.

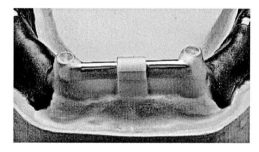

FIGURE 6.55.

- After the metal housing is cast and finished, insert a yellow hinge resilient matrix/clip (part # 430 0648 0) with an inserting tool inside the recipient site of the housing (Figures 6.56 and 6.57).

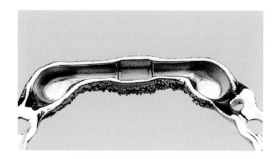

FIGURE 6.56.

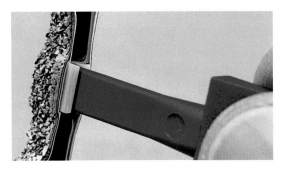

FIGURE 6.57.

- Follow Steps 12–15 of the rigid bar.

Verification of Passive Seat of the Bar

When the bar is finished and ready to be inserted, the following steps should be taken:

1. Perform the Sheffield test. (Refer to Chapter 7.) If the bar does not pass the Sheffield test perform following steps:
   - Cut and solder the bar.
   - Send it for the spark erosion process (Refer to Chapter 7).
2. After all of the retaining screws have been inserted, they should be flush with or below the top of the bar to minimize the chance of a screw loosening or damage to the head of a retaining screw.
3. Verify complete seating of the bar with a panoramic x-ray.

Incorporation of the Bar Assembly into the Denture

The final overdenture should be fabricated after the permanent bar has been delivered, instead of making it before the bar is placed. Fabricating the overdenture afterwards makes it easier to have the entire attachment assembly within the confinement of the overdenture, which maximizes the biomechanical properties of the overdenture. Some laboratories fabricate the denture first, index the teeth position with silicone, and then fabricate the bar. Since there are certain design specifications for the bar, the denture teeth should be set based on the position of the ideally fabricated bar.

REFERENCES AND ADDITIONAL READING

Academy of Prosthodontics. (1999). *The Glossary of Prosthodontic Terms* (7th edition). *Journal of Prosthetic Dentistry*, 81, 41–110.

Albrektsson, T. & Zarb, G. A. (1998). Determinants of correct clinical reporting. *International Journal of Prosthodontics*, 11, 517–521.

Albrektsson, T. & Zarb, G. A. *The Branemark Osseointegrated Implant.* Chicago: Quintessence Publishing, 1989.

Brewer, A. A. & Marrow, R. M. *Overdentures* (Second Edition). C. V. Mosby Company, 1980.

Carr, A. B. (1998). Successful long-term treatment outcomes in the field of osseointegrated implants: Prosthodontic determinants. *International Journal of Prosthodontics*, 11, 502–512.

Cochran, D. L. (1999). A comparison of endosseous dental implant surfaces. *Journal of Periodontology*, 70, 1523–1539.

Cochran, D. L. (2001). The scientific basis for and clinical experiences with Straumann implants including the ITI Dental Implant System: A consensus report. *Clinical Oral Implants Research*, 11(supplement 1), 33–58.

Devlin, H., et al. (1988). Overdentures for the general dental practitioner. *Quintessence International*, July 19(7), 501–504.

Dolder, E. J. (1961). The bar-joint mandibular denture. *Journal of Prosthetic Dentistry*, July–Aug, 11(4), 689–707.

Dolder, E. J. & Durrer, G. T. *The Bar-Joint Denture.* Chicago: Quintessence Publishing, 1978.

English, C. E. (1990). An overview of implant hardware. *Journal of the American Dental Association*, Sept, 121(9), 360–368.

English, C. E. (1990). Removable prosthodontics as first-line treatment. *Practical Periodontics and Aesthetic Dentistry*, Oct–Nov, 2(5), 33–36.

English, C. E. (1990). Use of the Steri-Oss PME abutment with a bar-retained overdenture. *Trends & Techniques in the Contemporary Dental Laboratory*, Jan–Feb, 7(1), 75–80.

Ericsson, I., Randow, K., Nilner, K., Peterson, A. (2000). Early functional loading of Branemark implants. 5-year clinical follow-up study. *Clinical Implant Dentistry and Related Research*, 2, 70–77.

Espositio, M., Coulthard, P., Worthington, H. V., & Jokstad, A. (2000). Quality assessment of randomized controlled trials of oral implants. *International Journal of Oral & Maxillofacial Implants*, 16, 783–792.

Fargan, M. J., Jr. *Implant Prosthodontics—Surgical and Prosthetic Techniques for Dental Implants*. Year Book Medical Publishers, Inc., 1990.

Fourmousis, I. & Bragger, U. (1999). "Radiographic interpretation of peri-implant structures." In *Proceedings of the 3rd European Workshop on Periodontology-Implant Dentistry*, ed. Lang, N. P., Karring, T., & Lindhe, J. Chicago: Quintessence Publishing, 228–241.

Friberg, B., Sennerby, L., Linden, B., Grondahl, U. K., & Lekholm, U. (1999). Stability measurements of one-stage Branemark implants during healing in mandibles. A clinical resonance frequency analysis study. *International Journal of Oral & Maxillofacial Surgery*, 28, 266–272.

Hobo, S., Ichida, E., & Garcia, L. T. *Osseointegration and Occlusal Rehabilitation*. Chicago: Quintessence Publishing, 1990.

Jemt, T., Chai, J., Harnett, J., et al. (1996). A 5-year prospective multicenter follow-up report on overdentures supported by osseointegrated implants. *International Journal of Oral & Maxillofacial Implants*, 11, 291–298.

Jumber, J. F. *An Atlas of Overdentures and Abutments*. Chicago: Quintessence Publishing, 1981.

Lekholm, U. & Zarb, G. A. (1985). "Patient selection and preparation." In *Proceedings of the 3rd European Workshop on Periodontology-Implant Dentistry*, ed. Branemark, P. I., Zarb, G. A., & Albrektsson, T. Chicago: Quintessence Publishing, 199–210.

Mason, M. E., Triplett R. G., & Alfonso, W. F. (1990). Life-threatening hemorrhage from placement of a dental implant. *Journal of Oral & Maxillofacial Surgery*, 48(2), 204–208.

Mckinney, R. V., Jr. *Endosteal Dental Implants*, Year Book Medical Publishers, Inc., 1991.

Meffert, R. M. (1990). The importance of periodontal maintenance for the dental implant. *Practical Periodontics and Aesthetic Dentistry*, Oct–Nov, 2(5), 19–22.

Mentag, P. J., et al. (1988). IMZ overdenture using the Stern ERA attachment. *General Dentistry*, Sept–Oct, 36(5), 390–392.

Mericske-Stern, R. (1998). Treatment outcomes with implant-supported overdentures: Clinical considerations. *Journal of Prosthetic Dentistry*, 79, 66–73.

Naert, I., Gizani, S., Vuylskeke, M., & van Steenberghe, D. (1999). A 5-year prospective randomized clinical trial on the influence of splinted and unsplinted oral implants retaining a mandibular overdenture: Prosthetic aspects and patient satisfaction. *Journal of Oral Rehabilitation*, 26, 195–202.

Payne, A. G. T., Solomons, Y. F., & Lownie, J. F. (1999). Standardization of radiographs for mandibular implant-supported overdentures: Review and innovation. *Clinical Oral Implants Research*, 10, 307–319.

Payne, A. G. T., Solomons, Y. F., Lownie, J. F., Tawse-Smith, A. (2001). Inter-abutment and peri-abutment mucosal enlargement with mandibular implant overdentures. *Clinical Oral Implants Research*, 13, 179–187.

Payne, A. G. T., Tawse-Smith, A., Duncan, W. J., & Kumara R., (2002). Conventional and early loading of unsplinted ITI implants supporting mandibular ovedentures: Two-year results of a prospective randomized clinical trial. *Clinical Oral Implants Research*, 13, 603–609.

Payne, A. G. T., Tawse-Smith, A., Kumara, R., & Thomson W. M. (2001). One-year prospective evaluation of the early loading of unsplinted conical Branemark fixtures with mandibular overdentures: A preliminary report. *Clinical Implant Dentistry and Related Research*, 3, 9–18.

Schmitt, A. & Zarb, G. A. (1998). The notion of implant-supported overdentures. *Journal of Prosthetic Dentistry*, 79, 60–65.

Sul, Y. T., Johansson, C. B., Jeong, Y., Wennerberg, A., & Albrektsson, T. (2002). Resonance frequency and removal torque analysis of implants with turned and anodized surface oxides. *Clinical Oral Implants Research*, 13, 252–259.

Szmukler-Moncler, S., Piattelli, A., Favero, G. A., & Dubruille, J. H. (2000). Considerations preliminary to the application of early and immediate loading protocols in dental implantology. *Clinical Oral Implants Research*, 11, 12–25.

Tawse-Smith, A., Duncan, W., Payne, A. G. T., Thomson, W. M., & Wennstrom, J, L. (2002). Effectiveness of electric toothbrushes in peri-implant maintenance of mandibular implant overdentures. *Journal of Clinical Periodontology*, 29, 275–280.

Tawse-Smith, A., Payne, A. G. T, Kumara, R., & Thomson W. M. (2001). A one-stage operative procedure using 2 different implant systems: A prospective study on implant overdentures in the edentulous mandible. *Clinical Implant Dentistry and Related Research*, 3, 185–193.

Tawse-Smith, A., Payne, A. G. T., Kumara, R., & Thomson, W. M. (2002). Early loading of unsplinted implants supporting mandibular overdentures using a one-stage operative procedure with two different implant systems: A 2-year report. *Clinical Implant Dentistry and Related Research*, 4, 33–42.

Watson, G., Payne, A. G. T., Purton, D. G., & Thomson W. G. (2002). Mandibular implant overdentures: Comparative evaluation of the prosthodontic maintenance during the first year of service using three different systems. *International Journal of Prosthodontics*, 15, 259–266.

Wismeijer, D., van Waas, M. A. J., Mulder, J., Vermeeren, J. I. J. F., & Kalk, W. (1999). Clinical and radiological results of patients treated with three treatment modalities for overdentures on implants of the ITI Dental Implant System. *Clinical Oral Implants Research*, 10, 297–306.

Zarb, G. A. (1983). The edentulous milieu. *Journal of Prosthetic Dentistry*, 49, 825–831.

7
Spark Erosion

Hamid Shafie
Eduard Eisenmann
Günter Rübeling

One of the most important factors in the long-term success of fully implant-supported overdenture is passive fitting of the metal substructure of the attachment assembly over the supporting implants or supporting abutments. An ill-fitting substructure will cause excessive stress on the supporting implants, which eventually will cause crestal bone loss. Another common problem caused by an ill-fitting metal substructure is breakage of retaining screws or abutments, and in the most severe case, the implant itself can be fractured.

The most common method to verify the passive fit of the metal substructure is the Sheffield test.

SHEFFIELD TEST

In order to perform this test, the metal substructure/bar should be inserted over the supporting implants or abutments. Then the most distal retaining screw should be tightened and the rest of the retaining screw should be kept out. If a

gap appears between the remaining supporting implants or supporting abutments and the metal substructure, it indicates that the metal framework does not fit passively. Tightening the remaining retaining screws in an ill-fitting metal substructure will cause unwanted strain to the supporting implants.

Sheffield Test
1. Only one of the terminal retaining screws is tightened before spark erosion and milling of the metal substructure (Figure 7.1).

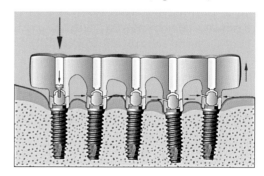

FIGURE 7.1.

2. Remove the terminal screw, which was used in Step 1 and then tighten only a middle retaining screw before spark erosion and milling of the metal substructure (Figure 7.2).

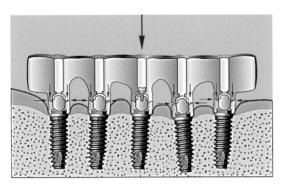

FIGURE 7.2.

3. Tighten all of the retaining screws before spark erosion and milling of the metal substructure (Figure 7.3).

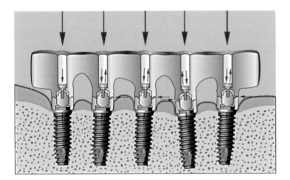

FIGURE 7.3.

4. After finishing the spark erosion process but before milling the screw access holes of the metal substructure, tighten only one of the terminal retaining screws to verify the passive fit of the metal substructure (Figure 7.4).

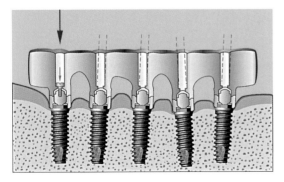

FIGURE 7.4.

5. After finishing the spark erosion process, if all of the retaining screws are tightened without milling the screw access holes, there will be a load concentration throughout the retaining screws (Figure 7.5).

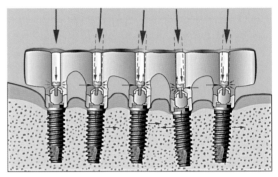

FIGURE 7.5.

6. Tighten only one of the terminal retaining screws and then start milling the screw access holes (Figure 7.6).

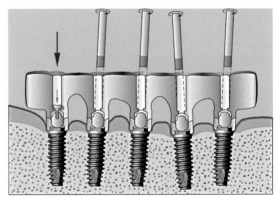

FIGURE 7.6.

Each screw access hole should be milled exactly with the trajectory of the supporting implant, as described in the following steps:
- Mount the master cast on the cast holder of the milling machine. Screw a guide sleeve over one of the terminal implants. Insert a guide pin into the drill holder of the milling machine (Figure 7.7).

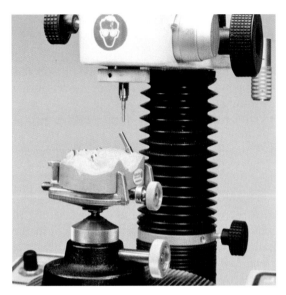

FIGURE 7.7.

- Completely loosen the stabilizing screw of the cast holder's ball joint (Figure 7.8).

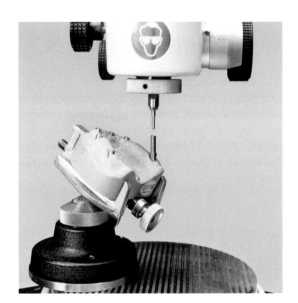

FIGURE 7.8.

- Insert the guide pin completely into the guide sleeve. Tighten the stabilizing screw of the cast holder's ball joint to lock the appropriate position of the master cast for the milling process (Figure 7.9).

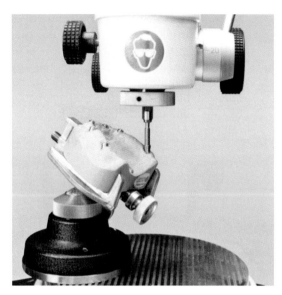

FIGURE 7.9.

- Replace the guide pin with an end-cutting carbide bur. Verify the milling position by lowering the carbide bur until it reaches the guide sleeve. This position should be considered as position zero for the milling machine and used to adjust the milling depth (Figure 7.10).

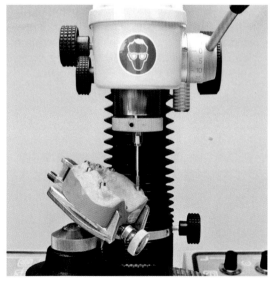

FIGURE 7.10.

- Screw the metal substructure firmly over the supporting implants. Insert the carbide bur into the first screw access hole and start the milling process at the appropriate depth. The milling depth can be adjusted by changing the measurements on the milling machine's micrometer (Figure 7.11).

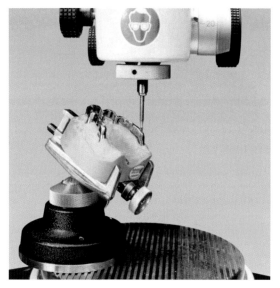

FIGURE 7.11.

7. When the spark erosion process and milling of the screw access holes is complete, tighten all of the retaining screws. The suprastructure has a perfect passive fit with no load concentration on the retaining screws (Figure 7.12).

MOST COMMON REASONS FOR ILL FIT

- Inaccurate impression technique or material
- Dimensional changes in stone model during setting
- Dimensional changes during casting procedures
- Dimensional changes after porcelain veneering in cases of fixed bridges

One way to achieve a passive fit in the metal substructure is to make the substructure in multiple segments, connect these pieces in the patient's mouth, and make an index of the whole piece. Use the index to solder or weld all of the pieces together. This step can also lead to new inaccuracies. In some fully implant-supported fixed denture designs, porcelain is applied to the metal substructure. The shrinkage of the porcelain during firing introduces some stress to the metal substructure, which can ultimately cause an ill fit again.

SPARK EROSION PROCESS

All of the discrepancies resulting from the above laboratory techniques can be corrected after fabrication of the metal substructure by utilizing the SAE Secotec spark erosion technique (Figure 7.13). Günter Rübeling introduced this technique to the field of implant dentistry in the mid 1990s.

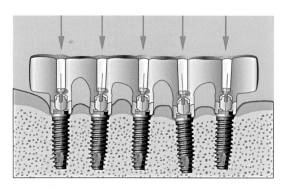

FIGURE 7.12.

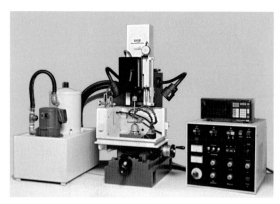

FIGURE 7.13.

The spark erosion process creates a short-circuit electrical field between the electrodes, which are similar to and interchangeable with lab analogs and the metal substructure. This process erodes very small metal particles from the inside of the metal substructure, starting from the areas that first come into contact with the lab analogs. The process is continued until all of the premature contacts are spark-eroded and the whole metal substructure has a 360-degree passive contact with the prosthetic table of lab analogs. This technique can be used for any electro-conductive metal.

Clinical Steps

1. Insert the pick-up impression copings into the implants (Figure 7.14).

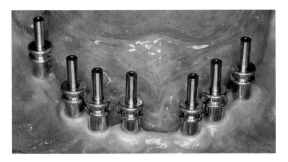

FIGURE 7.14.

2. Make the pick-up impression with a rigid impressing material such as polyether or rigid vinyl polysiloxane. Always use a custom tray; avoid using a stock tray, because it will contribute to inaccuracy (Figure 7.15).

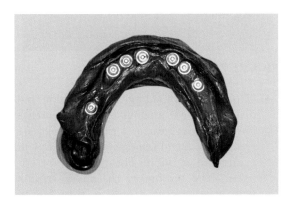

FIGURE 7.15.

3. After completion of laboratory steps 1, 2 and 3 (presented following these clinical steps) the dentists receive an acrylic assembly with matching impression copings embedded in it and the selected original implant abutments.
4. Install the abutments from the model into the implants (Figure 7.16).

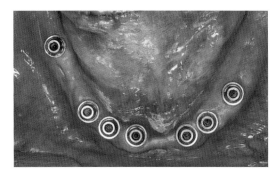

FIGURE 7.16.

5. Insert the acrylic assembly in the patient mouth over the supporting implant abutments and perform the Sheffield test to verify the passive fit of the assembly.
6. If the assembly does not fit passively, cut the acrylic joints near the ill-fitting coping with a thin diamond disk to make sure all of the copings are fitting passively (Figure 7.17).

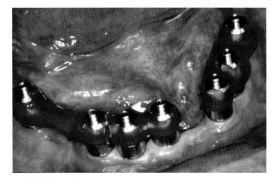

FIGURE 7.17.

7. Reconnect all of the sliced acrylic pieces with pattern resin in the mouth.
8. Use a custom tray and a rigid impression material such as polyether to make the final master impression (Figure 7.18). After this step, send the impression to the lab. The technician

should continue the laboratory procedures from Step 4.

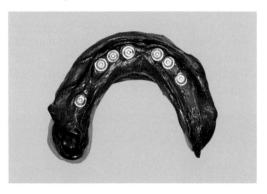

FIGURE 7.18.

9. After completion of laboratory Step 12 and receiving the wax record base, screw the record base into the supporting implant abutments and register vertical dimension as well as centric relation. Send the record to the lab for denture teeth setup.

Laboratory Steps

1. Screw the matching lab analogs of the implant system (the Ankylos implant system is shown in Figure 7.19), which has been utilized into the impression copings. Apply a soft tissue model material around the impression copings and their junctions with lab analogs. Use a class IV die stone to pour the impression.

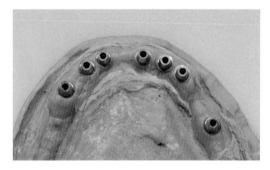

FIGURE 7.19.

2. Choose the final abutments and fix them in the lab analogs (Figure 7.20). Then choose the corresponding impression copings and screw them over the abutments on the first master model. Link all of the impression copings with self-curing resin (e.g. GC pattern resin). After the completion of polymerization, section the acrylic joints with a thin diamond disk.

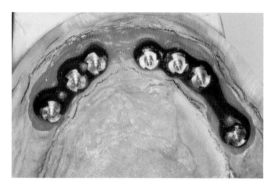

FIGURE 7.20.

3. Without unscrewing the impression copings from the cast, reconnect the acrylic pieces with pattern resin and leave the acrylic assembly for 12 hours (Figure 7.21). This step minimizes the strain generated from shrinkage of the pattern resin. After this step send the acrylic assembly to the dentist for intraoral try in.

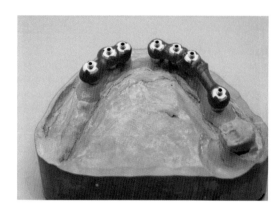

FIGURE 7.21.

4. Choose corresponding spark erosion implant abutment analogs with the patient's implants. The heads of these analogs are identical to the abutments made by implant manufactures, but the bottom portion is different. The bottom of the spark erosion implant abutment analog is threaded so the analog can be screwed into an electro-conducting copper sleeve (Figure 7.22).

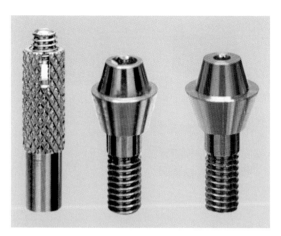

FIGURE 7.22.

5. Screw each analog into an electro-conducting sleeve. Insert the head of the analog into the impression coping and secure its position by tightening the retaining screw of the impression coping (Figures 7.23 and 7.24).

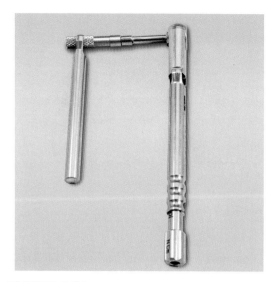

FIGURE 7.24.

6. Put resilient soft tissue model material into the impression and around lab analogs. Ensure that this material does not come into contact with electro-conducting sleeves. These sleeves should be covered and supported by hard stone to make sure that there are no micro movements of the analogs. Any movement will cause inaccuracy in the master cast, and in the end, the metal substructure will not be accurate.

7. Connect all of the electro-conducting sleeves with copper ribbons (Figures 7.25 and

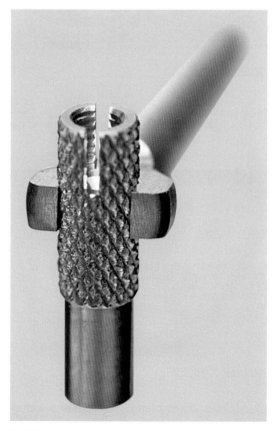

FIGURE 7.23.

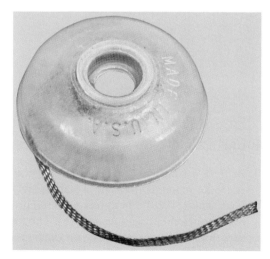

FIGURE 7.25.

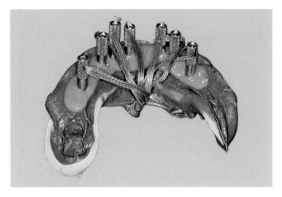

FIGURE 7.26.

7.26). These sleeves will form the positive terminal (anode), and the metal substructure will be the negative terminal (cathode).

8. Box the implant section of the impression with boxing wax.
9. Apply silver powder (Wieland Dental + Technik, Germany) on the soft tissue model material to create a separating layer between the soft tissue model material and the epoxy resin, which will be poured in the next step (Figure 7.27).

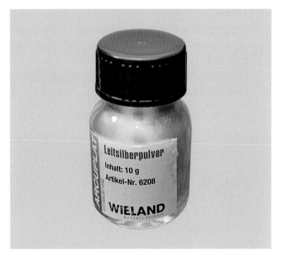

FIGURE 7.27.

10. Pour 0.5–1mm of low-contracting epoxy resin die material over the isolating silver layer (Figure 7.28). The epoxy resin requires 8–12 hours of curing time at 18°C. The setting time can vary depending on the actual room temperature and humidity.

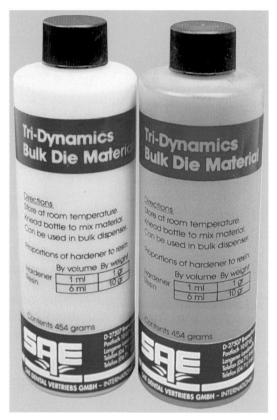

FIGURE 7.28.

11. Remove all of the boxing waxes and pour the rest of the impression with type IV die stone (Figure 7.29).

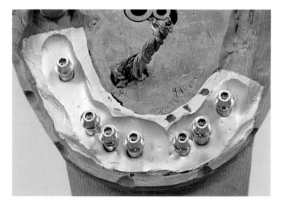

FIGURE 7.29.

12. Make a three points (triangular position) screw-retained wax record base and send it

to the dentist for a jaw relationship registration (Figure 7.30).

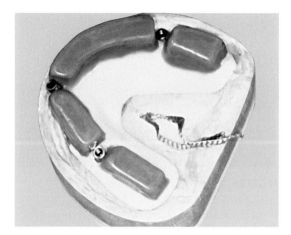

FIGURE 7.30.

13. After completion of clinical Step 9, mount the casts in a semi-adjustable articulator and set up the denture teeth (Figure 7.31). After the dentist has tried the teeth and approved the setup, make a silicone index on the teeth. This silicone index will be a guide for the positing and boundaries of the resin pattern of the metal substructure.

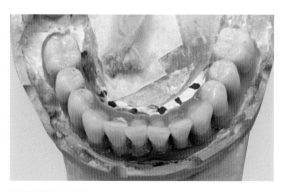

FIGURE 7.31.

14. Fabricate the resin pattern of the metal substructure from a resin that will not leave any residual after the burn-out step. Obviously, during this step the master cast should be mounted in the articulator at the proper vertical dimension of occlusion and centric

relation position. The relationship of the upper and lower casts and inter-ridge space are important factors in the design and contour of the metal substructure. Verify the position and orientation of the substructure pattern with the silicone index (Figures 7.32 and 7.33).

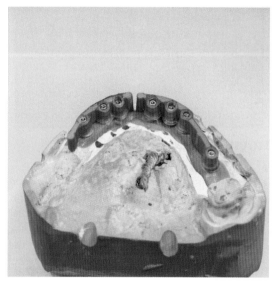

FIGURE 7.32.

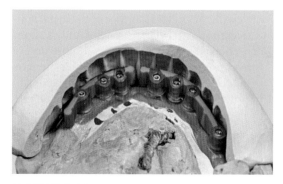

FIGURE 7.33.

15. Cast the metal substructure and then finish, mill, and polish it.
16. Remove the soft tissue model from the master cast. This provides better visibility to inspect the passive fit of the metal substructure over the lab analogs (Figure 7.34).

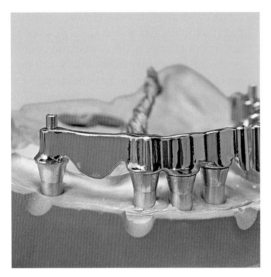

FIGURE 7.34.

17. Insert the finished metal substructure on the master cast over the implant abutment analogs. Mount the master cast on the cast holder of the spark erosion unit. Insert the cast holder on the magnetic table of the spark erosion unit. The cast holder is secured in its final position by activating the magnetic field of the magnetic table.

18. Use pattern resin to connect the metal substructure with the finger extensions of the spark erosion unit. The connection should be with the occlusal surface of the metal substructure. After the resin is set and the connection is secured, lift the metal substructure from the master cast by elevating the axis that is connected to the finger extensions.

19. Unscrew the lab abutment analogs and replace them with identical implant abutment electrodes. Use an 18Ncm torque wrench to secure implant electrodes. Then insert the cast holder and the master cast into the dielectric fluid bath (Figure 7.35).

20. Lower the metal substructure connected to the finger extensions of the spark erosion unit until it fits over the implant electrodes.

21. There are two alligator clips connected to the spark erosion unit. One is the positive terminal (anode) and the other is the negative terminal (cathode). Connect the positive (anode) alligator clip to the copper ribbons,

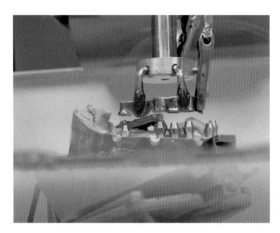

FIGURE 7.35.

which are connected to each electro-conducting sleeve and implant electrode. Then connect the negative (cathode) alligator clip to the metal substructure.

22. Pour dielectric coolant fluid over the metal substructure and close the dielectric bath.

23. Begin the first cycle of the spark erosion process. This cycle usually lasts for approximately 10–20 minutes. However, the duration of this cycle depends on the type of the metal that has been used to fabricate the substructure, as well as the degree of misfit and inaccuracy. Most erosion happens during this cycle.

24. After completion of the first cycle, elevate the metal substructure from the master cast (Figure 7.36). Unscrew all of the

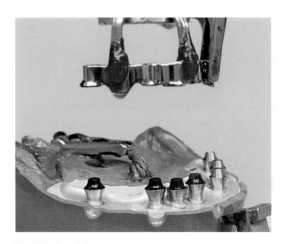

FIGURE 7.36.

used implant electrodes and replace them with new ones. This is an important step, because after completion of the first cycle, the implant electrodes are not smooth anymore, and they are eroded, too.

25. Start the second cycle similar to the first cycle, but this cycle usually lasts for one to two minutes. If necessary, a third cycle can be performed to achieve the desirable precise and passive fit. The third cycle usually is performed to smooth the contact surface of metal substructure with the implant abutment electrodes. For each cycle, new sets of electrodes must be used to achieve a precise and passive fit. The final surface roughness is approximately 4–6 microns. However electrodes from the second and third cycle can be used again for the first cycle of a next case (Figures 7.37 and 7.38).

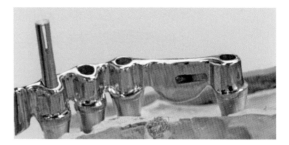

FIGURE 7.39.

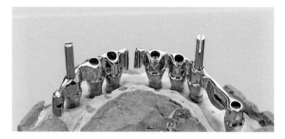

FIGURE 7.40.

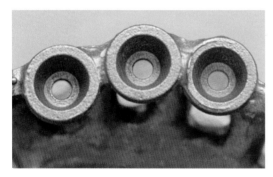

FIGURE 7.37.

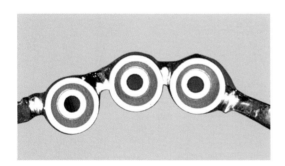

FIGURE 7.38.

26. After completion of the spark erosion process, elevate the metal substructure and replace the implant abutment electrodes with implant abutment analogs (Figures 7.39 and 7.40). The metal substructure should seat

and fit completely and passively over the analogs. Verify the precision of fit with the Sheffield test (Figures 7.41–7.48). Even with a passive and precise fit of the metal substructure over the implant abutment analogs, if the screw access holes are not parallel after tightening the retaining screws, there will be some residual stress on the supporting implants. Tensile and compressive loads generated by the head of retaining screws and screw access hole walls cause this stress. Always use an end- and side-cutting carbide bur to parallel all of the screw access holes to eliminate undesirable stress.

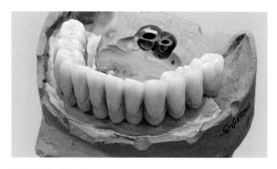

FIGURE 7.41.

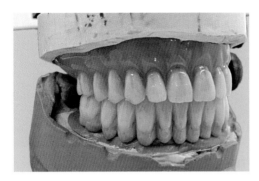

FIGURE 7.42.

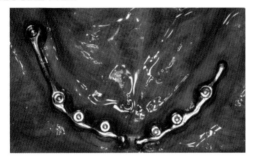

FIGURE 7.43.

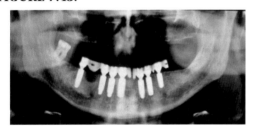

FIGURE 7.44.

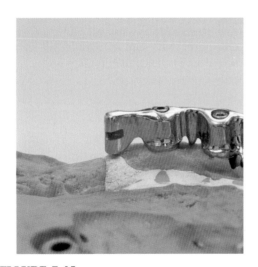

FIGURE 7.45.

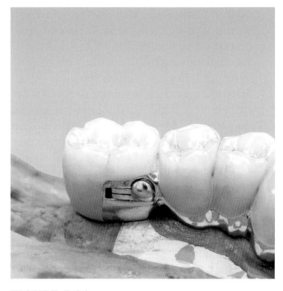

FIGURE 7.46.

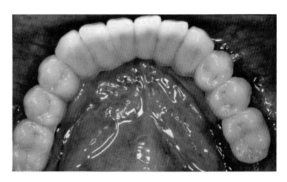

FIGURE 7.47.

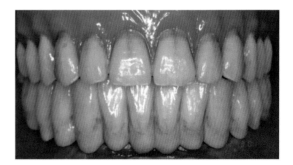

FIGURE 7.48.

Second Case

1. The first impression is made utilizing a rigid impression material (Figure 7.49).

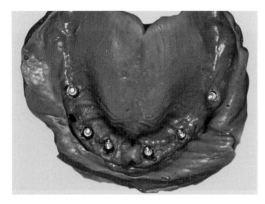

FIGURE 7.49.

2. The Secotec-System impression copings are screwed onto the master cast and connected with pattern resin. The resin sets for 12 hours to ensure that the thermosetting of the resin is complete. Using a very thin diamond abrasive disk, the acrylic is cut between the impression copings and the pieces are reconnected with pattern resin (Figures 7.50 and 7.51).

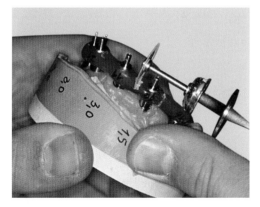

FIGURE 7.50.

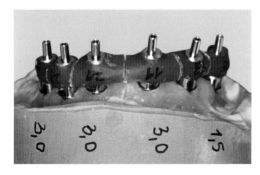

FIGURE 7.51.

3. Impression copings embedded in the acrylic block are screwed into the patient's mouth, and the Sheffield test is performed. If the acrylic block and impression copings do not fit passively over the implants, the acrylic is sectioned and then the sections are reconnected intra-orally (Figure 7.52).

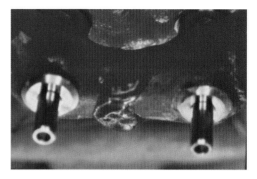

FIGURE 7.52.

4. The second impression is made by picking up the acrylic block and the Secotec-System impression copings (Figure 7.53).

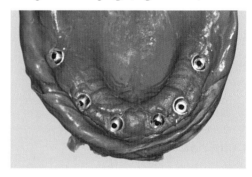

FIGURE 7.53.

5. Copper wire connects all of the electro-conducting sleeves (Figure 7.54).

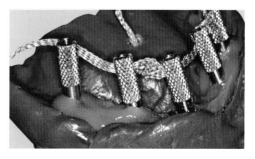

FIGURE 7.54.

6. The spark erosion master cast (Figure 7.55).

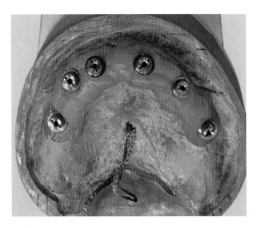

FIGURE 7.55.

7. Screw retained bite registration wax rim (Figure 7.56).

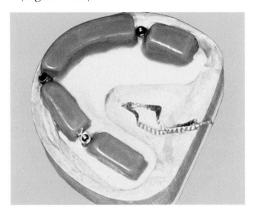

FIGURE 7.56.

8. The teeth are set up in the wax (Figure 7.57).

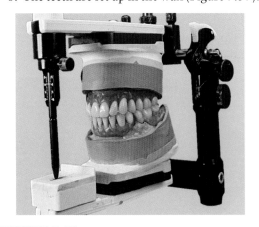

FIGURE 7.57.

9. The teeth are tried in (Figure 7.58).

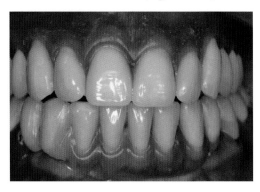

FIGURE 7.58.

10. The resin pattern of the metal sub-structure is made and milled to an appropriate shape and taper (Figure 7.59).

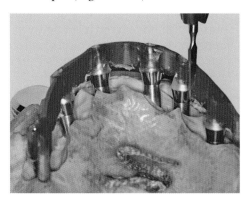

FIGURE 7.59.

11. The silicone index of the teeth setup is made and is used to verify the contour of the sub-structure acrylic pattern (Figure 7.60).

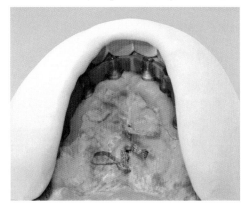

FIGURE 7.60.

12. The acrylic pattern is cast (Figure 7.61).

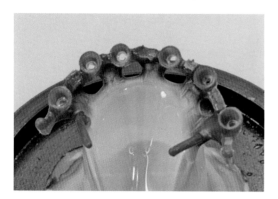

FIGURE 7.61.

13. The metal substructure is made immediately after the casting (Figure 7.62).

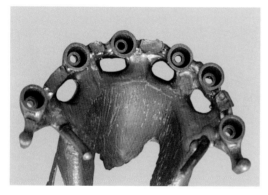

FIGURE 7.62.

14. The Sheffield test is performed on the finished and polished metal substructure. If the metal substructure is ill fitting, it will be visible (Figures 7.63 and 7.64).

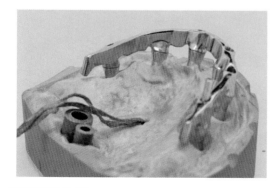

FIGURE 7.63.

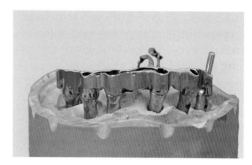

FIGURE 7.64.

15. The master cast is mounted on the cast holder and inserted in the spark erosion machine (Figure 7.65).

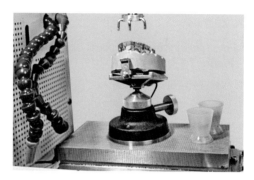

FIGURE 7.65.

16. Finger extensions of the spark erosion machine are connected to the metal substructure with pattern resin, and then the metal substructure is raised from the master cast (Figure 7.66).

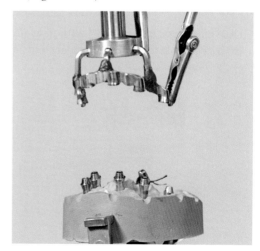

FIGURE 7.66.

17. Identically shaped spark erosion electrodes replace the regular prosthetic abutments. A torque wrench is used to tighten the retaining screws (Figure 7.67).

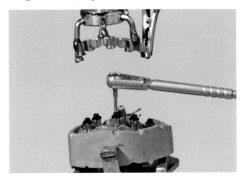

FIGURE 7.67.

18. The spark erosion process is in progress (Figure 7.68).

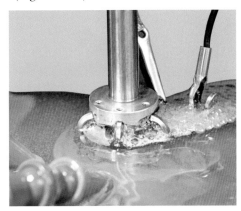

FIGURE 7.68.

19. Used electrodes are replaced with new electrodes before starting the next spark erosion cycle (Figures 7.69 and 7.70).

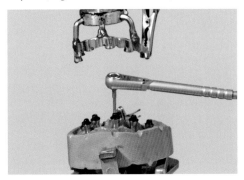

FIGURE 7.69.

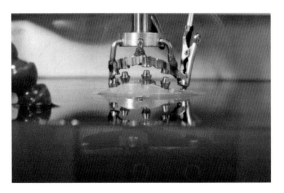

FIGURE 7.70.

20. After the spark erosion cycles are complete, the metal substructure is inserted back on the master cast, and the Sheffield test is repeated to verify the passive fit of the substructure (Figures 7.71 and 7.72).

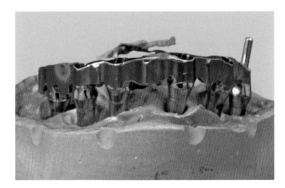

FIGURE 7.71.

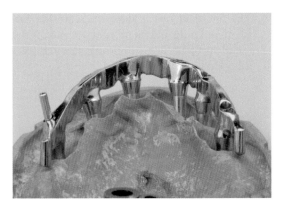

FIGURE 7.72.

21. The finished metal substructure is designed for friction pins and swivel latches (Figure 7.73).

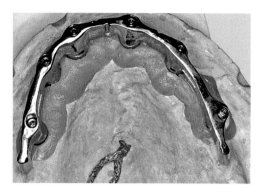

FIGURE 7.73.

22. The cast titanium superstructure is made to support the individual ceramic teeth, which will be unified with the superstructure using acrylic (Figures 7.74 and 7.75).

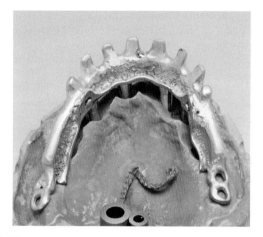

FIGURE 7.74.

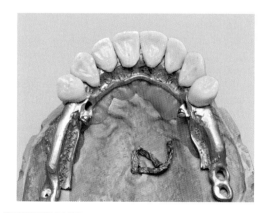

FIGURE 7.75.

23. The finished maxillary prosthesis with opened and closed latches (Figures 7.76 and 7.77).

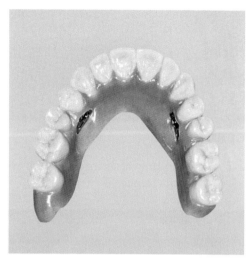

FIGURE 7.76.

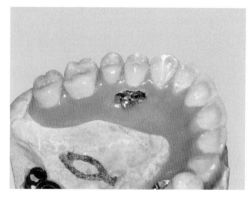

FIGURE 7.77.

24. The Sheffield test is performed intra-orally (Figures 7.78 and 7.79).

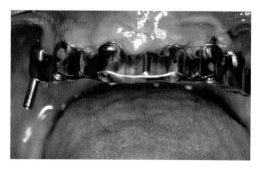

FIGURE 7.78.

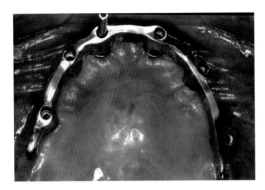

FIGURE 7.79.

25. The finished prosthesis in the mouth with closed latches (Figures 7.80 and 7.81).

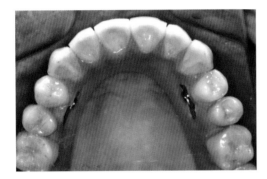

FIGURE 7.80.

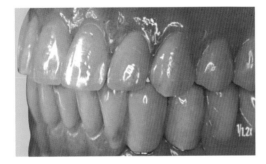

FIGURE 7.81.

REFERENCES AND ADDITIONAL READING

Adell, R., Lekholm, U., Rockler, B., & Branemark, P. (1981). A 15-year study of osseointegrated implants in the treatment of the edentulous jaw. *International Journal of Oral Surgery*, 10, 387–416.

Carr, A. B., Gerard, D. A., & Larsen, P. E. (1996). The response of bone in primates around unloaded dental implants supporting prostheses with different levels of fit. *Journal of Prosthetic Dentistry*, 76, 500–509.

Eisenman, E. & Rubeling, G. (1997). Die monometallische, spannungsfreie Versorgung auf Implantaten. Berlin: *Quintessenz Zahntechnik, Implantologie*, 12, 1440.

Isa, Z. M. & Hobkirk, J. A. (1995). The effects of superstructure fit and loading individual implant units: Part 1. The effects of tightening the gold screws and placement of a superstructure with varying degrees of fit. *European Journal of Prosthodontics & Restorative Dentistry*, Dec, 3(6), 247–53.

Jemt T. (1991). Failures and complications in 391 consecutively inserted fixed prostheses supported by Branemark implants in edentulous jaws: A study of treatment from the time of prosthesis placement to the first annual checkup. *International Journal of Oral & Maxillofacial Implants*, 6, 270–276.

Jemt T. (1996). In-vivo measurements of precision of fit involving implant-supported prosthesis in the edentulous jaw. *International Journal of Oral & Maxillofacial Implants*, 11, 151–158.

Jemt, T. & Lekholm, U. (1998). Measurements of bone and frame-work deformations induced by misfit of implant superstructures. A pilot study in rabbits. *Clinical Oral Implants Research* 9, 272–280.

Kallus, T. & Bessing, C. Loose gold screws frequently occur in full-arch fixed prostheses supported by osseointegrated implant after 5-years. *International Journal of Oral & Maxillofacial Implants*, 1994, 9, 169–178.

Kan, A., et al. (1999). Clinical methods for evaluating implant framework fit. *Journal of Prosthetic Dentistry*, 81, 7–31.

May, B., et al. (1997). The precision of fit at implant prosthodontic interface. *Journal of Prosthetic Dentistry*, 77, 497–502.

Millingington, N. D. & Leung, T. (1995). Inaccurate fit of implant superstructures. Part 1: Stresses generated on the superstructure relative to the size of fit discrepancy. *International Journal of Prosthodontics*, 8, 511–516.

Mokabberi, H. (1998). Spannungsophtische und raster-elektronenmikroskopische Untersuchungen zum passiven Sitz mit Hilfe der Funkenero-sion hergestellten implantatgetragenen Meso-und Suprastrukturen. Dissertation: FU Berlin.

Naert, I., Quirynen, M., van Steenberghe, D., & Darius, P. (1992). A study of 589 consecutive implants supporting complete fixed prostheses. Part III: Prosthetic aspect. *Journal of Prosthetic Dentistry*, 68, 949–959.

Rubeling G. (1997). "Titanverarbeitung mittels Funkenerosion." In *Titan in der Zahnmedizin*, Hrsg. Wirz J. & Bischoff, H. Berlin: Quintessenz Verlag, 231.

Rubeling, G. (1999). Metallkeramisch verblendeter Bruckenzahnersatz aus Titan mit passivem Sitz nach funkenerosiver Behandlung. *Implantologie*, 7, 279–294.

Rubeling, G., Eisenmann, E., Stiller, M., et al. (2002). Meso- und Suprastruktur auf Balance-Basisaufbauten des Ankylos-Implantat-Systems. *Zahntech Mag*, 6, 22–31.

Rubeling, G., Klar, A., Rubeling, F., et al. "Das expan-sionsfreie Modell als Grundlage fur den passiven Sitz der Implantatmeso- und Suprastrukturen." In *Implantatprothetische Therapiekonzepte*, ed. We-ber, H. P. & Monkmeyer, U. R. Berlin: Quintessenz Verlag, 1999, 171–180.

Skalak, R. (1983). Biomechanical considerations in osseointegrated prostheses. *Journal of Prosthetic Dentistry*, 49, 843–848.

Sullivan, D. Y. & Rubeling, G. (1997). Der Pas-sive Sitz von implantatgetragenen Meso- Supra-trukuren. *Dental Labor*, 45, 2.

Weber, H. P. & Monkmeyer, U. R. *Implantat-prothe-tische Therapiekonzepte*. Berlin: Quintessenz, 1999.

White, G. E. *Implantat-Zahntechnik*. Berlin: Quintes-senz, 1993.

Willers, H. H. & Rubeling, G. Vergleichsstudie: Gipse fur formstabile Implantatmodelle. Marburger Gipstagung, 2002.

8
Treatment Success with Implant Overdenture

Hamid Shafie

IMPLANT SURVIVAL

Most studies available on mandibular overdentures report a success rate of 90 to 100 percent. Neither the number of supporting implants nor the type of attachment assembly has been found to affect the rate of survival.

In contrast, the results of implants placed in the edentulous maxilla, particularly in conjunction with overdentures, are less favorable. Multiple studies have shown a higher failure rate for implants placed in the edentulous maxilla. If a distinction between the degree of atrophy in the maxilla and the bone quality is made, the results show that failure in the maxilla is a result of short implants, poor bone quality, and an inadequate number of implants.

Although bone grafting is often recommended for patients with advanced atrophy, this surgical procedure typically results in a high percentage of implant losses and increased bone resorption.

PROSTHETIC SUCCESS

Evaluation of prosthetic success can be challenging, since a clear distinction among normal maintenance, repairs, and adjustment of the prosthesis is not made. Maintenance due to normal wear can become excessive and a biased criteria for assessment of success. Complications can vary widely from requiring a simple adjustment to a remake of the entire prosthesis.

Clinically, the overdenture is simpler, and its initial treatment is less expensive compare to fixed prosthesis. However, since overdenture has more components (abutments, clips, bars, anchors, and female retainers), it carries a higher chance of complication.

A five-year longitudinal study comparing two resilient attachment assemblies showed more complications with bars than with ball attachments. Another study compared rigid and resilient attachment assemblies for mandibular overdentures supported by two implants during 5–15 year periods. This study showed no significant difference between the incidents of complications between the two groups. However, replacement of the entire attachment assembly was more common with stud attachments and round bars than with rigid bars.

PATIENT RELATED FACTORS

Treatment success should not be evaluated only on the implant and prosthesis survival and success. The psychological and physiological impacts of overdenture treatment on a patient's quality of life should be considered as well. The treatment cost and financial status of the patient are also important factors in deciding a treatment strategy. The average person may accept implant overdentures supported by two or four implants over the fixed prosthesis because they are less expensive.

BIOMECHANICAL RISK FACTORS FOR UPPER IMPLANT OVERDENTURE

- An upper implant overdenture attachment assembly design is an ideal solution that has minimum biomechanical risk. One clip/rider should be used for each bar (Figure 8.1).

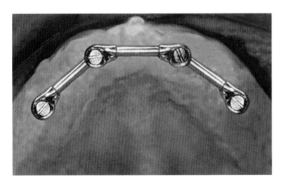

FIGURE 8.1.

- This design is mechanically less favorable than previous designs since the lateral forces will not distribute among all four implants. However, this design provides a better anterior aesthetic compared to previous designs (Figure 8.2).

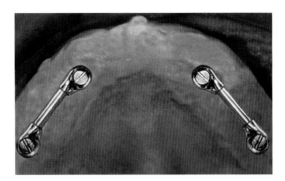

FIGURE 8.2.

- This design has a higher biomechanical risk compare to the previous two designs. This design is a completely non-resilient attachment assembly with cantilever components. It is very important to consider the Anterior–Posterior spread in this design. Generally, the distal cantilever should not exceed half of the Anterior–Posterior spread (Figure 8.3).

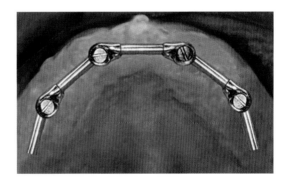

FIGURE 8.3.

- This design represents a moderate biomechanical risk when the supporting implants are not parallel (Figure 8.4).
- This design creates a high biomechanical risk, especially if the palatal coverage has been eliminated and the flanges are reduced. This design should only be used with an upper complete denture and maximum tissue coverage in cases in which the patient has severe bone loss, but there is still enough bone quantity to place two implants in the canine areas. If the patient is willing to consider a bone

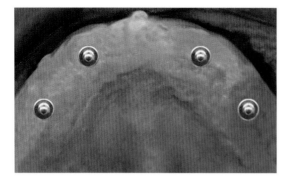

FIGURE 8.4.

graft procedure, then this treatment option should be avoided (Figure 8.5).

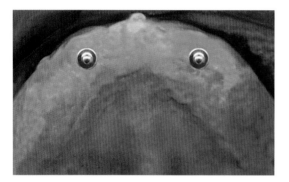

FIGURE 8.5.

From experimental points of view, maxillary overdentures are best supported by multiple implants connected by a rigid bar and reinforced with a metal framework to enhance rigidity of the superstructure.

BIOMECHANICAL RISK FACTORS FOR LOWER IMPLANT OVERDENTURE

- The lower implant overdenture is an ideal design in regard to biomechanical aspects. The bar should provide at lease hinge resiliency for the prosthesis. More resilient bars will provide more load relief on the supporting implants (Figure 8.6).
- This design is very simple and practical and will provide significant biomechanical advan-

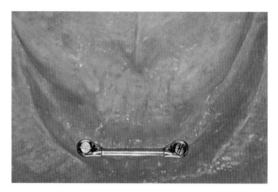

FIGURE 8.6.

tages to the supporting implants. A more resilient stud attachment provides more load relief for the implants (Figure 8.7).

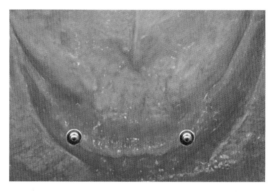

FIGURE 8.7.

- This design represents a significant biomechanical risk to the supporting implants. It carries a high risk of fracture and bending mode of failure for the cantilever distal extensions (Figure 8.8).

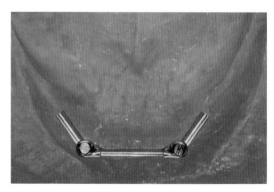

FIGURE 8.8.

- This design provides less biomechanical risk compared to previous designs. However, it is very important to design the distal extension cantilevers based on the Anterior–Posterior spread measurement (Figure 8.9).

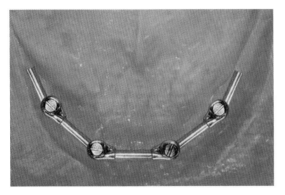

FIGURE 8.9.

- This design presents a significant biomechanical risk when the implants are short, narrow, and do not have enhanced surface characteristics. With this design, the attachment assembly does not provide any resiliency for the prosthesis or load relief to the supporting implants. The prosthesis is fully implant borne and not enough implants are available to support a fully implant-borne prosthesis (Figure 8.10).

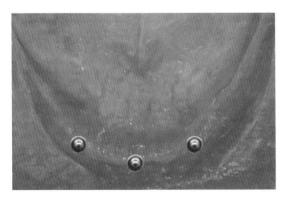

FIGURE 8.10.

- The attachment assembly in this design is rigid non-resilient. This assembly creates a significant biomechanical risk if the supporting implants are not parallel. However, if the supporting implants are long and wide and have been placed in a perfect parallel position, this design can be predictable (Figure 8.11).

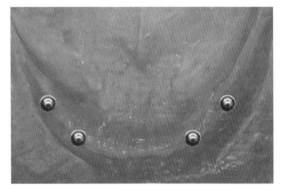

FIGURE 8.11.

The key purpose of the implants in the mainly tissue supported implant overdenture is to improve the retention of the denture, not support all of the chewing forces. In order to reduce the amount of load transfer to the supporting implants, the prosthesis should be made like a conventional complete denture with respect to support and stabilization criteria.

SHAPE OF THE MANDIBLE AND ITS EFFECT ON THE LOADING OF THE SUPPORTING IMPLANTS

Shape of the mandible has a significant influence on the location of the supporting implants and biomechanical properties of the overdenture. If the anterior mandible is ovoid, a relatively high resistance to the lever arm will exist (Figure 8.12).

If the anterior mandible has a square shape, it will create an unfavorable biomechanical situation, because there is a minimum resistance to the lever arm (Figure 8.13).

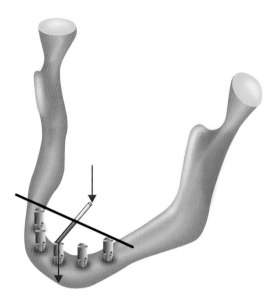

FIGURE 8.12.

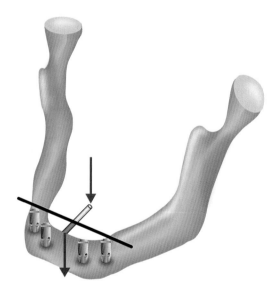

FIGURE 8.13.

REFERENCES AND ADDITIONAL READING

Academy of Prosthodontics. (1999). *The Glossary of Prosthodontic Terms* (7th edition). *Journal of Prosthetic Dentistry*, 81, 41–110.

Adell, R., Eriksson, B., Lekholm, U., Branemark, P. I., & Jemt T. (1990). A long-term follow- up study of osseointegrated implants in the treatment of totally edentulous jaw. *International Journal of Oral & Maxillofacial Implants*, 5, 347–359.

Adell, R., Lekholm, U., Rockler, B., & Branemark, P. I. (1981). A 15-year study of osseointegrated implants in the treatment of the edentulous jaw. *International Journal of Oral Surgery*, 10, 387–416.

Albrektsson, T. & Zarb, G. A. Determinants of correct clinical reporting. (1998). *International Journal of Prosthodontics*, 11, 517–521.

Andersson, Odman P., Boss, A., Jorneus, L. (1994). Mechanical testing of superstructures on the CeraOne abutment in the Branemark System. *International Journal of Oral & Maxillofacial Implants*, 9, 665–672.

Balshi, T. J. & Wolfinger, G. J. (1997). Two-implant-supported single molar replacement: Interdental space requirements and comparison to alternative options. *International Journal of Periodontics & Restorative Dentistry*, 17, 427–435.

Balshi, T. J., Hernandez, R. E., Pryszlak, M. C., & Rangert, B. (1996). A comparative study of one implant versus two replacing a single molar. *International Journal of Oral & Maxillofacial Implants*, 11, 372–378.

Becker, W. & Becker, B. (1995). Replacement of maxillary and mandibulary molars with single endosseous implant restorations: A retrospective study. *Journal of Prosthetic Dentistry*, 74, 51–55.

Branemark, P. I., Hansson, B., Adell, R., Breine, U., Lindstrom, J., Hallen, O., & Ohman A. (1977). Osseointegrated implants in the treatment of the edentulous jaw. Experience from a 10-year period. *Scandinavian Journal of Plastic and Reconstructive Surgery and Hand Surgery*, 16, 1–132.

Carr, A. B. (1998). Successful long-term treatment outcome in the field of osseointegrated implants: Prosthodontic determinants. *The International Journal of Prosthodontics*, 11, 502–512.

Chan, M. F., Narhi, T. O., de Baat, C., & Kalk, W. (1998). Treatment of the atrophic edentulous maxilla with implant-supported overdentures. A review of the literature. *International Journal of Prosthodontics*, 11, 207–215.

Cochran, D. L. (1999). A comparison of endosseous dental implant surfaces. *Journal of Periodontology*, 70, 1523–1539.

Cochran, D. L. (2001). The scientific basis for and clinical experiences with Straumann implants including the ITI Dental Implant System: A consensus report. *Clinical Oral Implants Research*, 11(supplement 1), 33–58.

Dudic, A., Mericske-Stern, R. (2002). Retention mechanism and prosthetic complications of implant-supported mandibular overdentures: long-term results. *Implant Dentistry and Related Research*, 4, 212–219.

Engleman, M. J. *Clinical Decision Making and Treatment Planning in Osseointegration*. Chicago: Quintessence Publishing, 1997.

Ericsson, I., Randow, K., Nilner, K. & Peterson, A. (2000). Early functional loading of Branemark implants. 5-year clinical follow-up study. *Clinical Implant Dentistry and Related Research*, 2, 70–77.

Espositio, M., Coulthard, P., Worthington, H. V., Jokstad, A. (2000). Quality assessment of randomized controlled trials of oral implants. *International Journal of Oral & Maxillofacial Implants*, 16, 783–792.

Fourmousis, I. & Bragger, U. (1999). "Radiographic interpretation of peri-implant structures." In *Proceedings of the 3rd European Workshop on Periodontology-Implant Dentistry*, ed. Lang, N. P., Karring, T., Lindhe, J. Chicago: Quintessence Publishing, 228–241.

Friberg, B., Sennerby, L., Linden, B., Grondahl, U. K., & Lekholm, U. (1999). Stability measurements of one-stage Branemark implants during healing in mandibles. A clinical resonance frequency analysis study. *International Journal of Oral & Maxillofacial Surgery*, 28, 266–272.

Gotfredsen, K., Holm, B. (2000). Implant-supported mandibular overdentures retained with ball or ball attachments: A randomized prospective 5-year study. *The International Journal of Prosthodontics*, 13, 125–130.

Henry, P., Laney, W., Jemt, T., Harris, D., Krogh, P., Polizzi, G., Zarb, G., & Herrmann, I. (1996). Osseointegrated implants for single-tooth replacement: A prospective multicenter study. *International Journal of Oral & Maxillofacial Implants*, 11, 450–455.

Higuchi, K., Folmer, T., & Kultje, C. (1995). Implant survival rates in partially edentulous patients. A 3-year prospective multicenter study. *Journal of Oral and Maxillofacial Surgery*, 53, 264–268.

Hobo, S., Ichida, E., Garcia, L. T. *Osseointegration and Occlusal Rehabilitation*. Chicago: Quintessence Publishing, 1990.

Hutton, J. E., Heath, R., Chai, J. Y., et al. (1995). Factors related to success and failure rates at 3-year follow-up in a multicenter study of overdentures supported by Branemark implants. *International Journal of Oral & Maxillofacial Implants*, 10, 33–42.

Jemt, T. & Lekholm, U. (1993). Oral implant treatment in the posterior partially edentulous jaw: A 5-year follow-up report. *International Journal of Oral & Maxillofacial Implants*, 8, 635–640.

Jemt, T. & Lekholm, U. (1995). Implant treatment in edentulous maxillae: A 5-year follow-up report on patients with different degrees of jaw resorption. *International Journal of Oral & Maxillofacial Implants*, 10, 303–311.

Jemt, T., Chai, J., Harnett, J., et al. (1996). A 5-year prospective multicenter follow-up report on overdentures supported by osseointegrated implants. *International Journal of Oral & Maxillofacial Implants*, 11, 291–298.

Jemt, T., Lekholm, U., & Grondahl. (1990). A 3-year follow-up study of early single implant restorations ad modum Branemark. *International Journal of Periodontics & Restorative Dentistry*, 10, 341–349.

Laney, W., Jemt, T., Harris, D., Henry, P., Krogh, P., Polizzi, G., Zarb, G., & Herrmann, I. (1994). Osseointegrated implants for single-tooth replacement: Progress report from a multicenter prospective study after 3 years. *International Journal of Oral & Maxillofacial Implants*, 9, 49–54.

Lekholm, U. & Zarb, G. A. (1985). "Patient selection and preparation." In *Tissue Integrated Prostheses: Osseointegration in Clinical Dentistry*, ed. Branemark, P. I., Zarb, G. A., & Albrektsson, T. Chicago: Quintessence Publishing, 199–210.

Lekholm, U., van Steenberghe, D., Heerman, I., Boledner, C., Folmer, T., Gunne, J., Henry, P., et al. (1994). Osseointegrated implants in the treatment of partially edentulous jaws: A prospective 5-year multicenter study. *International Journal of Oral & Maxillofacial Implants*, 9, 627–635.

Lundqvist, S., Haraldson, T., & Lindblad, P. (1992). Speech in connection with maxillary fixed prostheses on osseointegrated implants: A three-year follow-up study. *Clinical Oral Implants Research*, 3, 176–180.

Lundqvist, S., Lohmander-Agerskov, A., & Haraldson, T. (1992). Speech before and after treatment with bridges on osseointegrated implants in the edentulous. *Clinical Oral Implants Research*, 3, 57–62.

Mericske-Stern, R. (1998). Treatment outcomes with implant-supported overdentures: Clinical considerations. *Journal of Prosthetic Dentistry*, 79, 66–73.

Naert, I., Gizani, S., Vuylskeke, M., & van Steenberghe, D. (1999). A 5-year prospective randomized clinical trial on the influence of splinted and unsplinted oral implants retaining a mandibular overdenture: Prosthetic aspects and patient satisfaction. *Journal of Oral Rehabilitation*, 26, 195–202.

Naert, J., Quirynen, H., van Steenberghe, D., & Darius, P. (1992). A six-year prosthodontic study of 509 consecutively inserted implants for the treatment of partial edentition. *Journal of Prosthetic Dentistry*, 67, 236–245.

Nevins, M. & Langer, B. (1993). The successful application of osseointegrated implants to the posterior jaw: A long-term retrospective study. *International Journal of Oral & Maxillofacial Implants*, 8, 428–432.

Nevins, M. & Mellongi, J. T. *Implant Therapy: Clinical Approaches and Evidence of Success*, vol 2. Chicago: Quintessence Publishing, 1998.

Palacci, P., Ericsson, I., Engstrand, P., & Rangert, B. *Optimal Implant Positioning & Soft Tissue Management for the Branemark System*. Chicago: Quintessence Publishing, 1995.

Parel, S. M. & Sullivan, D. Y. *Esthetics and Osseointegration*. Dallas, TX: Osseointegration Seminars, 1989.

Parel, S. M. *The Smiline System*. Dallas, TX: Stephen M. Parel, 1991.

Payne, A. G. T., Solomons, Y. F., Lownie, J. F. (1999). Standardization of radiographs for mandibular implant-supported overdentures: Review and innovation. *Clinical Oral Implants Research*, 10, 307–319.

Payne, A. G. T., Solomons, Y. F., Lownie, J. F., Tawse-Smith, A. (2001) Inter-abutment and peri-abutment mucosal enlargement with mandibular implant overdentures. *Clinical Oral Implants Research*, 13, 179–187.

Payne, A. G. T., Tawse-Smith, A., Duncan, W., Kumara, R., (2002). Early loading of unsplinted ITI implants supporting mandibular overdentures: Two-year results of a randomized controlled trial. *Clinical Oral Implants Research*, 13, 603–609.

Payne, A. G. T., Tawse-Smith, A., Kumara, R., & Thomson, W. M. (2001). One-year prospective evaluation of the early loading of unsplinted conical Branemark fixtures with mandibular overdentures: A preliminary report. *Clinical Implant Dentistry and Related Research*, 3, 9–18.

Pestipino, V., Ingber, A., & Kravitz, J. (1998). Clinical and laboratory considerations in the use of a new all-ceramic restorative system. *Practical Periodontics & Aesthetic Dentistry*, 10, 567–575.

Petropoulos, V. C., Woollcott, S., & Kousvelari, E. (1997). Comparison of retention and release periods for implant overdenture attachments. *International Journal of Oral & Maxillofacial Implants*, 12, 176–185.

Schmitt, A. & Zarb, G. A. (1998). The notion of implant-supported overdentures. *Journal of Prosthetic Dentistry*, 79, 60–65.

Strub, J. R., Witkowski, S., & Einsele, F. "Prosthodontic aspects of implantology." In *Endosseous Implants: Scientific and Clinical Aspects*, ed. Watzek, G. Chicago: Quintessence Publishing, 1996.

Sul, Y. T., Johansson, C. B., Jeong, Y., Wennerberg, A., & Albrektsson, T. (2002). Resonance frequency and removal torque analysis of implants with turned and anodized surface oxides. *Clinical Oral Implants Research*, 13, 252–259.

Szmukler-Moncler, S., Piattelli, A., Favero, G. A., & Dubruille, J. H. (2000). Considerations preliminary to the application of early and immediate loading protocols in dental implantology. *Clinical Oral Implants Research*, 11, 12–25.

Tawse-Smith, A., Duncan, W., Payne, A. G. T., Thomson, W. M., & Wennstrom, J. L. (2002). Effectiveness of electric toothbrushes in peri-implant maintenance of mandibular implant overdentures. *Journal of Clinical Periodontology*, 29, 275–280.

Tawse-Smith, A., Payne, A. G. T., Kumara, R., & Thomson, W. M. (2001). A one-stage operative procedure using 2 different implant systems: A prospective study on implant overdentures in the edentulous mandible. *Clinical Implant Dentistry and Related Research*, 3, 185–193.

Tawse-Smith, A., Payne, A. G. T., Kumara, R., & Thomson, W. M. (2002). Early loading of unsplinted implants supporting mandibular overdentures using a one-stage operative procedure with two different implant systems: A 2-year report. *Clinical Implant Dentistry and Related Research*, 4, 33–42.

Tolman, D. & Laney, R. (1992). Tissue-integrated prosthesis complications. *International Journal of Oral & Maxillofacial Implants*, 7, 477–484.

Tulasne, J. F. (1988). Implant treatment of missing posterior dentition. In *The Branemark*

Osseointegrated Implants, ed. Albrektsson, T. & Zarb, G. A. Chicago: Quintessence Publishing.

Watson, G., Payne, A. G. T., Purton, D. G., & Thomson, W. G. (2002). Mandibular implant overdentures: Comparative evaluation of the prosthodontic maintenance during the first year of service using three different systems. *International Journal of Prosthodontics*, 15, 259–266.

Wismeijer, D., van Waas, M. A. J., Mulder, J., Vermeeren, J. I. J. F., & Kalk, W. (1999). Clinical and radiological results of patients treated with three treatment modalities for overdentures on implants of the ITI Dental Implant System. *Clinical Oral Implants Research*, 10, 297–306.

Zarb, G. A. & Schmitt, A. (1990). The longitudinal clinical effectiveness of osseointegrated dental implants. Part III. Problems and complications encountered. *Journal of Prosthetic Dentistry*, 64, 185–194.

Zarb, G. A. (1983). The edentulous milieu. *Journal of Prosthetic Dentistry*, 49, 825–831.

9
Occlusion and Implant-Supported Overdenture

Hamid Shafie
Frank Luaciello

Occlusion is a key factor in the success of any implant treatment. It is very important to establish an occlusal scheme that minimizes the lateral forces on supporting implants without compromising chewing efficiency.

Establishing an ideal occlusal scheme for edentulous patients is more challenging, since it is very difficult to remove all of the lateral forces from supporting implants, because no natural teeth are available to share the occlusal forces. Choosing the proper denture teeth and occlusal scheme are important factors in the long-term success of osseointegration in implant-supported overdenture.

DIFFERENT OCCLUSAL SCHEMES FORMED BY DENTURE TEETH

(Figures 9.1 and 9.2)

In the anatomic scheme, denture teeth have cusp angles of 30 degrees or more. They have

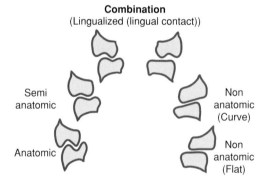

Combination
(Lingualized (lingual contact))

Semi anatomic

Non anatomic (Curve)

Anatomic

Non anatomic (Flat)

FIGURE 9.1.

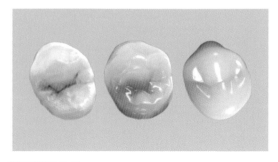

FIGURE 9.2.

112

been designed to intercuspate similar to the natural teeth occlusion. The steep cusp angles facilitate bilateral balanced occlusion and anterior disclusion (Figures 9.3 and 9.4).

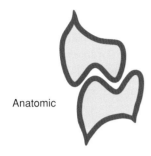

Anatomic

FIGURE 9.3.

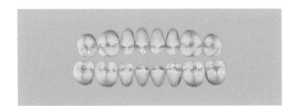

FIGURE 9.4.

Advantages
- Natural tooth anatomy
- Enhanced food penetration
- Cusp angles can achieve bilateral balanced occlusion
- Cusp angles allow for anterior disclusion, which is an advantage especially for those patients who require significant anterior vertical overlap to satisfy their esthetic needs (Figure 9.5)

Disadvantages
- Greater potential for destructive lateral forces
- Limited intercuspation relationship. For example, the anterior teeth must be arranged in a class I relationship; otherwise, distemas and/or tooth modifications are necessary to keep the first premolars positioned next to the canines
- Greater need for occlusal adjustment after processing

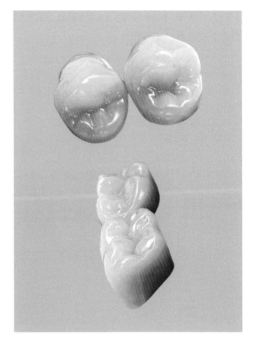

FIGURE 9.5.

SET-UP PROCEDURE FOR THE BALANCED OCCLUSION UTILIZING VITA PHYSIODENS TEETH

Setting Up the Premolars

SETTING UP THE 1ST UPPER PREMO-LAR Refer to Figure 9.6.

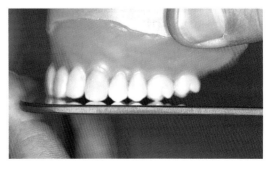

FIGURE 9.6.

- The buccal cusp touches the occlusal plane and is perpendicular to it.
- The palatal cusp does not.

SETTING UP THE 1ST LOWER PREMOLAR   Refer to Figure 9.7.

- Its labial surface is positioned above the vestibule.
- The vertical axis is upright or slightly mesially inclined.
- It is slightly inclined lingually.
- It will be slightly below the occlusal plane.

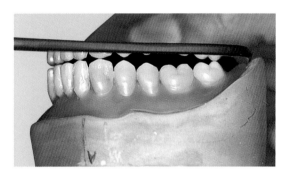

FIGURE 9.7.

OCCLUSAL CONTACTS BETWEEN THE UPPER AND LOWER 1ST PREMOLARS
Refer to Figure 9.8.

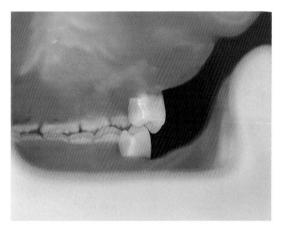

FIGURE 9.8.

Contact between the upper and lower first premolars is mainly on the inner slopes of the working cusps. Non-working contacts are infrequent, but if they do occur they do so more usually on the non-working cusps of the upper premolar. The working cusps of the lower first premolar may be in contact with the disto-palatal surface of the upper canine or the mesial marginal ridge of the upper first premolar or both. The lower first premolar should be in normal intercuspation with its long axis between the upper canine and the first premolar. It may be displaced a little mesially or distally depending on the amount of space taken up by the lower anterior setup (Figures 9.9 and 9.10).

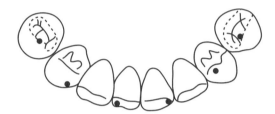

FIGURE 9.9.

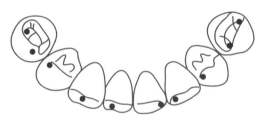

FIGURE 9.10.

SETTING UP THE UPPER 2ND PREMOLAR   Refer to Figures 9.11 and 9.12.

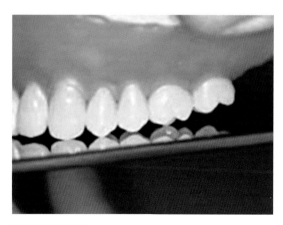

FIGURE 9.11.

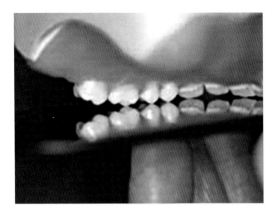

FIGURE 9.12.

- Both cusps touch the occlusal plane.
- The tooth is set perpendicular to the plane.
- If viewed from the buccal, its axial inclination should be similar to the upper canine and premolar.
- It is positioned in the arch so that the ellipse formed by the buccal outline and the central fissure (when viewed from the occlusal) is paralleled to the crest of the alveolar ridge.
- The proximal contact is a spherical interdental contact area, not a contact point.

OCCLUSAL CONTACTS OF THE UPPER 2ND PREMOLAR   Refer to Figures 9.13 and 9.14.

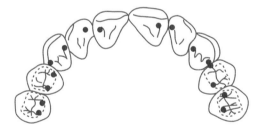

FIGURE 9.13.

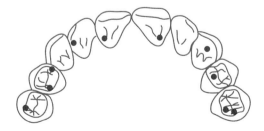

FIGURE 9.14.

- Contacts are mainly on the inner slopes of the working cusps.
- The outer slopes of the working cusps are mostly out of contact.
- Non-working cusps are mostly out of contact.
- Some marginal ridge contacts are acceptable as with the first premolar.

SETTING UP THE LOWER 2ND PREMOLAR   Refer to Figures 9.15–9.18.

- This tooth will be a little below the occlusal plane compare the lower first premolar.
- Its buccal surface should not be over the vestibule.

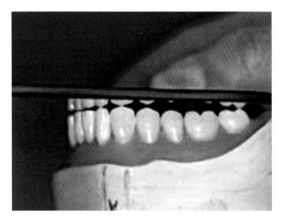

FIGURE 9.15.

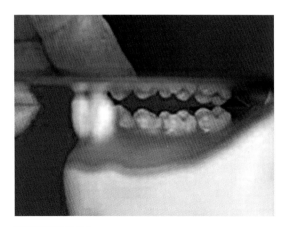

FIGURE 9.16.

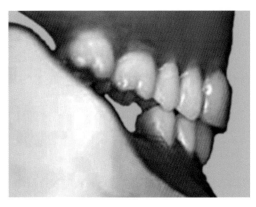

FIGURE 9.17.

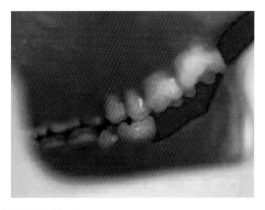

FIGURE 9.18.

- Its central fissure should be set on the canine-retromolar line.
- Its position should follow the mandibular arch.
- It should not incline lingually as much as the first premolar.
- The lingual (non-working) cusp should be out of contact but closer to the occlusal plane compared to the first premolar.
- Its long axis is mesially inclined (but not so much as the first premolar).

OCCLUSAL CONTACTS OF THE LOWER 2ND PREMOLAR   Refer to Figures 9.19 and 9.20.

- Contacts are mainly on the inner slopes of the working cusps.
- The buccal non-working contacts (upper) are more frequent than lingual (lower) non-working contacts.

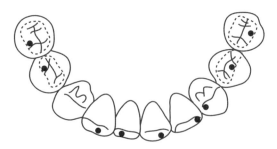

FIGURE 9.19.

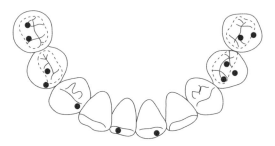

FIGURE 9.20.

Note: It is a good practice when setting up the upper and lower premolars to leave a small space, perhaps 1mm, behind the canines, so that the anterior teeth setup can be altered as needed at a later time. This space also allows the lab technician to modify the posterior teeth setup to improve the intercuspation.

Setting Up the Molars

The molars are set up so that their cusps are in contact with the transverse Wilson, and the anterior-posterior compensating curves of the occlusion.

SETTING UP THE UPPER 1ST MOLAR
Refer to Figures 9.21 and 9.22.

- Only its mesio-palatal cusp forms contact with the occlusal plane.
- The disto-palatal cusp starts rising up and away from the occlusal plane.
- The buccal cusps are out of contact with the occlusal plane and positioned about 1mm above the occlusal plane.

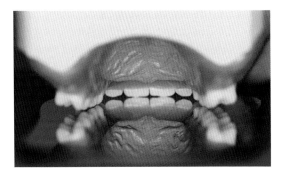

FIGURE 9.21.

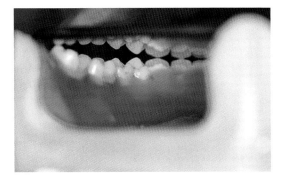

FIGURE 9.22.

- If the patient's upper posterior teeth are viewed from frontal aspect, less and less buccal surface of the teeth should be visible starting from the first upper premolar and going back toward the second molar. This transition in the contour and positioning of the upper posterior teeth forms the *buccal corridor* (Figures 9.23 and 9.24).

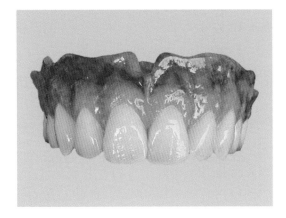

FIGURE 9.23.

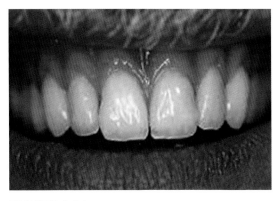

FIGURE 9.24.

OCCLUSAL CONTACTS OF THE UPPER 1ST MOLAR   Refer to Figures 9.25 and 9.26.

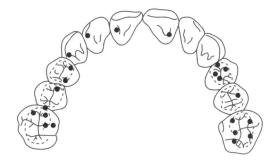

FIGURE 9.25.

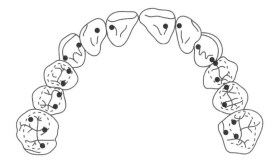

FIGURE 9.26.

- Contacts are located mainly on the inner slopes of the working (palatal) cusps.
- There are few marginal ridge contacts.
- There are few non-working contacts.
- The non-working contacts are located more on the molars than on the premolars.

- The first molars (upper and lower) have more points of contact than any other occluding teeth.

SETTING UP THE LOWER 1ST MOLAR
Refer to Figures 9.27–9.29.

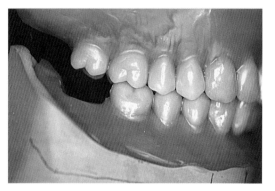

FIGURE 9.27.

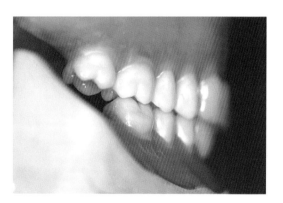

FIGURE 9.28.

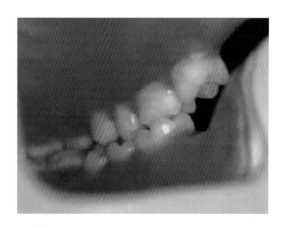

FIGURE 9.29.

- It is usually positioned at the lowest part of the anterior-posterior compensating curve.
- Its occlusal surface is lingually inclined and rises distally to accommodate the formation of the compensating curve.
- Its long axis is inclined mesially.

OCCLUSAL CONTACTS OF THE LOWER 1ST MOLAR   Refer to Figures 9.30 and 9.31.

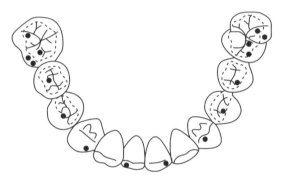

FIGURE 9.30.

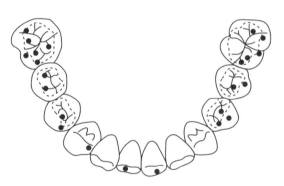

FIGURE 9.31.

- The contacts are mainly located on the lingual slopes of the buccal cusps.
- There are few marginal ridge contacts.
- There are few non-working contacts.
- Its mesio-buccal and mesio-lingual cusps are in contact with the distal of the upper 2nd premolar.

SETTING UP THE UPPER 2ND MOLAR
Refer to Figures 9.32 and 9.33.

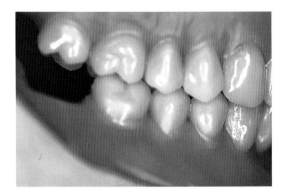

FIGURE 9.32.

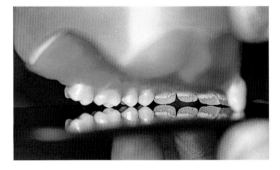

FIGURE 9.33.

- Neither palatal cusps are touching the occlusal plane, and the buccal cusps, like the upper first molar, are about 1mm above the occlusal plane.
- Disto-palatal cusp starts rising up and away from the occlusal plane.

OCCLUSAL CONTACTS OF THE UPPER 2ND MOLAR Refer to Figures 9.34 and 9.35.

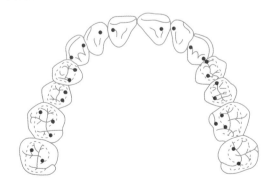

FIGURE 9.34.

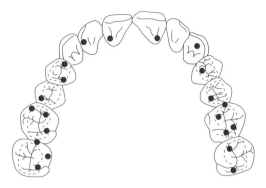

FIGURE 9.35.

- The contacts are mainly on the inner slopes of the working (palatal) cusps.
- There are few marginal ridge contacts.
- There are few non-working contacts.

SETTING UP THE LOWER 2ND MOLAR
Refer to Figures 9.36–9.38.

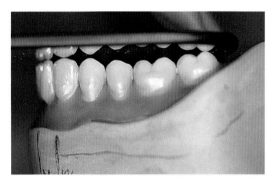

FIGURE 9.36.

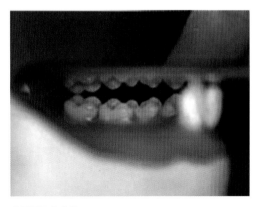

FIGURE 9.37.

- Its occlusal surface is inclined lingually.
- Its mesio-buccal cusp is located approximately at the level of the occlusal plane.

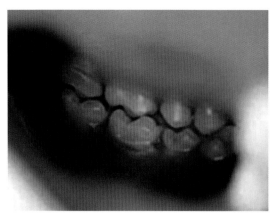

FIGURE 9.38.

- Its distal cusps are slightly above the occlusal plane.
- Its long axis is inclined mesially.

OCCLUSAL CONTACTS OF THE LOWER 2ND MOLAR Refer to Figures 9.39 and 9.40.

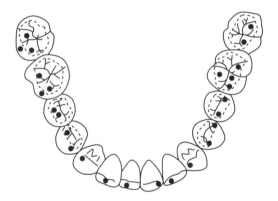

FIGURE 9.39.

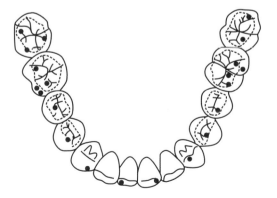

FIGURE 9.40.

- The contacts are mainly on the inner (lingual) slopes of the working cusps.
- There are few marginal ridge contacts (point 4 *centric relation*).
- There are few non-working contacts (point 5 *centric relation*).

IMPORTANT POINTS TO REMEMBER DURING THE OCCLUSAL ADJUSTMENT

- Any grinding must not alter the occlusal surface to the extent that the anatomy is changed.
- Assuming that the occlusal adjustment is necessary, if the contacts are few or are uneven in their intensity, the first contacts should be reduced (with respect to the tooth anatomy) until simultaneous and harmonious contacts are established throughout the occlusion.
- Contacts on mesial slopes will be against opposing distal slopes.
- Contacts on the inner slopes of working cusps will be against the inner slopes of opposing working cusps.
- Contacts on the outer slopes of non-working cusps will be against the inner slopes of non-working cusps.

Note: Positive stabilization in occlusion only occurs in centric relation and this is the only occlusal balance that should be sought.

Semi-Anatomic

These teeth are modified versions of anatomic teeth with shallower cusp angles. Cusp angles generally range from 10–20 degrees, and the teeth occlude similar to anatomic teeth and create a precise intercuspation. However, these teeth typically have a more "forgiving" intercuspation (Figures 9.41–9.43).

Non-Anatomic

These teeth have a zero-degree cusp angle. It is difficult to achieve balanced occlusion with them due to lack of cusp angles, unless the teeth are

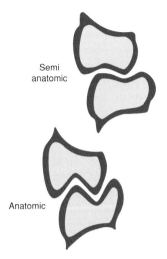

FIGURE 9.41.

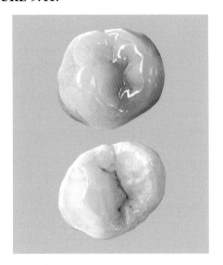

FIGURE 9.42.

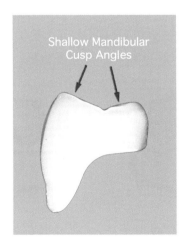

FIGURE 9.43.

arranged with a balancing ramp (Figures 9.44–9.46).

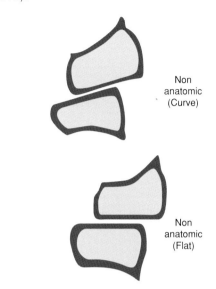

FIGURE 9.44.

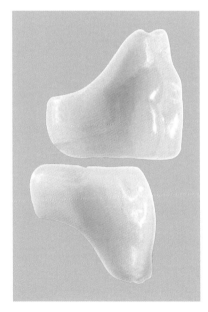

FIGURE 9.45.

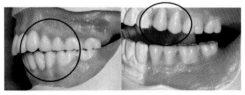

FIGURE 9.46.

ADVANTAGES   Refer to Figure 9.47.

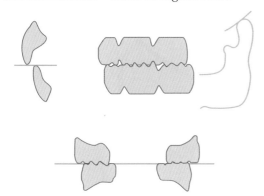

FIGURE 9.47.

- Minimal lateral forces
- Easy to set up
- Easy to adjust

DISADVANTAGES   Refer to Figure 9.48.

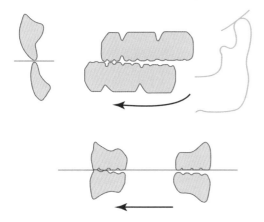

FIGURE 9.48.

- Unnatural tooth anatomy
- Require more vertical forces to penetrate food
- Difficult to adjust in eccentric movements unless set on a balancing ramp
- Elimination of incisal guidance
- Vertical overlap must be eliminated due to the lack of cusp angles

Lingualized

Steep maxillary lingual cusps, shallow mandibular teeth cusp angles, and an uncomplicated central fossa characterize these teeth. These teeth can accommodate balanced and non-balanced occlusal schemes. Historically, there are two variations of "lingual contact occlusion." These variations depend on the cusp angles of the mandibular teeth and whether the plane of occlusion is flat or curved. If bilateral balanced occlusion is planned, lower posterior teeth should have cusp angles of 10–20 degrees, and the plane of occlusion should be arranged on a curve. If maximum freedom in lateral excursions is desired and there is no plan to achieve eccentric bilateral balanced occlusion, then the lower posterior teeth can be at zero degrees, and the plane of occlusion should be flat.

To establish a lingualized occlusion, the maxillary posterior teeth should have relatively steep cusp angles, preferably 30 degrees or more. The maxillary lingual cusps should be in contact with the mandibular central fissure. The maxillary buccal cusps should be eliminated with a progressive increase in clearance from the first premolar to the second molar. With this arrangement, the occlusal forces during working side excursion are directed lingual to the crest of the residual ridges. In comparison, with anatomic occlusion, the maxillary buccal cusps will be in contact with lower posterior teeth during working side excursion, which will direct the occlusal forces to the crest of the ridges resulting in a destabilizing situation. The lingualized occlusal scheme is more stable than anatomic occlusion (Figures 9.49–51).

Combination
(Lingualized (lingual contact))

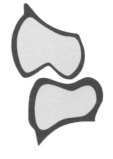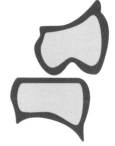

FIGURE 9.49.

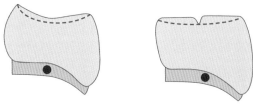

Uncomplicate mandibular central fossa

FIGURE 9.50.

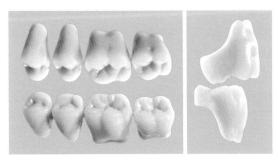

FIGURE 9.51.

BIOMECHANICAL ADVANTAGES

- During centric occlusion, occlusal forces will be transferred to the center of residual ridge.
- During working side excursion, occlusal forces will be transferred more lingual to the residual ridge, which results in greater stability.
- This occlusal scheme minimizes the occlusal contact area, provides more efficient penetration of teeth through food, provides a better escape way for food, and minimizes destabilizing contacts.

CLINICAL AND TECHNICAL ADVANTAGES

- Prevents cheek biting by eliminating occlusal contacts with maxillary buccal cusps.
- Minimizes occlusal disharmonies that resulted from error in the jaw relationship record and dimensional changes during processing.

- Simplifies setting the denture teeth and subsequent occlusal adjustments and eliminates the precise intercuspation, which often complicates the arrangement of anatomic denture teeth.

HISTORY OF LINGUALIZED (LINGUAL CONTACT) OCCLUSION

In 1927, Gysi of Switzerland introduced the concept of a lingualized occlusal scheme. In 1941, Payne published the "modified posterior setup" concept. This occlusal scheme consisted of prominent maxillary lingual cusps that occlude with relatively flat and uncomplicated mandibular occlusal surfaces. Only the maxillary lingual cusps are in contact with mandibular teeth. The occlusal forces are transferred lingual to the mandibular ridge. Because of this pattern of loading, it is called "lingualized occlusion." Recently the term was changed to "lingual contact occlusion" to eliminate the suggestion that the teeth are set more lingual to the lower ridge, which can limit the tongue space. This occlusal scheme has become more popular because of its aesthetics, biomechanics, simplicity, and higher patient satisfaction.

SET-UP PROCEDURE FOR LINGUALIZED OCCLUSION UTILIZING IVOCLAR ORTHOLINGUAL TEETH

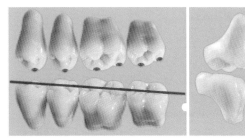

FIGURE 9.52.

Sequence of Tooth Arrangement
1. Position mandibular teeth.
2. Position maxillary teeth.
3. Eliminate maxillary buccal cusp interferences.
4. Eliminate anterior interferences.
5. Eccentric balance on inclined planes of mandibular posteriors.

1: Position Mandibular Teeth

Several anatomical landmarks such as retromolar pads, buccal shelf, and mylohyoid ridge, which guide the arrangement of denture teeth, are located on the mandibular cast. Therefore, it is recommended that the mandibular teeth be set first.

HEIGHT OF OCCLUSAL PLANE The retromolar pad is an excellent guide for establishing the height of the occlusal plane. The occlusal surface of the last molar should be placed at a level that is two-thirds of the height of the retromolar pad (Figure 9.53).

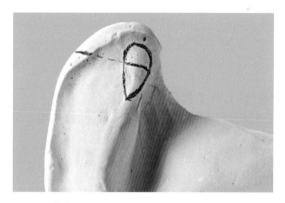

FIGURE 9.53.

BUCCOLINGUAL POSITION There are two popular guides for buccolingual positioning of mandibular posterior teeth:

• Placing the central fossa of the mandibular posterior teeth on a line that extends from

the mesial proximal contact of the canine to the middle of retromolar pad (Figure 9.54).

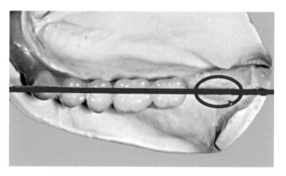

FIGURE 9.54.

• Utilizing Pound's Triangular. Mandibular lingual cusps should be located within this triangular. The buccal and lingual side of the retromolar pad and the mesial proximal contact of the canine form Pound's Triangular (Figure 9.55).

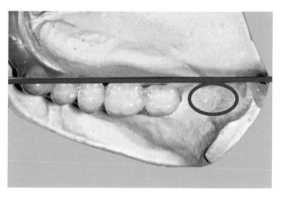

FIGURE 9.55.

OCCLUSAL PLANE (CURVED VS. NON-CURVED) If bilateral balanced occlusal contact is desired, it is recommended that the mandibular teeth be set with anterior-posterior and mediolateral compensating curves (Figures 9.56 and 9.57).

Set premolars and mesial cusp of 1st molar on a plane from the tip of the canine to two-thirds up the retomolar pad (Figure 9.58).

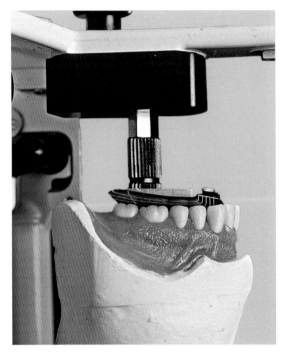

FIGURE 9.56.

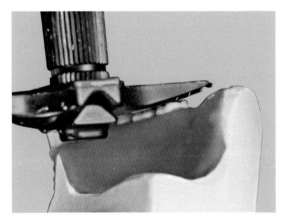

FIGURE 9.57.

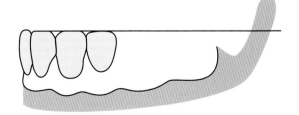

FIGURE 9.58.

Progressively set the distal of the 1st molar and the 2nd molar above the plane to create an anterior-posterior compensating curve (curve of Spee). Note that the distal of the 2nd molar should not exceed two-thirds of retromolar pad's height (Figure 9.59).

Compensating Curve

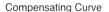

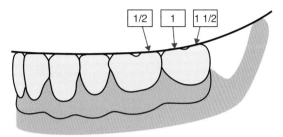

Curve of Spee

FIGURE 9.59.

The buccal and lingual cusp tips are set on a bilateral flat plane (no mediolateral curve of Wilson) (Figure 9.60).

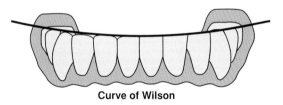

Curve of Wilson

FIGURE 9.60.

2: Position Maxillary Teeth

Position the maxillary lingual cusps into the central fossa of the mandibular teeth. The lingual cusp can occlude anywhere along the V-shaped central channel of the mandibular teeth. This concept simplifies and expedites the process of arranging the maxillary teeth (Figure 9.61).

The only points of contact in centric occlusion are the maxillary lingual cusp tips and their opposing contacts in the central grooves of the mandibular teeth. These contacts are easily

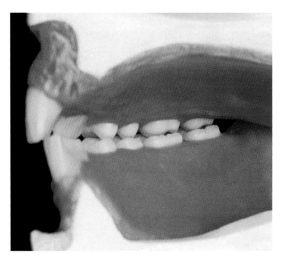

FIGURE 9.61.

established and identified with articulating paper (Figure 9.62).

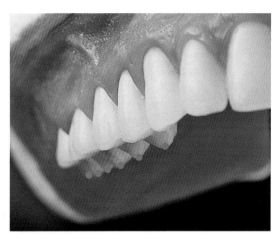

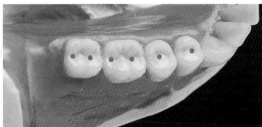

FIGURE 9.62.

Maxillary and mandibular arrangement should be in centric occlusion position. Note

that the maxillary buccal cusps are not in contact with opposing teeth (Figure 9.63).

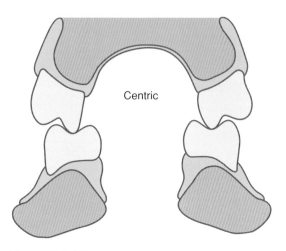

FIGURE 9.63.

3: Eliminate Maxillary Buccal Cusp Interferences

Maxillary buccal cusp contacts can be eliminated by selectively removing the inclined surface of the maxillary buccal cusp, and/or by tipping the long axis of the tooth. However, the easiest way is to utilize upper posterior teeth such as Ortholingual by Ivoclar. These teeth have been designed specifically for lingual contact occlusion, and have a progressive anterior-posterior decrease in maxillary buccal cusp height (Figures 9.64 and 9.65).

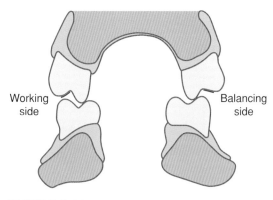

FIGURE 9.64.

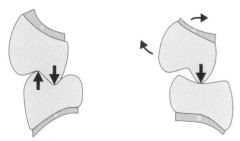

Eliminate maxillary buccal cusp contacts

FIGURE 9.65.

4: Eliminate Anterior Interferences

Anterior tooth contacts can be a destabilizing factor and should be eliminated by reducing the vertical overlap and/or increasing the horizontal overjet (Figure 9.66).

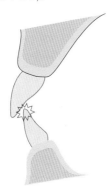

FIGURE 9.66.

Repositioning the maxillary and/or the mandibular anterior teeth in eccentric movements until all contacts are eliminated can decrease vertical overlap (Figure 9.67).

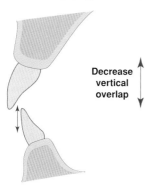

Decrease vertical overlap

FIGURE 9.67.

Increasing the horizontal overlap to provide room for functional movements can also eliminate anterior tooth contacts. For most patients, 2mm horizontal overlap is adequate (Figure 9.68).

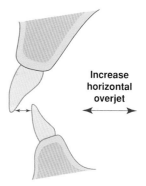

Increase horizontal overjet

FIGURE 9.68.

5: Eccentric Balance

WORKING SIDE In working excursion, the maxillary lingual cusps contact the buccal inclines of the mandibular lingual cusps. Note that the maxillary buccal cusps are not in contact (Figures 9.69 and 9.70).

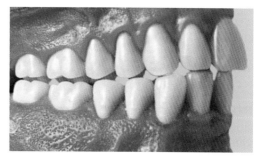

FIGURE 9.69.

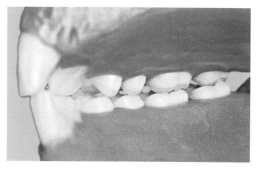

FIGURE 9.70.

BALANCING SIDE In balancing side excursion, the maxillary lingual cusps contact the lingual inclines of the mandibular buccal cusps (Figures 9.71 and 9.72).

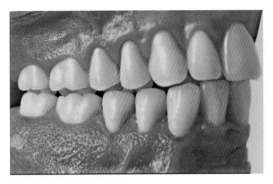

FIGURE 9.71.

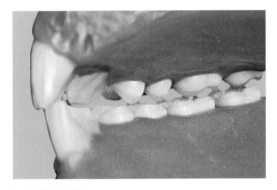

FIGURE 9.72.

PROTRUSION Protrusive contacts typically follow the working side inclinations (buccal inclines of the mandibular lingual cusps) (Figures 9.73 and 9.74).

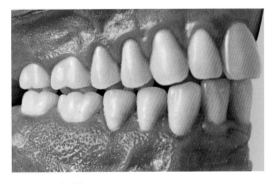

FIGURE 9.73.

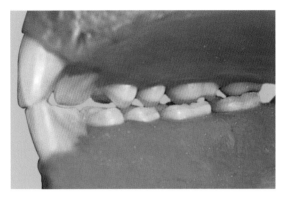

FIGURE 9.74.

EQUILIBRATION AFTER PROCESSING

Dentures routinely require occlusal adjustment after processing to correct possible inaccuracies of jaw relationship records as well as dimensional changes during processing.

Sequence of Equilibiration
1. Re-establish centric occlusion contacts.
2. Eliminate maxillary buccal cusp and/or anterior interferences.
3. Complete the equilibration by adjusting only the incline planes of the mandibular teeth.

1: Re-Establish Centric Occlusion Contacts

The occlusal marks in centric position are adjusted until the maximum number of contacts between the upper lingual cusps and the central grooves of the mandibular teeth are achieved. The maxillary lingual cusps should *NEVER* be adjusted. Once the centric contacts are re-established, they are marked and require no further adjustment. To prevent the inadvertent adjustment of the centric stops, it is recommended that they be marked with a permanent marker after they are re-established. After completion of equilibration, the permanent marks can be removed with fine pumice and a small cotton wheel (Figure 9.75).

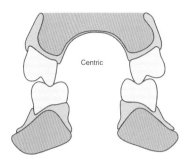

FIGURE 9.75.

2: Eliminate Maxillary Buccal Cusp and/or Anterior Interferences

Move the articulator into eccentric relationships. Mark and remove any contacts on the maxillary buccal cusps and/or anterior teeth by selective adjustment. If the teeth were set properly, this adjustment should not be necessary or should at least be minimal (Figures 9.76 and 9.77).

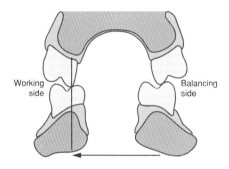

FIGURE 9.76.

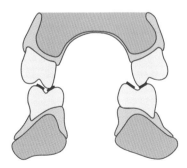

FIGURE 9.77.

3: Complete Equilibration by Adjusting Only the Incline Planes of the Mandibular Posterior Teeth

Once the centric contacts are re-established and the anterior interferences are removed, the remainder of the eccentric equilibration should be concentrated only on the incline planes of the mandibular posterior teeth. As previously mentioned, the *maxillary lingual cusps* and the *re-established mandibular centric stops* should not be adjusted (Figure 9.78).

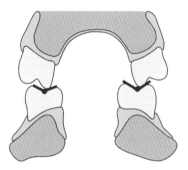

FIGURE 9.78.

ECCENTRIC JAW MOVEMENTS

It is desirable to achieve as many centric and eccentric contacts as possible. The lingualized occlusal scheme greatly simplifies interpretation of the various occlusal markings (Figure 9.79).

- In *working* (black) excursion, the maxillary lingual cusps contact the buccal inclines of the mandibular lingual cusps.
- In *balancing* (blue) side excursion, the maxillary lingual cusps contact the lingual inclines of the mandibular buccal cusps.
- *Protrusive* (red) contacts follow a steeper angle on the buccal inclines of the mandibular lingual cusps compared to working contacts.

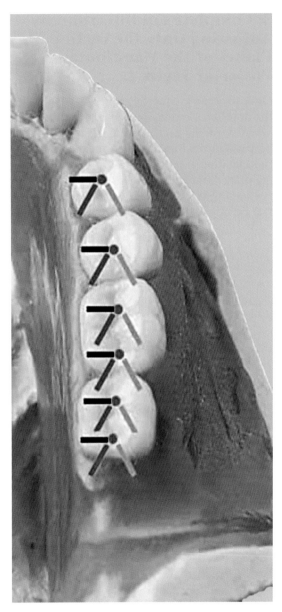

FIGURE 9.79.

REFERENCES AND ADDITIONAL READING

Bascom, P. W. (1962). Masticatory efficiency of complete dentures, *Journal of Prosthetic Dentistry*, 12, 453–459.

Becker, C. M., Swoope, C. C., & Guckes, A. D. (1977). Lingualized occlusion for removable prosthodontics. *Journal of Prosthetic Dentistry*, 38(6), 601–607.

Brewer, A. A., Reibel, P. R., & Nassif, N. J. (1967). Comparison of zero degree teeth and anatomic teeth on complete dentures. *Journal of Prosthetic Dentistry*, 17, 28–35.

Clough, H. E., et al. (1983). A comparison of lingualized occlusion and monoplane occlusion in complete dentures. *Journal of Prosthetic Dentistry*, 50, 176–179.

Folz, S. & Byars, B. (1980). Lingualized bilateral balanced occlusion complete dentures constructed on fixed articulators. *Texas Dental Journal*, 99(10), 12–17.

Garg, A. *Practical Implant Dentistry*. Dallas: Taylor Publishing, 1997.

Haraldson, T. & Zarb, G. (1988). A 10-year follow-up study of the masticatory system after treatment with osseointegrated implant bridges. *Scandinavian Journal of Dental Research*, 96, 243–52.

Kelly, E. (1977). Centric relation, centric occlusion, and posterior tooth forms and arrangements. *Journal of Prosthetic Dentistry*, 37, 5–11.

Khamis, M. M., Hussein, S. Z., & Rudy, T. E. (1998). A comparison of the effect of different occlusal forms in mandibular implant overdentures. *Journal of Prosthetic Dentistry*, 79, 422–429.

Koyama, M., Inaba, S., & Yokoyama, K. (1972). Quest for ideal occlusal patterns for complete dentures. *Journal of Prosthetic Dentistry*, 27, 269–274.

Kydd, W. L. (1956). Complete denture base deformation with varied occlusal tooth form. *Journal of Prosthetic Dentistry*, 6, 714–718.

Lang, B. R. & Kelsey, C. C. (ed.) (1973). International Prosthodontic Workshop on Complete Denture Occlusion. Ann Arbor, The University of Michigan School of Dentistry.

Lang, B. R. & Razzoof, M. E. (1983). A practical approach to restoring occlusion for edentulous patients: Part II. Arranging the functional & rational mold. *Journal of Prosthetic Dentistry*, 50, 599–606.

Lang, B. R. & Razzoog, M. E. (1983). A practical approach to restoring occlusion for edentulous patients: Part I. Arranging the functional & rational mold. *Journal of Prosthetic Dentistry*, 50, 455–458.

Lang, B. R. & Razzoog, M. E. (1992). Lingualized integration: tooth molds and an occlusal scheme for edentulous implant patients. *Implant Dentistry*, (3), 204–211.

Lundgren, D., Laurell, L., Falk, H., & Bergendal, T. (1987). Occlusal force pattern during mastication in dentitions with mandibular fixed partial dentures. *Journal of Prosthetic Dentistry*, 58(2), 197–203.

Lundquist, L. W., Carlsson, G. E., & Hedegard, B. (1986). Changes in bite force and chewing efficiency after denture treatment in edentulous patients with denture adaptation difficulties. *Journal of Oral Rehabilitation*, 13, 21–29.

Manly, RS, Vinton P. (1951). Factors influencing denture function, *Journal of Prosthetic Dentistry* 1, 578–586.

Massad, J. & Connelly, M. (2000). A simplified approach to optimizing denture stability with lingualized occlusion, *Compendium of Continuing Education in Dentistry*, 21, No 7, 555–571.

Mehringer, E. J. (1973). Function of steep cusps in mastication with complete dentures. *Journal of Prosthetic Dentistry*, 30, 367–372.

Murrell, G. A. (1974). The management of difficult lower dentures. *Journal of Prosthetic Dentistry*, 32, 243–250.

Ortman, H. R. (1988). "Complete denture occlusion." In *Essentials of Complete Denture Prosthodontics* (2nd edition), ed. Winkler, S. St Louis: Mosby–Year Book, 217–249.

Parr, G. R. & Ivanhoe, J. R. (1996). Lingualized occlusion: an occlusion for all reasons. *Dental Clinics of North America*, 40(1), 103–112.

Parr, G. R. & Loft, G. H. (1982). The occlusal spectrum and complete dentures. *Compendium of Continuing Education in Dentistry*, Vol III.

Payne, S. H. (1952). A comparative study of posterior occlusion. *Journal of Prosthetic Dentistry*, 2, 661–666.

Payne, S. H. (1958). Posterior occlusion. *Journal of the American Dental Association*, 57, 174–176.

Pound, E. & Murrell, G. A. (1973). An introduction to denture simplification, Phase I. *Journal of Prosthetic Dentistry*, 29, 570.

Pound, E. & Murrell, G. A. (1970). An introduction to denture simplification, Phase II. *Journal of Prosthetic Dentistry*, 29, 598.

Pound, E. (1966). Utilizing speech to simplify a personalized denture on chewing efficiency. *Journal of Prosthetic Dentistry*, 16, 34–43.

Sauser, C. W. & Yurkstas, A. A. (1957). The effect of various geometric occlusal patterns on chewing efficiency. *Journal of Prosthetic Dentistry*, 7, 634–645.

Swoope, C. C., Kydd, W. L. (1966). The effect of cusp form and occlusal area on denture base deformation, *Journal of Prosthetic Dentistry*, 16, 34–43.

Yurkstas, A. A. & Manly, R. S. (1950). Value of different test foods in estimating masticatory ability. *Journal of Applied Physiology*, 3, 45–53.

10

Surgical Considerations for Implant Overdenture

Richard Green
George Obeid
Roy Eskow
Hamid Shafie

PRESURGICAL INSTRUCTIONS

Prior to embarking on the surgical treatment of an elderly patient, a complete medical history is required. While many abnormalities may be noted, specific disease processes can adversely affect the outcome of implant surgery. Many elderly patients take medications that can affect the coagulation process. Clopidogrel (Plavix), warfarin (Coumadin), and aspirin are common medications that can have a profound effect on homeostasis after surgery. Preoperative evaluation by the prescribing physician is needed to ascertain the reason for the anticoagulant, and the possibility of withholding the medication prior to surgery. If warfarin is taken, measurement of the International Normalized Ratio (INR) is needed to determine the level of anticoagulation.

Many elderly surgical patients take steroids for treatment of systemic disorders. Steroids can affect the patient's ability to withstand the stress of surgery and heal after surgery. Prednisone, dexamethasone, and betamethasone are common examples of corticosteroids. While many patients are on sub-physiologic doses of corticosteroids (less that 20mg of cortisol per day), others may be on doses that suppress the adrenal gland's ability to release cortisol. A decision, in conjunction with the patient's primary care physician, will need to be made as to the need for steroid supplementation.

Diabetes is a disease that affects glucose metabolism. While many patients only require adjustments in lifestyle, the majority of patients will be placed on either oral or injectable form of medications. While a well-controlled diabetic is a good surgical candidate, a poorly controlled patient is at risk for an infection and other microvascular damage. If the glucose control of a patient is unknown, a Hemoglobin A1C will provide a gauge of the previous three months of control. If the patient takes insulin, a preoperative (that morning) glucose level is needed to ensure the patient does not become hypoglycemic during the procedure.

Hypertension is common in the elderly surgical patient. While hypertension is not a contraindication to surgery, uncontrolled hypertension can result in cardiovascular accident. It is important to confirm that patients are taking their medication as prescribed by their physician. A blood pressure reading prior to surgery is certainly desirable.

Inhalation analgesia is generally avoided due to the awkwardness of the nasal hood when positioning surgical stents and orienting pilot drills to the horizontal plane. Premedication with Ibuprofen 600mg and Xanax 0.25–0.5mg P.O. one hour before appointment is useful if intravenous sedation is not used. Intravenous sedation is advisable for highly apprehensive patients, but if the immediate implant-supported overdenture techniques are being utilized, the IV sedation is contraindicated, because these techniques require patient cooperation during the operation. A one-minute preoperative rinse with 0.12 percent chlorhexidine or other oral antiseptic rinse is also advisable to reduce levels of oral microflora.

Treatment Room Preparation and Utilization Protocol

The treatment room should have a large table covered by sterile drapes on which to organize all the sterile equipment. The sterile area is accessed only by those who are using sterile gloves. The aseptic chain must not be broken.

All the people involved in surgery should prepare as follows:

- *Protective Cover:* Clean gown, cap, protective glasses, and facemask must be worn.
- *Gloves:* Use only disposable sterile gloves.
- *Surgical Hand Disinfection:* Disinfect hands and forearms by regular scrubbing or by using medical based skin sanitizer.

Patient

- *Mouth:* Clean patient's mouth with chlorhexidine 0.12 percent mouthwash.
- *Draping:* Use a sterile surgical drape.

Instruments

Arrange the instruments in the surgical cassette and then sterilize them, or place individually sterilized instruments on a surgical tray covered with a sterilized surgical drape. Only individuals with sterilized gloves are allowed to handle the instruments. Make sure that you have additional spare sterile instruments, gloves, and implants available to deal with any unforeseen circumstances.

INCISIONS AND FLAP DESIGN

Block- and infiltration-anesthesia is obtained using local anesthetics containing vasoconstrictor 1:100,000 epinephrine. A number 15 Bard-Parker blade on a round handled scalpel holder is the ideal blade for making incisions on the fully edentulous alveolar ridge. The blade is drawn from posterior to anterior making firm contact with the underlying bone severing the periosteum. An Orban number 1/2 knife is passed through the incision line to ensure the periosteum is completely severed before reflecting the mucoperiosteal flap using a Prichard elevator.

Incision and Flap Design Objectives

- Providing ease of access to visualize the underlying osseous structures
- Preserving existing crestal gingival tissue
- Avoiding critical neurovascular structures
- Allowing stable positioning of the surgical stent

Basic Flap Designs

Three basic flap designs are considered in the edentulous arch. All of these flaps are full thickness, and the selection depends on the number and location of implants being placed.

ANTERIOR CRESTAL INCISION WITH OR WITHOUT VESTIBULAR RELEASE

This flap design permits access for implant placement in the inter-canine region of either the maxilla or mandible. This design is used when two to four implants are being placed. The incision is intended to split the keratinized mucosa at the ridge crest in order to provide each flap margin with durable keratinized tissue for suturing and post-operative primary closure. The flap is reflected full thickness and affords the surgeon the ability to assess the alveolar ridge width and contour. This is important as apical concavities and irregularities are often masked by the overlying mucosal tissue giving a false impression of available bone to support the dental implant. The anterior vertical releasing incisions leave the posterior alveolar ridge unaffected, providing a stable base to position the surgical stent and mark the osteotomy sites. Care must be taken in the mandibular arch to identify the position of the mental foramina. The mental artery, vein and nerve are often near or at the alveolar crest in the atrophic mandible. Localization and avoidance of this structure with both the crestal and vertical releasing incisions is required to prevent nerve injury resulting in post-surgical lip paresthesia. The surgeon may likewise elect not to disrupt or sever the nasopalatine artery, vein, and nerve at the incisive foramen when operating in the maxillary arch. Although not as critical a structure as the mental neurovascular bundle, severing the nasopalatine artery can result in excessive intraoperative bleeding causing an otherwise avoidable surgical complication. A modification of this incision and flap design relies upon "mini" flaps placed directly at the site of the desired implant location. This technique is minimally invasive and preserves keratinized tissue for the facial tissue margin.

FULL ARCH EXTENDED CRESTAL INCISION   The full arch crestal incision and flap design is performed when six implants are being placed for a hybrid fixed detachable overdenture or fully implant-supported bar overdenture. The flap is reflected full thickness, and the maxillary or mandibular ridge is effectively "degloved" or exposed. This flap preserves keratinized tissue at the margin but lacks stability for the surgical stent. This is especially true in the mandible.

VESTIBULAR INCISION   This incision is placed lateral to the crest of the ridge. The aim

of this design is to archive closure of the flap that is away from the crest of the ridge, providing full coverage of the cover screws. It is important to note that this incision can risk injuring superficially positioned mental nerves. There are no similar concerns in the maxilla.

MANDIBULAR SURGERY

1: Crestal Incision

WITHOUT RELEASING INCISIONS The crestal incision without releasing incisions is indicated for placement of overdenture implants as well as uncovering submerged implants during second-stage surgery (Figure 10.1).

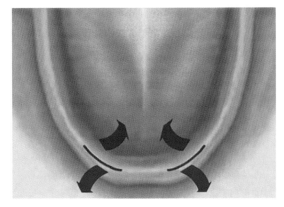

FIGURE 10.1.

WITH VESTIBULAR RELEASING INCISIONS   When multiple regular restorative implants are being placed, it is important to have a clear view of the crest of the ridge as well as width of the bone. This incision design permits visualization of alveolar ridge topography including crestal ridge width and vestibular or lingual concavities when tomograms are not available to assess the ridge dimensions. Vertical releasing incisions must be shallow or be placed well anterior or posterior to the mental foramina (Figures 10.2 and 10.3).

2: Extended Crestal Incision

This incision is indicated when the treatment plan involves implant placement distal to the

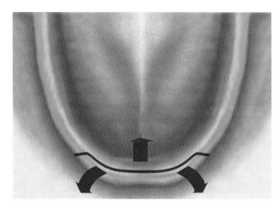

FIGURE 10.2.

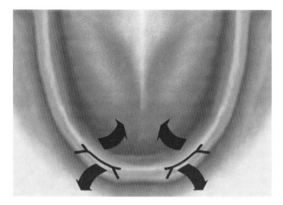

FIGURE 10.3.

mental foramina. Care should be taken to assess the position of the mental foramen. In Class C and D bone quantity cases advanced alveolar ridge atrophy often results in the mental neurovascular bundle exiting the mandible at the crest of the ridge (Figures 10.4 and 10.5).

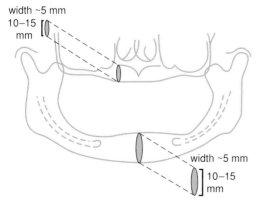

FIGURE 10.4.

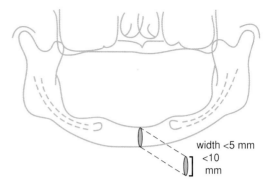

FIGURE 10.5.

If you can paltate the foramen, avoid it by locating your incision to the lingual of this structure. If you are unsure of the nerve position, you must carefully reflect the flap with blunt dissection until the structure is localized. One can then protect the mental nerve from improperly placed incisions or implant osteotomy (Figure 10.6).

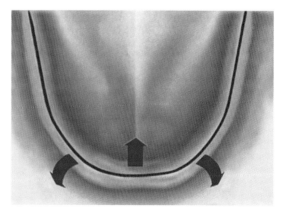

FIGURE 10.6.

3: Vestibular Incision

The vestibular incision is indicated when multiple submerged implants are being placed between the mental foramina and the crestal gingiva is narrow (Figure 10.7). This approach creates a lingually reflected flap and provides complete coverage of the implants. With this type of incision, the mental nerve is at a higher risk for injury. Care should be taken to localize and avoid this structure.

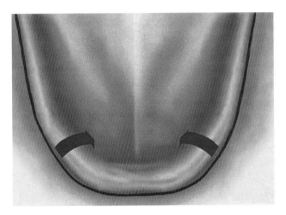

FIGURE 10.7.

MAXILLARY SURGERY

1: Crestal Incision

The crestal incision is ideal for single-stage over-denture implants as well as the second-stage uncovering step. A generous band of keratinized mucosa is retained in the buccal flap (Figures 10.8 and 10.9).

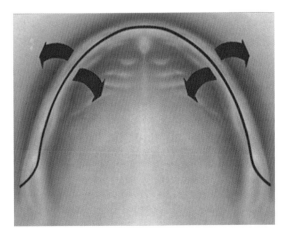

FIGURE 10.8.

2: Palatal Incision

The primary incision is palatal to the crest of the ridge with two releasing incisions toward the buccal vestibule (Figure 10.10). The flap will be reflected buccally. This design provides very good visual access.

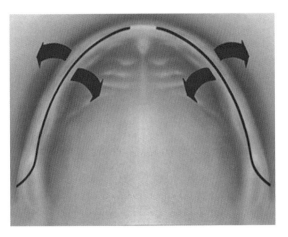

FIGURE 10.9.

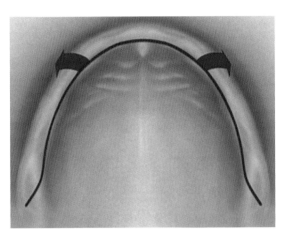

FIGURE 10.10.

3: Buccal Incision

The primary incision is buccal to the crest of the ridge. The flap will be reflected palatally. This design provides very good visual access as well as easy use of traditional as well CT generated surgical guide (Figure 10.11). With this flap, the patient may experience more postoperative edema and discomfort.

Tissue Punch Technique

The alternative tissue punch or "flapless" implant placement procedure often obliterates all keratinized tissue, requiring an otherwise unnecessary gingival grafting procedure to reestablish a margin of keratinized tissue around

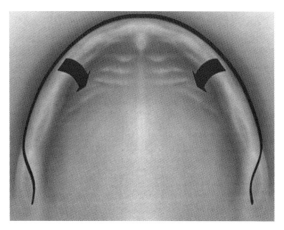

FIGURE 10.11.

the implant (Figure 10.12). This technique is indicated when the width of keratinized tissue is at least 6–8mm and the ridge is wide. This will leave 1–2mm of peri-implant gingiva when conventional diameter implants are being used. The

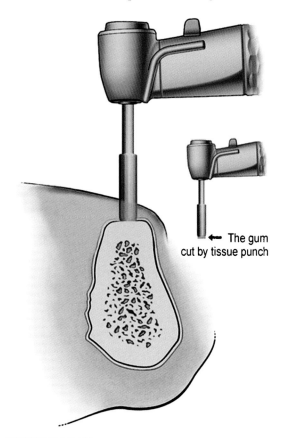

← The gum cut by tissue punch

FIGURE 10.12.

disadvantage of this technique lies in the inability of the clinician to visualize alveolar ridge concavities when aligning the implant drills for the osteotomy. The surgeon may inadvertently perforate the buccal or lingual plate, bringing the successful implant integration into jeopardy.

OSTEOTOMY AND IMPLANT PLACEMENT

The patient should be positioned such that the clinician is comfortable and can visualize the surgical site and the horizontal plane related to the maxillary or mandibular occlusal plane. The first implant placed is often used as a reference to parallel subsequent implants in an overdenture case. If the first implant is not perpendicular to the path of denture insertion, then subsequent implants will also be misaligned, compromising the function of the overdenture attachment. The attachment design dictates the implant positioning. In the case of a bar overdenture, a minimum of 18–20mm is required between the implants to permit adequate space for the bar and sleeve attachment. Surgical stents should be used to their fullest potential, as spatial orientation in the edentulous patient is difficult.

The osteotomy should always be prepared according to the implant manufacturer's guidelines regarding drill rpm and drill sequencing. Sharp surgical drills are mandatory to prevent trauma while preparing the osteotomy. This is especially true in type I and type II bone where excessive speed or force on the implant drill creates heat and bone necrosis. The surgeon should also abide by insertion torque limits on threaded implants. Dense bone sites should be pre-tapped for threaded implant designs, as excessive insertion torque can damage or fracture the internal or external attachment design on the implant.

PROCEDURAL CONSIDERATIONS DURING THE SURGERY

Every instrument must be used only for its specific and intended purpose. Keep the surgical burs free from dry blood throughout the procedure by dipping them in saline or Ringer's solution. Dry blood can prevent you from correctly reading the marking on the burs. Bone particles that become attached to the cutting blades of the burs should be collected and preserved for possible use at the conclusion of implant placement.

SUTURING TECHNIQUES USED FOR IMPLANT OVERDENTURE SURGERIES

1: Simple Interrupted

The interrupted suturing technique is simple and efficient in closing most wounds. It is particularly helpful in uneven and irregular wounds. Multiple knotted sutures make the security of closure very good, as the flap will not displace if one knot unties or if it pulls through the tissue. This technique is slightly more time-consuming than a continuous suture (Figure 10.13).

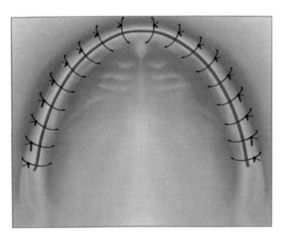

FIGURE 10.13.

2: Continuous (Locking or Non-Locking)

The continuous suture provides a uniform distribution of tension across the length of the suture and wound margin (Figures 10.14 and 10.15). It is fast and simple. It provides rapid closure

of a long incision with a single knot placed at the beginning and another at the end of the suture. Generous bites greater than 4mm should be made while suturing to reduce tearing at the tissue margin and loss of suture tension. Long incisions are best managed using continuous suturing techniques.

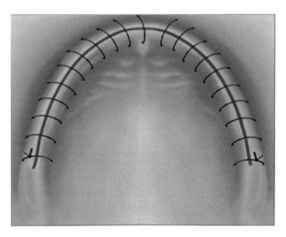

FIGURE 10.14.

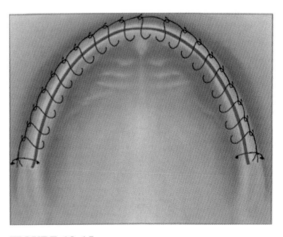

FIGURE 10.15.

Disadvantages
- The disadvantage of the continuous suture technique is that if the suture unties or if one or more passes of the material tears through, the flap tension is lost across the entire wound margin, allowing the displacement of the flap and healing by secondary intention.

- Minor bleeding under the flap will generally seep through the edges of the flap or migrate through the muscle planes, causing bruising or swelling at a site distant to the wound.
- Continuous locking sutures may add more pressure on the edges of the wound, compromising the vascularity of the wound edges and increasing the chance of necrosis.

3: Horizontal Mattress

The objective of this suturing technique is to evert the wound edges, maximizing their contact and providing a more secure tension-free closure (Figure 10.16). This is particularly helpful when graft material has been placed. In these cases, a combination of the periosteal-releasing incision, which provides flap mobility for closure over regenerative barriers, and the horizontal mattress suture is recommended. The wide bite of this suture permits the use of secondary continuous or interrupted suturing at the incision line for added security.

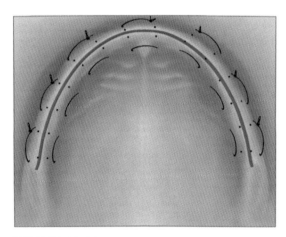

FIGURE 10.16.

Most Common Suturing Techniques for Implant-Supported Overdenture Cases

Selection of the easiest and most reliable suture technique depends upon the length of the incision requiring closure. A short incision is easily managed with interrupted sutures, whereas a long incision is managed best with a continuous suture supplemented with isolated interrupted sutures at critical points requiring more security if the continuous suture should fail.

Suture Material

Options of sutures materials for implant overdenture cases include the following:

RESORBABLE MATERIAL

- Chromic gut
- Vicryl

NON-RESORBABLE MATERIAL

- Silk
- Monofilament (prolene, nylon)
- PFTE polytetrafluoroethylene

A resorbable suture is one that the clinician should not have to remove and should remain for the appropriate period of time to achieve wound stability. Wounds that require longer stabilization benefit from the use of non-resorbable monofilament materials. They generally remain clean and last for very long time. 4–0 or 5–0 with a 3/8- or 1/2-round cutting needle are the usual sizes.

POST-SURGICAL CARE

After suturing is complete, the patient's existing denture must be generously relieved over the location of the dental implants. This will minimize premature loading of the implants in uncontrolled variable directions. Following this adjustment, the dentures should be relined with a tissue conditioner such as Coe-Comfort. The patient is instructed not to remove the denture for 48 hours as postoperative swelling may prevent reinsertion of the prosthesis. The tissue conditioner is replaced at one week and maintained for one additional week. At that time, a soft denture liner is placed. The patient should be seen every 3–4 weeks thereafter to monitor healing around the implants.

Post-Healing Criteria for Successful Integration of the Implant with Surrounding Tissues

- Patient with no subjective symptoms
- No peri-implant inflammation with suppuration
- Stable implant with light percussion
- No peri-implant radiolucency

Procedural Considerations after Surgery

Residue of blood, saliva, tissue, or bone must be removed from the instruments immediately.

Note: Do not allow blood, saliva, tissue, or bone to dry on the instruments. Dismantle multi-piece instruments, such as ratchets. Place the dirty instruments in a suitable medium for disinfection.

Note: Used instruments must always be disinfected before being cleaned. Place dirty instruments only on the intended surface, either the cassette lid or in the appropriate dish. Damaged instruments must be sorted and separately disinfected, cleaned, and discarded.

The careful handling of all drills and burs is of the utmost importance. Damage to the drill tip can occur when the drill is "thrown" into a dish of water. Damage to the drill tip greatly impairs its cutting ability. With proper care, the high quality of the material ensures that the drills and taps can be used repeatedly up to the number of surgeries recommended by the manufactures. Discard your surgical drills after reaching the maximum number of uses recommended by the manufactures.

Note
- Treat drills and burs carefully.
- Never allow instruments to land on their tips.
- Do not mix implant surgery instruments with other instruments during ultrasonic cleaning.
- Separate stainless steel instruments from titanium instruments when cleaning them in the ultrasonic cleaner.

SITE PREPARATION FOR OVERDENTURES

Overdentures and the implants that support them require solid osseous profiles. This is especially true where the implants are going to be placed for the eventual overdenture. The basic principles of pre-surgical medical analysis, clearances, and management apply. Likewise, all standard surgical techniques must be rigorously adhered to. However, insufficient ridge height, width, depth and/or inadequate bone quality can be a recipe for failure. Careful planning based on sound occlusal and force distribution principles will greatly enhance long-term success. Therefore, the restorative dentist must determine the ideal position for the placement of the implants. Subsequently, this information must be conveyed to the surgeon. In turn, the surgeon must strive to create adequate housing, both dimensionally as well in terms of quality, for proper placement, retention, and long-term maintenance of the implants.

Techniques for Site Development

- Ridge preservation upon extraction
- Ridge expansion
- Ridge enhancement
- Onlay grafting
- Distraction osteogenesis

Materials used to achieve these goals include osseous grafting materials, membranes, and devices, such as osseotomes and expanders, which can reshape or modify the dimensions of the bone, as well as create ideal positioning for the implants.

Bone Grafting Materials

- *Autograft*
- *Allograft*: Freeze dried, FDBA, demineralized bone, DFDBA
- *Xenograft*: BioOss, osteograft
- *Alloplast*: Calcium phosphate ceramics (HANTCP), bio-active plast, calcium sulphate, HTR
- *RH-BMP2 and Growth Factors*

Refer to Table 10.1 and Figures 10.17–10.23.

TABLE 10.1. Bone Grafting Materials

Category	Product (Company)	Comments	Applications
Allogeneic Bone	DBM Particles (Figures 10.17 and 10.18)	Osteoinductive (usually)	Require membrane Periodontal intrabony defects Extraction sites Alveolar reconstruction
	DynaGraft (GenSci) (Figure 10.19)	Matrix forms use a collagen sponge to carry DBM Gel/putty forms use a reverse phase copolymer to carry DBM	Periodontal intrabony defects Extraction site Alveolar reconstruction Coverage of exposed implants Implant Salvage procedures Gel as bone expander for sinus augmentation Putty as bone expander for ridge augmentation
	Grafton (Osteotech) (Figures 10.20–10.22)	Available in four forms: gel, putty, flexible sponge and the matrix; all using glycerol to carry DBM	Extraction sites Alveolar reconstruction
Xenogeneic Bone	Bio-Oss (Osteohealth) (Figure 10.23)	Bovine-derived anorganic bone matrix (particles) Recommended to use with a membrane	Extraction site Alveolar reconstruction Implant related procedures Used as bone expander
	Osteograft (Ceramed)	Bovine-derived HA	Extraction sites Alveolar reconstruction Implant-related procedures

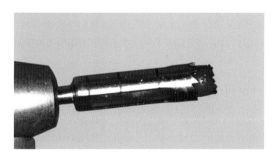

FIGURE 10.17.

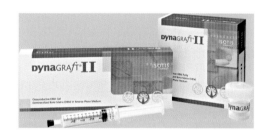

FIGURE 10.19.

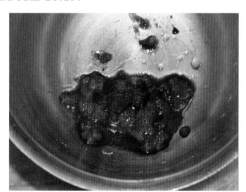

FIGURE 10.18.

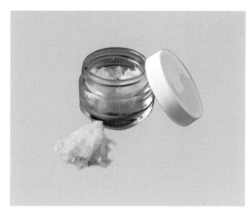

FIGURE 10.20.

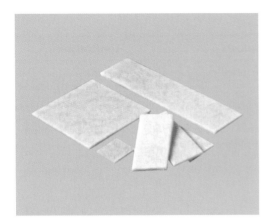

FIGURE 10.21.

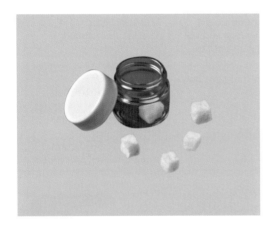

FIGURE 10.22.

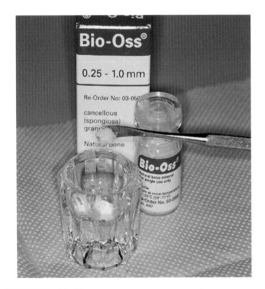

FIGURE 10.23.

In addition to grafting materials, membranes are widely used to allow osseous maturation to maximize following surgery. The soft tissue, connective tissue, and epithelium mature at a much more rapid pace—approximately ten weeks—versus bone maturation, which takes about six months. Therefore, the use of membranes allows sufficient time for this maturation process. This can be critical in establishing ideal position, volume, and topography for subsequent implant placement and retention.

Numerous products exist, but they fall into two basic categories: non-resorbable and resorbable. Non-resorbable membranes are fabricated of polytetrafloralethylene (ePTFE), which is extremely biocompatible and malleable for making space. Certain configurations come embedded with titanium skeletons that assist in maintaining shape or encouraging enhanced growth. Two management concerns are complete closure of soft tissue over these membranes at the time of placement and the necessity for their subsequent removal at the Stage II procedure, prior to placement of the implants. Some clinicians state that these membranes provide a higher incidence of postoperative infections as the tissue may open. The most commonly utilized and recognizable trade name is Gore-Tex.

Resorbable membranes are somewhat easier to handle and come in various rates of resorbability. Some resorb relatively quickly, and others last up to six months, depending on their composition and type of collagen used. Still, all of them are quite malleable when saturated and are easily adapted to ridge configurations. However, none are available with reinforcing skeletons. Likewise, many resorb relatively quickly, not allowing osseous maturation or tissue re-engineering to proceed as predictably as it does with a non-resorbable membrane.

Available Resorbable Membranes

- *BioMend:* Type I collagen which resorbs in eight weeks (Zimmer)

- *BioMend Extend:* Type I collagen which resorbs in 18 weeks (Zimmer) (Figure 10.24)

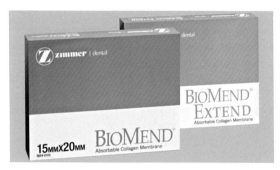

FIGURE 10.24.

- *Bio-Gide:* Types I and III collagen which resorb in 24 weeks (Osteohealth) (Figures 10.25 and 10.26)

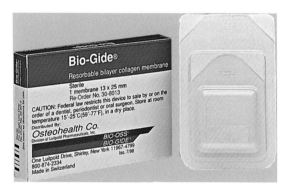

FIGURE 10.25.

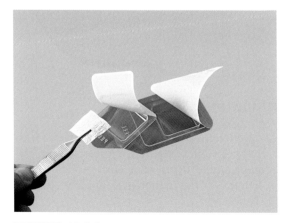

FIGURE 10.26.

- *Neomem:* Type I bovine collagen which resorbs in 26–38 weeks (Innova, Inc.) (Figure 10.27)

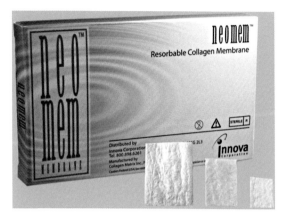

FIGURE 10.27.

Regardless of the type of membrane used, recent research indicates that bone, if grown outside of what were the original borders of the maxilla or mandible, may not retain the newly formed configurations long-term, and in turn may remodel to the earlier shapes. Often membrane success is enhanced by use of fixation tacks or pins. These help to more predictably seal the borders of the membrane with the surrounding bone by minimizing pouching and open avenues for the ingress of connective tissue.

Also, various devices exist, while others are being formulated, that aid in mechanically reshaping the bone. Primarily, these devices change the buccal/palatal-lingual dimensions by expanding or splitting the ridges, thus allowing the newly created void to be filled in with bone material. Osseotomes increase vertical dimensions via sinus reconstructions. Also, they can be utilized in the maxilla for ridge spreading and distraction.

Surgical microsaws (Frios) can be utilized to harvest autogenous blocks for onlay grafts which are stabilized with screws until fixation to the host/recipient site is achieved (Figures 10.28 and 10.29).

Even advanced surgical techniques such as distraction osteogenesis (Ace) can be performed to develop bone in certain deficient sites.

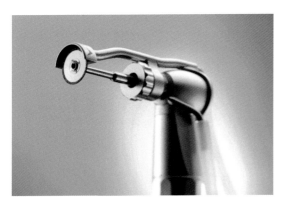

FIGURE 10.28.

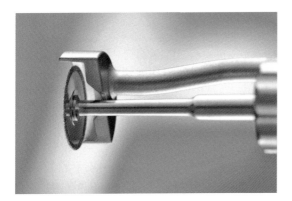

FIGURE 10.29.

SPLIT-CONTROL SYSTEM

The split-control system is a bone spreading and condensing system developed by Dr. Streckbein and Dr. Hassenpflug. The split-control system is a minimally invasive alternative to the ridge expansion by osteotomes. Bone spreading and condensing are achieved by utilizing a series of the special screw-like instruments called *spreaders*. Using spreaders allows the clinician to achieve a controlled and standardized expansion of the horizontally resorbed alveolar ridge as well as a gentle condensation of the cancellous bone. The alveolar ridge can be optimally prepared for the subsequent process of implant insertion while maintaining the existing bone substance without complicated horizontal or vertical bone grafting.

Advantages

- Minimally invasive alternative to osteotomes
- Provides a controlled expansion of the horizontally resorbed alveolar ridge
- In most cases eliminates the need for the horizontal ridge augmentation
- Increases the firmness of the alveolar bone at the osteotomy site
- Enhances the primary stability of the implant through bone condensation
- Can be used in combination with any implant system

Bone-Spreading Sequence

1. Start drilling the osteotomy with initial bur. This will prevent slippage of the pilot bur (Figures 10.30 and 10.31).

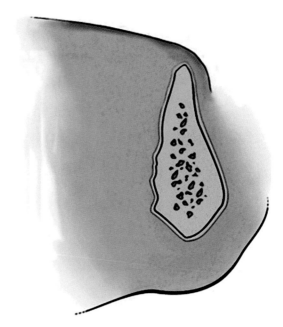

FIGURE 10.30.

2. Continue the drilling of the osteotomy with the pilot bur. Prepare the osteotomy to the appropriate depth that corresponds to the length of the designated implant (Figure 10.32).
3. Use the osteotomy disk and make a horizontal cut on the crest of the ridge. This will enhance the bone spreading (Figure 10.33).

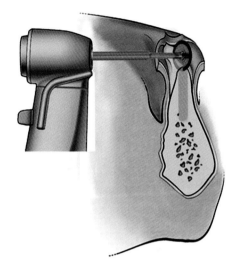

FIGURE 10.33.

4. Start utilizing the spreaders beginning with the narrowest spreader and ending with the spreader that has similar diameter to the designated implant. The sequential use of spreaders leads to bone spreading and expansion of the alveolar ridge. The spreaders can be driven into the osteotomy by a finger driver or a wretch. In bone density D1 and D2, use the expansion bur after the pilot drill before starting to use the spreaders (Figures 10.34 and 10.35).

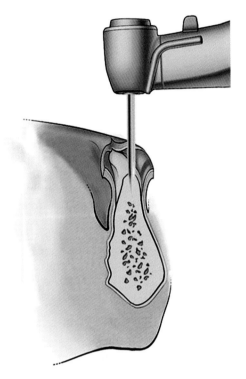

FIGURE 10.31.

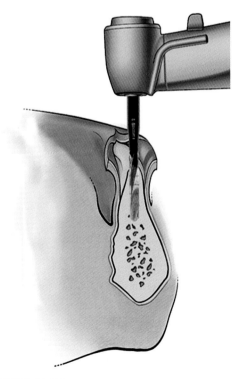

FIGURE 10.32.

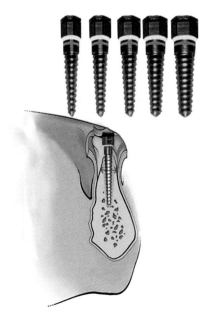

FIGURE 10.34.

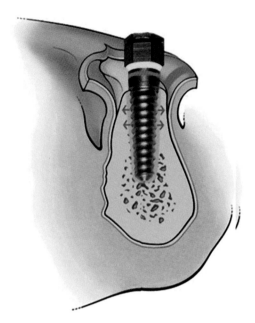

FIGURE 10.35.

5. After achieving the desirable expansion, insert the designated implant into the osteotomy. This technique not only expands the ridge but also increases the bone firmness by bone condensation. It ultimately will enhance the primary stability of the implant (Figure 10.36).

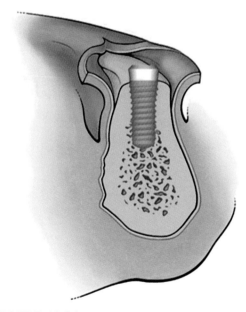

FIGURE 10.36.

SURGRY RELATED PROBLEMS

Problem: Hemorrhaging during drilling.

Possible Causes: Lesion or injury of an artery (blood vessel).

Solutions: Localize the position and depth of the initial pilot drill by radiograph if operating in the vicinity of the mandibular canal. Make necessary adjustments in drilling technique to avoid vascular and nerve injury. Other bleeding complications can be treated with local pressure and hemostatic agents. Bleeding within the osteotomy site will generally stop with implant placement.

Problem: Implant mobility after placement.

Possible Causes: Soft bone, imprecise preparation of the osteotomy.

Solutions: Remove the implant and replace it with a larger diameter implant. If the mobility is minimal, extend the healing time.

Problem: Exposed implant threads.

Possible Causes: Crest is too narrow.

Solution: Cover the threads with osseous coagulum or suitable bone graft material in conjunction with a barrier regenerative membrane.

Problem: Lingual swelling immediately after implant placement in anterior mandible.

Possible Causes: Injury of a blood vessel in the floor of the mouth.

Solutions: *This is an emergency.* Send the patient to a hospital. Bleeding vessels should be identified and tied or cauterized, and hematoma should be evacuated.

Problem: Substantial postoperative pain remaining after a few days.

Possible Causes: Osteitis due to aggressive preparation of the osteotomy, such as the use of high rpm's and inadequate irrigation, or a bacterial contamination.

Solution: Remove the affected implant and allow site to repair.

Problem: Sensory disturbance of lower lip in the immediate postoperative period.

Possible Causes: Injury of the inferior alveolar nerve.

Solutions: Map out and document the location and quality of the sensory deficit. Use radiographs to determine if any portion of the implant is within the canal space and remove it if necessary. Follow the patient weekly during the first month to document and track symptomatic improvement. Minor paresthesis generally resolve over one to eight months.

Problem: Sensory disturbance of lower lip that starts several weeks after surgery.

Possible Causes: Osteomyelitis of the mandible.

Solutions: Determine which implant is causing the problem and remove it. Debride bone if necessary, and place patient on long-term antibiotics. CT scan of the mandible is recommended.

Problem: Exposed cover screw after a few weeks.

Possible Causes: Superficial placement of the implant, thin mucosa, loose cover screw, pressure on the tissue from the transitional prosthesis.

Solution: Try to retighten the cover screw. Prescribe rigorous oral hygiene. Avoid the transitional prosthesis.

Problem: Abscess around a cover screw after a few weeks.

Possible Causes: Implant is not integrating (low probability). Infection around loose cover screw or incomplete primary closure.

Solutions: Tighten cover screw if loose. If the implant is mobile, remove it. Substitute healing abutment for the cover screw to open tissue environment.

Problem: Slightly painful and mobile implant.

Possible Causes: Lack of integration.

Solutions: Remove the implant.

Problem: Slightly sensitive but perfectly immobile implant.

Possible Causes: Inadequate osseo-integration.

Solutions: Cover the implant for additional two to three months and test again.

Problem: Difficulty inserting a transfer screw, gold screw, or healing cap.

Possible Causes: Damaged inner thread of the abutment screw, or the inner thread of the implant is damaged.

Solutions: Change the abutment screw. Freshen the internal implant threads using repair tap from implant manufacturer. If the damage is beyond repair, the implant should be removed. Remove the implant with the appropriate diameter trephine, graft the site, and place a new implant at a later date.

Problem: Inability to perfectly connect the abutment to the implant.

Possible Causes: Crestal bone interfering with abutment seating.

Solutions: Inject local anesthesia, use a mill with guide, remove the bone, clean with saline solution, and replace the abutment.

Problem: Granulation tissue around the implant head.

Possible Causes: Traumatic placement of the implant, compression from the transitional prosthesis.

Solutions: Open the area and disinfect with chlorhexidine. If the lesion is too large, consider a bone regeneration or grafting technique.

Problem: Fracture of the overdenture implant during insertion in the osteotomy.

Possible Cause: Bone quality is type I, and the bone tap was not used before implant insertion. This problem is more common with implants less than 3.5mm in diameter.

Solutions: Always use the bone tap for type I bone. If the fracture piece cannot be removed from the bone, leave it in the bone and place a new implant in another site.

Problem: Failure of an implant that has been placed in the anterior mandible. At the time of surgery the implant had perfect primary stability and there was no obvious etiology for the failure.

Possible Cause: Pressure necrosis. This problem is more common with a tapered screw type implant that has been placed in type I bone without tapping the bone.

Solutions: Remove the failed implant, let the site heal for eight weeks, and make another attempt. Always tap type I bone before placing implant.

REFERENCES AND ADDITIONAL READING

Alloderm Universal Soft Tissue Graft Manual. Woodland, TX: LifeCell Corporation.

Anitua, E. (1999). Plasma rich in growth factors: preliminary results of use in the preparation of future sites for implants. *International Journal of Oral & Maxillofacial Implants*, 14, 529.

Anson, D. (1996). Calcium sulfate: a 4-year observation of its use as a resorbable barrier in guided tissue regeneration of periodontal defects. *Compendium of Continuing Education in Dentistry*, 17, 895.

Babbush, C. A. (1999). The use of platelet rich plasma with implant reconstructive procedures. Buenos Aires, Argentina, International College of Oral Implants; World Congress.

Babbush, C. A. (2000). The use of platelet rich plasma with implant reconstruction using SMARTPReP™ technology. New Delhi, India, Pre-Congress Seminar, 54th Commonwealth International Congress.

Babbush, C. A. (2000). The use of platelet rich plasma with implant reconstruction use of SMARTPReP™ technology, Atlanta, Pre-Congress Seminar, Annual Meeting of the Academy of Osseointegration.

Babbush, C. A. (1998). Porous hydroxyapatite and autograft. Report of the sinus consensus conference 1996. *International Journal of Oral & Maxillofacial Implants*,13, 33.

Bartee, B. K. (1995). The use of high-density polytetrafluoroethylene membrane to treat osseous defects: clinical reports. *Implant Dentistry*, 4(1), 21.

Becker, W., et al. (1996). A prospective multi-center study evaluating periodontal regeneration for class II furcation invasions and intrabony defects after treatment with a bioabsorbable barrier membrane: 1-year results. *Journal of Periodontology*, 67, 641.

Betts, N. J. & Miloro, M. (1994). Modification of the sinus lift procedure for septa in the maxillary antrum. *Journal of Oral & Maxillofacial Surgery*, 52, 332.

BioMend Absorbable Collagen Membrane Manual. Calcitek, Colla-Tec, Inc, 1995.

Block, M. & Kent J. N. (1997). Sinus augmentation for dental implants. The use of autogenous bone. *Journal of Oral & Maxillofacial Surgery*, 55, 1281.

Block, M. S., Kent, J. N. (1995). "Maxillary sinus bone grafting." In *Endosseous Implants for Maxillofacial Reconstruction*, ed. Block, M., Kent, J. N. Philadelphia: W.B. Saunders.

Blumenthal, N. & Steinberg J. (1990). The use of collagen membrane barriers in conjunction with combined demineralized bone-collagen gel implants in human infrabony defects. *Journal of Periodontology*, 61, 319.

Blumenthal, N. M. (1993). A clinical comparison of collagen membranes with e-PTFE membranes in the treatment of human mandibular buccal class II furcation defects, *Journal of Periodontology*, 64, 925.

Boyne, P. J. & James R. A. (1980). Grafting of the maxillary sinus floor with autogenous marrow and bone. *Journal of Oral Surgery*, 38, 613.

Caffesse, R. G. & Quinones, C. R. (1992). Guided tissue regeneration: biologic rationale, surgical technique, and clinical results, *Compendium of Continuing Education in Dentistry*, 13(3), 166.

Caton, J. & Greenstein, G. (1993). Factors related to periodontal regeneration, *Periodontology 2000*, 1, 9.

Chanavaz, M. (1996). Sinus grafting related to implantology. Statistical analysis of 15 years of surgical experience (1979–1994). *Journal of Oral Implantology*, 22, 119.

Connolly, J. F., et al. (1987). Clinical and experimental studies of bone marrow infection to promote osteogenesis. Helsinki, Meeting of International Society of Fracture Repair.

Connolly, J. F., et al. (1989). Development of an osteogenic bone marrow preparation. *Journal of Bone and Joint Surgery—American Volume*, 71(5), 684.

Degenshoin, G., Hurwitz, A., & Ribaceff, S. (1963). Experience with regenerative oxidized cellulose. *NY State Journal of Medicine*, 63, 18.

Fleisher, N., Waal, H. D., & Bloom, A. (1988). Regeneration of lost attachment apparatus in the dog using Viryl® absorbable mesh (polyglactin 910), *International Journal of Periodontics & Restorative Dentistry*, 8, 45.

Fritz, M. E., Eke, P. L., Malmquist, J., & Hardwick, R. (1996). Clinical and microbiological observations of early polytetrafluoroethylene membrane exposure in guided bone regeneration. Case reports in primates. *Journal of Periodontology*, 67, 245.

Galgut, P. (1990). Oxidized cellulose mesh used as a biodegradable barrier membrane in the technique of guided tissue regeneration. A case report. *Journal of Periodontology*, 61, 766.

Garey, D. J., Whittaker, J. M., James, R. A., Lozada, J. L. (1991). The histologic evaluation of the implant interface with heterograft and allograft materials—an eight month autopsy report, Part II. *Journal of Oral Implantology*, 17, 404.

Gore-Tex Regenerative Material Manual. Flagstaff, AZ: W. L. Gore, 1986.

Gottlow, J., et al. (1992). New attachment formation in the monkey using Guidor, a bioresorbable GTR-device (abstract 1535). *Journal of Dental Research*, 71, 298.

Gottlow, J., et al. (1993). Treatment of infrabony defects in monkeys with bioresorbable and nonresorbable GTR devices (abstract 823). *Journal of Dental Research*, 72, 206.

Gottlow, J., et al. (1992). Clinical results of CTR-therapy using a bioabsorbable device (Guidor) (abstract 1537). *Journal of Dental Research*, 71, 298.

Gottlow, J. (1993). Guided tissue regeneration using bioresorbable and nonresorbable devices: initial healing and long-term results. *Journal of Periodontology*, 64, 1157.

Greenstein, G. & Caton, J. (1993). Biodegradable barriers and guided tissue regeneration. *Periodontology 2000*, 1, 36.

Hardwick, R., Hayes, B. K., & Flynn, C. (1995). Devices for dentoalveolar regeneration: an up-to-date literature review. *Journal of Periodontology*, 66, 495.

Hirsch, J. M. & Ericsson, I. (1991). Maxillary sinus augmentation using mandibular bone grafts and simultaneous installation of implants: a surgical technique. *Clinical Oral Implants Research*, 2, 91.

Holmes, R., et al. (1984). A coralline hydroxyapatite bone graft substitute. *Clinical Orthopaedics & Related Research*, 188, 252.

Hugoson, A., et al. (1995). Treatment of Class II furcation involvements in humans with bioresorbable and nonresorbable guided tissue regeneration barriers. A randomized multi-center study. *Journal of Periodontology*, 66, 624.

Hyder, P. R., Dowell, P., & Dolby, A. E. (1992). Freeze-dried, cross-linked bovine type I collagen: analyses of properties. *Journal of Periodontology*, 63, 182.

Jensen, O. T., Perkins, S., Van de Water, F. (1992). Nasal fossa and maxillary sinus grafting of implants from a palatal approach. *Journal of Oral & Maxillofacial Surgery*, 50, 415.

Jensen, O. T. (1990). Allogeneic bone or hydroxylapatite for the sinus lift procedure? *Journal of Oral & Maxillofacial Surgery*, 48, 771.

Jortikka, L., et al. (1998). Use of myoblasts in assaying the osteoinductivity of bone morphogenetic proteins. *Life Sciences*, 62, 2359.

Karring, T., Nyman, S., Gottlow, J., & Laurell, L. (1993). Development of the biological concept of guided tissue regeneration—animal and human studies, *Periodontology 2000*, 1, 26.

Kent, J. N. & Block, M. S. (1989). Simultaneous maxillary sinus floor bone grafting and placement of hydroxylapatite-coated implants. *Journal of Oral & Maxillofacial Surgery*, 47–238.

Kirsch, A., Acherman, K., Hurzeler, M., & Hutmacher, D. "Sinus grafting using porous hydroxylapatite." In *The Sinus Bone Graft*, ed. Jensen, O. T. Chicago: Quintessence Publishing, 1998.

Lang, N. P. & Karring, T. (1994). Proceedings of the 1st European Workshop on Periodontology, London.

Langer, B. & Langer, L. "Use of allografts for sinus grafting." In *The Sinus Bone Graft*, ed. Jensen, O. T. Chicago: Quintessence Publishing, 1998.

Laurell, L., et al. (1994). Clinical use of a bioresorbable matrix barrier in guided tissue regeneration therapy. Case series. *Journal of Periodontology*, 65, 967.

Laurell, L., et al. (1993). Gingival response to GTR therapy in monkeys using two bioresorbable devices (abstract 824). *Journal of Dental Research*, 72, 206.

Laurell, L., et al. (1992). Ginigival response to Guidor, a bioresorbable device in GTR-therapy (abstract 1536). *Journal of Dental Research*, 71, 298.

Leder, A. J., McElroy, J., & Deasy, M. J. (1993). Reconstruction of the severely atrophic maxilla with autogenous iliac bone graft and hydroxylapatite/decalcified freeze-dried bone allograft in the same patient: a preliminary report. *Periodontal Clinical Investigations*, Fall, 5.

Lidhe, A., et al. (1993). Osteopromotion: a soft-tissue exclusion principle using a membrane for bone healing and bone neogenesis. *Journal of Periodontology*, 64, 1116.

LifeCore Biomedical Manual. Woodland, TX: Life-Cell Corporation, 1995.

Livesey, S., et al. (1994). An acellular dermal transplant processed from human cadaver skin retains normal extracellular components and ultrastructural characteristics. Presented at the American Association of Tissue Banks Conference in New Orleans.

Lundgren, D., et al. (1995). The influence of the design of two different bioresorbable barriers on the results of guided tissue regeneration therapy. An intra-individual comparative study in the monkey. *Journal of Periodontology*, 66, 605.

Magnusson, I., Batic, C., & Collins, B. R. (1988). New attachment formation following controlled tissue regeneration using biodegradable membranes. *Journal of Periodontology*, 9, 290.

Magnusson, I., Stenberg, W. V., Batich, C., & Egelberg, J. (1990). Connective tissue repair in circumferential periodontal defects in dogs following use of a biodegradable membrane. *Journal of Clinical Periodontology*, 17, 243.

Marx, R. E., Garg, A. K. Bone graft physiology with use of platelet-rich plasma and hyperbaric oxygen. In *The Sinus Bone Graft*, ed. Jensen, O. T. Chicago: Quintessence Publishing, 1999.

Maze, G. I., Hinkson, D. W., Collins, B. H., & Garbin, C. (1994). Bone regeneration capacity of a combination calcium sulfate-demineralized freeze-dried bone allograft. Presented at the AAP meeting.

Meffert, R. (1986). Guided tissue regeneration/guided bone regeneration. A review of the barrier membranes, *Practical Periodontics and Aesthetic Dentistry*, 8, 142.

Melcher, A. H. (1976). On the repair potential of periodontal tissues. *Journal of Periodontology*, 47(5), 256.

Mellonig, J. T. & Triplett, R. G. (1993). Guided tissue regeneration and endosseous dental implants. *International Journal of Periodontics & Restorative Dentistry*, 13(2), 108-19.

Mishkin, D., Shelly, L. Jr., & Neville, B. (1993). Histologic study of a freeze-dried skin allograft in a human. A case report. *Journal of Periodontology*, 54, 534.

Moss-Salentijin, L. "Anatomy and embryology." In *Surgery of the Paranasal Sinuses*, ed. Bletzer, A., Lawson, W., & Freedman, W. H. Philadelphia: W.B. Saunders, 1991.

Moy, P. K., Lundgren, S., & Holmes, R. E. (1993). Maxillary sinus augmentation: histomorphometric analysis of graft materials for maxillary sinus floor augmentation. *Journal of Oral & Maxillofacial Surgery*, 51, 857.

Nowzari, H. & Slots, J. (1994). Microogranisms in polytetrafluoroethylene barrier membranes for guided tissue regeneration. *Journal of Clinical Periodontology*, 21, 203.

Nyman, S., Lindhe, J., Karring, T., Rylander, H. (1982). New attachment following surgical treatment of human periodontal disease. *Journal of Clinical Periodontology*, 9, 290.

Payne, J., et al. (1996). Migration of human gingival fibroblasts over guided tissue regeneration barrier materials. *Journal of Periodontology*, 67, 236.

Piecuch, J. F., et al. (1983). Experimental ridge augmentation with porous hydroxylapatite implants. *Journal of Dental Research*, 62, 148.

Pitaru, S., et al. (1991). Heparan sulfate and fibronectin improve the capacity of collagen barriers to prevent apical migration of the junctional epithelium. *Journal of Periodontology*, 62(10), 598.

Pitaru, S., et al. (1988). Partial regeneration of periodontal tissues using collagen barriers. Initial observations in the canine. *Journal of Periodontology*, 59, 380.

Pitaru, S., Tal, H., Soldinger, M., & Noff, M. (1989). Collagen membranes prevent apical migration of epithelium and support new connective tissue attachment during periodontal wound healing in dogs. *Journal of Periodontal Research*, 24, 247.

Polson, A. M., et al. (1995). Initial study of guided tissue regeneration in Class II furcation after use of a biodegradable barrier, *International Journal of Periodontics & Restorative Dentistry*, 15, 43.

Polson, A. M., et al. (1995). Periodontal healing after guided tissue regeneration with Atrisorb barriers in beagle dogs. *International Journal of Periodontics & Restorative Dentistry*, 15(6), 575.

Polson, A. M., et al. (1995). Guided tissue regeneration in human furcation defects after using a biodegradable barrier: a multi-center feasibility study. *Journal of Periodontology*, 66, 377.

Ricci, G., Rasperini, G., Silvestri, M., & Cocconcelli, P. S. (1996). In vitro permeability evaluation and colonization of membranes for periodontal regeneration by *Porphomonas gingivalis*. *Journal of Periodontology*, 67, 490.

Roccuzzo, M., Lungo, M., Corrente, G., & Gondolfo, S. (1996). Comparative study of a bioresorbable and non-resorbable membrane in the treatment of human buccal gingival recessions. *Journal Periodontology*, 67(1), 7–14.

Rowe, D., Leung, W., & DeCarlo, D. (1996). Osteoclast inhibition by factors from cells associated with regenerative tissue. *Journal of Periodontology*, 67, 414.

Scantlebury, T. (1993). 1982–1992: A decade of technology development for guided tissue regeneration. *Journal of Periodontology*, 64, 1129.

Schenk, R., Buser, D., Hardwick, W., & Dahlin, C. (1994). Healing pattern of bone regeneration in membrane-protected defects. *International Journal of Oral & Maxillofacial Implants*, 9, 13.

Seitz, W. H., Froimson, A. L., & Leeb, R. B. (1992). Autogenous bone marrow and allograft replacement of bone defects in the hand and upper extremities. *Journal of Orthopaedic Trauma*, 6(1), 36.

Selvig, K. A., et al. (1990). Scanning electron microscopic observations of cell population and bacterial contamination of membranes used for guided periodontal tissue regeneration in humans. *Journal of Periodontology*, 61, 515.

Shigeyama, Y., et al. (1995). Commercially prepared allograft material has biological activity in vitro. *Journal of Periodontology*, 66, 478.

Shulamn, J. (1996). Clinical evaluation of an acellular dermal allograft for increasing the zone of attached gingiva. *Practical Periodontics and Aesthetic Dentistry*, 8, 201.

Sigurdsson, T., Hardwick, W., Bogle, G., & Wilkesjo, U. (1994). Periodontal repair in dogs: space provision by reinforced ePTFE membranes enhances bone and cementum regeneration in large supra-alveolar defects. *Journal of Periodontology*, 65, 350.

Simion, M., Scarano, A., Gionso, L., Piatelli, A. (1996). Guided bone regeneration using resorbable and nonresorable membranes: a comparative histologic study in humans. *International Journal of Oral & Maxillofacial Implants*, 11, 735.

Smiler, D. G., Holmes, R. E. (1987). Sinus lift procedure using porous hydroxylapatite: a preliminary clinical report. *Journal of Oral Implantology*, 13, 239.

Sottosanti, J. (1997). Calcium sulfate: a valuable addition to the implant/bone regeneration complex. *Dental Implantology Update*, 8, 25.

Sottosanti, J. (1995). Calcium sulfate-aided bone regeneration. A case report. *Periodontal Clinical Investigations*, 17, 10.

Stankiewicz JA. "Endoscopic nasal and sinus surgery." In *Surgery of the Paranasal Sinuses*, ed. Bletzer, A., Lawson, W., & Freedman, W. H. Philadelphia: W.B. Saunders, 1991.

Tatum, O. H. Jr. (1986). Maxillary and sinus implant reconstructions. *Dental Clinics of North America*, 30, 207.

Tayapongsak, P., et al. (1994). Autologous fibrin adhesive in mandibular reconstruction with particulate cancellous bone and marrow. *Journal of Oral & Maxillofacial Surgery*, 52, 161.

Tinti C. & Vicenzi, G. (1993). Expanded polytetrafluoroethylene titanium reinforced membranes for regeneration of mucogingival recession defects. A 12-case report. *Journal of Periodontology*, 64, 1157.

Triplett, R. G. & Schow, S. R. (1996). Autologous bone grafts and endosseous implants: complementary techniques. *Journal of Oral & Maxillofacial Surgery*, 54, 486.

Vuddhakanok, S., et al. (1993). Histologic evaluation of periodontal attachment apparatus following the insertion of a biodegradable copolymer barrier in humans. *Journal of Periodontology*, 64, 202.

Wang, H., et al. (1994). Adherence of oral microorganisms to guided tissue membranes. An in vitro study. *Journal of Periodontology*, 65, 211.

Warrer, K., Karring, T., Nyman, S., & Gogolewski, S. (1992). Guided tissue regeneration using biodegradable membranes of polyactic acid or polyurethane. *Journal of Clinical Periodontology*, 19, 633.

Watzek, G. *Endosseous Implants: Scientific and Clinical Aspects*. Chicago: Quintessence Publishing, 1996.

Wetzel, A. C., Stich, H., & Caffesse, R. G. (1995). Bone apposition onto oral implants in the sinus area filled with different grafting materials. *Clinical Oral Implants Research*, 6, 155.

Wheeler, S. L., Holmes, R. E., & Calhoun, C. J. (1996). Six year clinical and histologic study of sinus-lift grafts. *International Journal of Oral & Maxillofacial Implants*, (11)1, 26.

Wheeler, S. L. (1997). Sinus augmentation for dental implants: the use of alloplast material. *Journal of Oral & Maxillofacial Surgery*, 55, 1287.

Whittaker, J. M., James, R. A., Lozada, J., Cordova, C., Garey, D. J. (1989). Histological response and clinical evaluation of heterograft and allograft materials in the evaluation of the maxillary sinus for the preparation of endosteal dental implant sites. Simultaneous sinus elevation and root form implantation: an eight-month autopsy report. *Journal of Oral Implantology*, 15, 141.

Wood, R. M. & Moore, D. L. (1988). Grafting of the maxillary sinus with intraorally harvested autogenous bone prior to implant placement. *International Journal of Oral & Maxillofacial Implants*, 3, 209.

Yukna, C. N. & Yukna, R. A. (1996). Multi-center evaluation of bioabsorbable collagen membrane for guided tissue regeneration in human Class II furcations. *Journal of Periodontology*, 67, 650.

Yumet, J. A. & Polson, A. M. (1985). Gingival wound healing in the presence of plaque-induced inflammation. *Journal of Periodontology*, 56, 107.

Zhang, M., et al. (1997). A quantitative assessment of osteoinductivity of human demineralized bone matrix. *Journal of Periodontology*, 68, 1076.

Zinner, I. D. & Small, S. A. (1996). Sinus-lift graft: Using the maxillary sinuses to support implants. *Journal of the American Dental Association*, 127, 51.

11
Straumann Implant System

Hamid Shafie

The Straumann® Dental Implant System has been on the market since 1974. Straumann pioneered the single-stage surgical procedure with implants ideally designed for non-submerged placement. With the evolution of Straumann's product range, the portfolio now consists of implants that are suitable for a non-submerged, semi-submerged, or fully submerged technique, or for immediate placement or immediate loading procedures. Standard implants are designed for non-submerged placement, while Standard Plus implants are optimal for esthetically demanding areas. The specially designed Tapered Effect implants are ideal for placement in immediate extraction sites. All Straumann implants are made of commercially pure titanium (grade 4-ISO 5832/II).

Standard implants (i.e. Straumann implants with a 2.8mm smooth collar height) are recommended for overdenture cases.

TWO SECTIONS OF STRAUMANN IMPLANTS

Rough Surface on the Implant Body

This portion should be completely embedded in the bone.

Polished Collar

This portion is a transgingival part on the implant that provides ultimate gingival health. The height of the smooth neck section of Straumann Standard implants is 2.8mm. Standard Plus and Tapered Effect implants have a shorter polished collar height of 1.8mm for aesthetic zone crown and bridge cases. Because overdenture cases do not require a submerged surgical placement, Standard implants are recommended for this indication (Figure 11.1).

Originally, the rough portion of the implant had TPS (Titanium Plasma Spray) surface

153

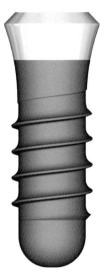

FIGURE 11.1.

characteristics to increase the surface area and enhance osseointegration. Based on the success of their TPS surface, Straumann developed an improved surface called SLA® (Sandblasted, Large grit, Acid-Etched). Both the TPS and SLA® surfaces consist chemically of titanium oxide. However, the SLA® surface does not have the semi-porous structure of the TPS surface. Also, it is not a coating but rather a surface treatment (Figure 11.2).

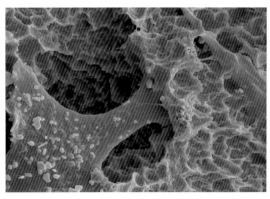

FIGURE 11.2.

The SLA® surface is produced by a coarse sandblasting process that leads to macro rough-

ness on the titanium and achieves outstanding bone fixation as a result. After this process, etching in acid produces micro-pits that can be seen on SEM images and promote cell activity on the surface.

The SLA® surface provides greater bone-to-implant contact, confirmed by high release moments that allow earlier functional loading. In healthy patients with good bone quality and quantity, this patented and proven surface allows the possibility of placing the attachment assembly and the overdenture only six weeks after the implant surgery.

ENDOSSEOUS DIAMETERS

Straumann implants are available in three different endosseous diameters in varying lengths. For implant-supported overdenture cases, the following implants are recommended:

- Standard implant, Ø 3.3mm, RN (Regular Neck)
  SLA length: 8, 10, 12, 14, 16mm (Figure 11.3)

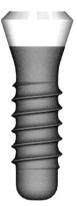

FIGURE 11.3.

- Standard implant, Ø 4.1mm, RN (Regular Neck)
  SLA length: 6, 8, 10, 12, 14, 16mm (Figure 11.4)

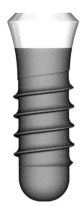

FIGURE 11.4.

- Standard implant, Ø 4.8mm, RN (Regular Neck)
  SLA length: 6, 8, 10, 12, 14mm (Figure 11.5)

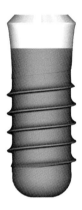

FIGURE 11.5.

RECOMMENDED ATTACHMENT ASSEMBLIES FOR STRAUMANN IMPLANTS

- Standard implant, Ø 3.3mm, RN (Regular Neck):
  – Single bar or multiple bar assemblies
- Standard implant, Ø 4.1mm, RN (Regular Neck):
  – Single bar or multiple bar assemblies
  – Retentive anchor abutment
- Standard implant, Ø 4.8mm, RN (Regular Neck):
  – Single bar or multiple bar assemblies
  – Retentive anchor abutment

SURGICAL STEPS FOR STANDARD IMPLANTS Ø 4.1MM RN (REGULAR NECK)

1: Preparation of the Implant Bed

After raising the flap, evaluate the width of the ridge. Typically, a bony wall of approximately 1.0mm is recommended both on the facial and lingual. To determine the minimum ridge width needed, add 2.0mm to the core diameter of the implant being used (Table 11.1).

TABLE 11.1. Minimum Ridge Width Requirements

Implant type	Core diameter	Minimum ridge width required
Ø 3.3 mm, RN	2.8 mm	≥ 4.8 mm
Ø 4.1 mm, RN	3.5 mm	≥ 5.5 mm
Ø 4.8 mm, RN	4.2 mm	≥ 6.2 mm

If the crest of the ridge is narrow, use a large round bur (Ø 3.1mm) and flatten the ridge as necessary. After preparing the ridge, mark the implantation site with a small round bur (Ø 1.4mm) and make the mark wider by using a medium round bur (Ø 2.3mm). *Slight pressure should be used with sufficient irrigation during the entire drilling sequence* (Figure 11.6).

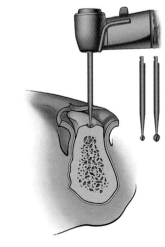

FIGURE 11.6.

2: Drilling Sequence for Standard Implants Ø 4.1mm RN (Regular Neck)

Start with a Ø 2.2mm pilot drill and initiate drilling to a depth of 6.0mm. Remove the pilot drill and insert the Ø 2.2mm alignment pin to verify the trajectory of the osteotomy. At this stage, an unsatisfactory implant axis can still be corrected. Continue drilling with the Ø 2.2mm pilot drill to the same depth as the selected implant.

Next, a Ø 2.8mm pilot drill is used to widen the osteotomy to the appropriate depth. Check the depth with a Ø 2.2/2.8mm depth gauge.

Then use a Ø 3.5mm twist drill to widen the osteotomy to the appropriate depth. The depth should be verified with a Ø 3.5mm depth gauge (Figure 11.7).

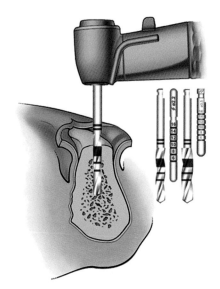

FIGURE 11.7.

3: Tapping the Implant Site

Use a Ø 4.1mm tap to cut the screw threads in the osteotomy. The thread can be cut manually or mechanically.

- *Manual Tapping:* Fit the top handle of the tap into the ratchet and then place the holding key over the tap handle. Cut the threads with

the entire length of the tap with slow rotation. During the process, the holding key acts as a stabilizer to maintain the direction of cutting (Figure 11.8).

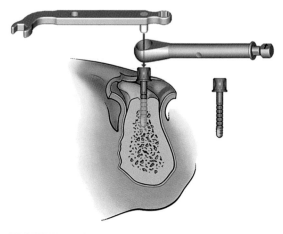

FIGURE 11.8.

- *Mechanical Tapping:* Insert the hand piece adapter over the mechanical tap *and* use a slow speed, 15rpm, to tap the osteotomy (Figure 11.9).

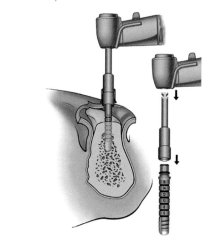

FIGURE 11.9.

4: Implant Insertion

The implant can be placed either manually or mechanically. The sequence of insertion is identical with both approaches. The only difference is that for manual insertion the ratchet and corresponding adapters and tools must be used, but for mechanical insertion the hand-piece and corresponding adapters must be used at 15rpm (Figure 11.10).

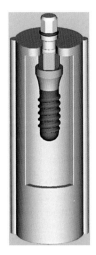

FIGURE 11.10.

1. Grasp the implant holder without touching the implant. Attach the adapter to the pre-mounted transfer part and ensure that it clicks into place (Figures 11.11 and 11.12).

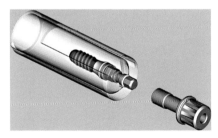

FIGURE 11.11.

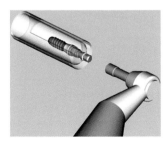

FIGURE 11.12.

2. To remove the implant from the holder, gently turn and pull the holder downward. Gently turn and lift the implant upwards at the same time (Figures 11.13 and 11.14).

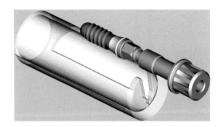

FIGURE 11.13.

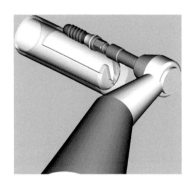

FIGURE 11.14.

3. Place the implant into the osteotomy using either a ratchet adapter or hand piece and adapter (Figures 11.15 and 11.16).

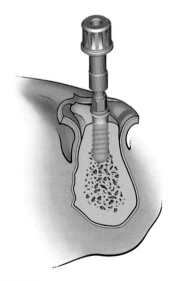

FIGURE 11.15.

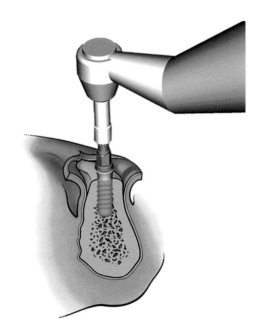

FIGURE 11.16.

For manual insertion execute following steps:
- Place the ratchet over the adapter (make sure that the arrow is pointing in the direction of insertion, clockwise). Use the holding key for stabilization while ratcheting the implant into its final position using slow movements (Figure 11.17).

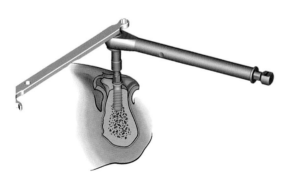

FIGURE 11.17.

- Remove the holding key and reverse the direction of the ratchet (pull arrow out and flip it over) (Figure 11.18).

For mechanical insertion execute following steps:
- After placing the implant into the osteotomy using a hand-piece and cor-

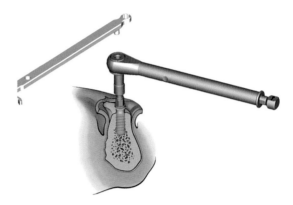

FIGURE 11.18.

responding adapter, insert the implant (clockwise) into its final position using a maximum speed of 15rpm. Stop when the bottom of the osteotomy has been reached. At this point, there will be some resistance (Figure 11.19).

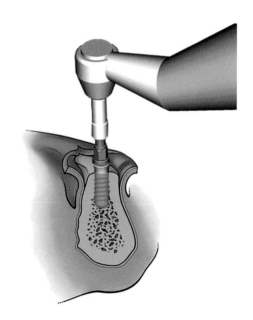

FIGURE 11.19.

4. Remove the transfer part.
Manual:
- Engage the hexagon of the transfer part with the holding key and then turn the ratchet counterclockwise (Figure 11.20).

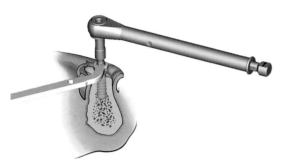

FIGURE 11.20.

- Remove the holding key. Hold the bottom of the adapter and remove the ratchet (Figure 11.21).

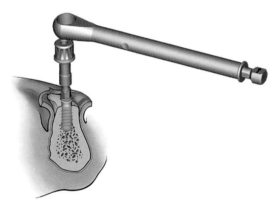

FIGURE 11.21.

- Completely remove the transfer part from the implant using the adapter for ratchet (Figure 11.22).

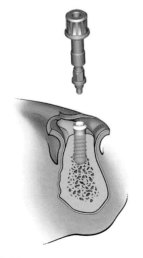

FIGURE 11.22.

Mechanical:
- Engage the hexagon of the transfer part with the holding key. Before removing the transfer part, set the surgical motor on reverse and unscrew the transfer part (Figure 11.23).

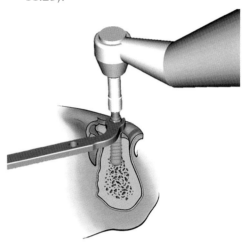

FIGURE 11.23.

- Remove the holding key and remove the transfer part completely from the implant (Figure 11.24).

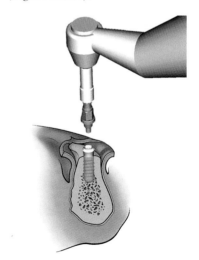

FIGURE 11.24.

WOUND CLOSURE

Adapt the gingiva around the smooth collar of the implant, and if necessary, perform a minor gingivectomy to idealize the soft tissue adaptation around the implant's neck. A non-resorbable suture material, such as polyamide or Teflon, is recommended.

HEALING PERIOD FOR STRAUMANN IMPLANTS WITH SLA SURFACE

In healthy patients with good bone density and adequate bone quality, the SLA surface makes it possible for the implant to be loaded after only six weeks. However, if bone augmentation techniques are used or the patient has poor bone quality, the healing time is at least 12 to 14 weeks. There is no fundamental difference between implants in the maxilla or the mandible. In implant-supported overdenture cases in which the attachment assembly design requires the supporting implants to be splinted rigidly, Straumann implants can be loaded immediately.

12
Endopore® Dental Implant System

Hamid Shafie

BASIC FACTS

The Endopore® dental implant was designed at the University of Toronto by Drs. Deporter, Watson, and Pilliar and was first used in humans in 1989. This implant has a five-degree truncated shape and is made of a high-strength Ti6Al4V alloy cone with a multi-layer porous surface over most of its length. The porous surface is achieved by sintering spherical particles, which create the possibility of three-dimensional bone ingrowths (Figure 12.1–12.3).

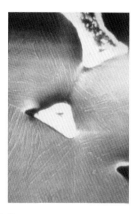

FIGURE 12.2.

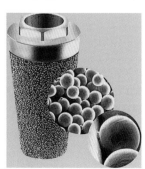

FIGURE 12.1.

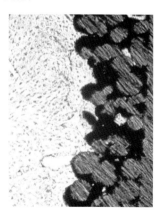

FIGURE 12.3.

The Endopore® dental implant is available in two different implant abutment connection forms.

External Connection

(Refer to Figure 12.4)

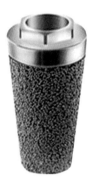

FIGURE 12.4.

- 1mm polished collar
- 2mm polished collar

A polished collar between the prosthetic platform and porous surface ensures the health of the gingiva. The Endopore® dental implant with a 2mm polished collar is the preferred choice.

Internal Connection

(Refer to Figure 12.5)

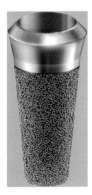

FIGURE 12.5.

- 1.8mm transgingival collar
- 2.8mm transgingival collar

Bone is directly opposed to and extends in between the sintered particles on the surface of the implant. The Endopore® dental implant engages with the alveolar crest by cortical bone growth into its porous surface. During function, the occlusal forces are transferred to the crestal bone area, and this eventually stimulates further cortical bone development.

Because the porous design greatly increases the surface area at the interface between the bone and the implant, a shorter implant can be used. A shorter implant helps the patient and clinician avoid some expensive bone augmentation procedures such as sinus lifts.

MECHANICAL RATIONAL FOR SHORT ENDOPORE® DENTAL IMPLANTS

The resulting mechanical interlocking of bone and implant at the interface provides a very effective means of force transfer between the implant and the peri-implant tissues, including the ability to effectively transfer the tensile forces. Both the axial and transverse force components (tensile, shear, and compressive) acting on the implant are effectively resisted, resulting in a more uniform distribution of mechanical stresses in the peri-implant bone. As a result, peak stresses next to the most coronal portion of the porous-surfaced implant are significantly lower than the stresses that would occur with a threaded implant, because the forces are distributed more uniformly with a porous implant.

The porous-surfaced implants possess a unique ability to effectively resist the tensile forces acting at the implant-bone interface, resulting in a more favorable response.

Advantages of the Endopore® Dental Implant System

- Three dimensional interlocking of the bone with the implant surface
- Predictable and minimal crestal bone remodeling

- Eliminates the need for bone grafting in the patient with compromised bone height
- Tapered design and press-fit insertion technique is ideal for patients with a split ridges technique treatment planned
- Uncomplicated surgical sequence; only two drills are used to prepare the implant bed
- Expanded overdenture attachment options

Surgical Steps

1. Based on the design of the surgical guide, you should start the drilling process before or after raising the flap. If the surgical guide has been made based on the impression of the residual ridge and sits over the gum, you have to start the drilling process before raising the flap; otherwise, after raising the flap you will not be able to insert the surgical guide in a stable manner. With this type of surgical guide, insert the guide in the patient's mouth, mark the location of each implant by using a 2mm pilot, and drill through the gum and supporting bone. The drill speed should be set at 1000rpm with constant irrigation. If the surgical guide has been made based on CT-scan data and fits over the underlying bone, you should raise the flap first to make sure the guide fits perfectly over the underlying bone and then start the drilling process.

2. Raise a full thickness flap. Refer to the section, "Incisions and Flap Design," in Chapter 10.

3. Identify the drilling marks from Step 1. Use the 2mm pilot again and drill until reaching the appropriate depth. The drill speed should be set at 1000rpm with constant irrigation. If the initial marks are not deep enough, they will not provide a good guide for the trajectory and parallelism of the supporting implants. In this case, either use the guide pins as a reference when drilling the osteotomy with the pilot bur to make sure all of them are parallel, or use a paralleling device to achieve ideal parallelism (Figures 12.6–12.8).

4. After preparing the implant beds with the pilot drill, choose a corresponding final taper implant bur that matches the length and diameter of the designated implant, and final-

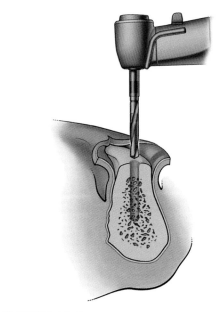

FIGURE 12.6.

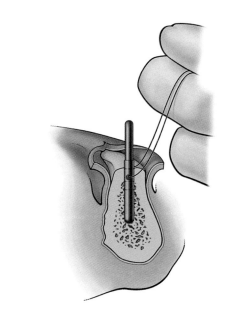

FIGURE 12.7.

ize the shape of the osteotomy to receive that particular implant. The drill speed should be set at 1000rpm with constant irrigation. For overdenture cases, never countersink the implant bed. The entire porous surface should be in the bone and the polished collar should stay above the crestal bone. If a 5.00mm

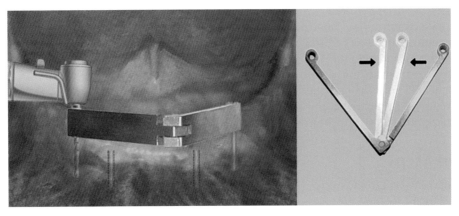

FIGURE 12.8.

diameter implant is being used, it is recommended to expand the osteotomy gradually by using an intermediate 4.1mm implant bur of the same length. Then finish the
site preparation by using the corresponding
length 5.00mm diameter implant bur (Figure 12.9).

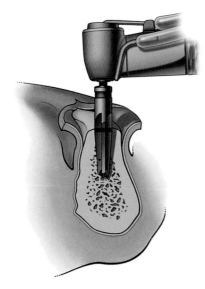

FIGURE 12.9.

Exception: If placing the implant in type IV
bone (such as the posterior maxilla), after
completion of Step 3, either use osteotome to
prepare the osteotomy instead of using corresponding implant bur with the designated
implant, or use a one-size-smaller diameter
implant bur with the same length to pre-

pare the osteotomy. These two techniques
will minimize the chance of unwanted widening of the osteotomy as well as ensuring a
good primary stability.

Note: Sharp burs are critical to avoid overheating of the bone and unwanted widening
of the osteotomy. Changing the implant burs
after approximately 10 to 15 uses is recommended, depending on bone density.

5. Generously irrigate the osteotomy with sterile saline solution to remove any bone chips
   or residue following preparation. Before implant placement, check the site by inserting
   the appropriately sized trial fit gage into the
   prepared site. Trial fit gauges have the same
   shape and dimensions as the corresponding
   implants. After insertion of the trial fit gage
   into the osteotomy, the shoulder of the cone-
   shaped portion of the gauge should be flush
   or just below the crest of the bone (Figure 12.10).

Note: Surgical gauze fibers can contaminate
the surface of the implant or osteotomy site
and increase the risk of implant failure; therefore, gauze should not be used near the surgical site or on the instruments used in site
preparation.

6. The height and width of the bone dictate the implant length and diameter. The
   thickness of the gingival tissue dictates the
   height of the polished collar. Implants with
   a 2mm polished collar are recommended for

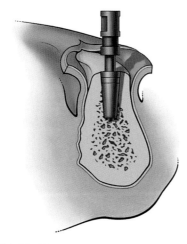

FIGURE 12.10.

overdenture cases. Remove the Endopore® dental implant from its sterile package and transfer it to the osteotomy by holding the plastic delivery handle. Press the implant with manual pressure into the osteotomy until it will not go any further down into the os-teotomy, and then remove the plastic handle and discard it.

Note: With this implant system, the cover screw is pre-inserted over the implant, and a white plastic delivery handle is attached to it (Figure 12.11).

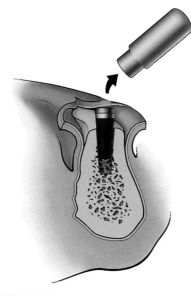

FIGURE 12.11.

Percussion: Avoid contact of the porous sur-face of the implant with anything prior to in-sertion of the implant into the osteotomy. If contact should occur, do not use that implant and open another one.

7. Drive the implant into its final position by using a mallet and one of the insertion handles. The surgical kit contains two inser-tion handles—straight and offset. Based on the location of the implant, choose the han-dle that provides the best access for tapping the implant. Apply several firm taps to se-cure and stabilize the implant in the bone. At the end, the entire porous surface should be embedded in the bone and the polished col-lar should stay above the crest of the bone. The implant should be completely immobile at this point (Figure 12.12).

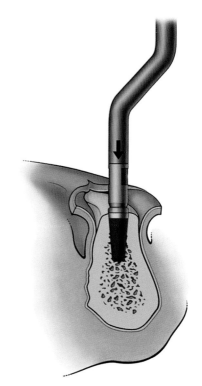

FIGURE 12.12.

8. Use a 0.050 inch hex driver to check the tight-ness of the cover screw and the stability of the implant. Tighten the cover screw if it is loose.

After the cover screw is completely tight, a stable and secure implant should resist any further torque movement (Figure 12.13).

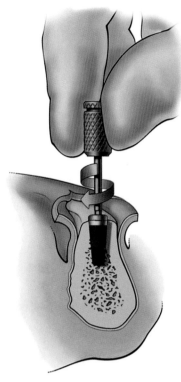

FIGURE 12.13.

9. Close the flap and suture the gum with the appropriate suturing technique (Figure 12.14). Refer to the section, "Suturing Techniques Used for Implant Overdenture Surgeries," in Chapter 10.

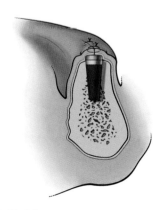

FIGURE 12.14.

Postsurgical Instructions

1. Preferably the transitional denture should not be worn for first week after the implant placement. However, if the patient cannot be without a transitional denture, relieve the inside of the transitional denture with an E-cutter bur (everyday cutting carbide bur) and reline the inside of the transitional denture with tissue conditioner (CO-Comfort GC) (Figure 12.15).

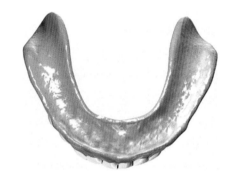

FIGURE 12.15.

The tissue conditioner will keep its properties for seven days. When the patient returns for the one-week post-surgery follow-up, remove the one-week-old tissue conditioner and reline the transitional denture with fresh tissue conditioner. Fourteen days after the implant surgery, replace the tissue conditioner with a soft liner. Soft liners can keep their resiliency for 30 to 60 days depending on the brand.

2. Instruct the patient to rinse with 2 percent chlorhexidine mouthwash twice a day.
3. Remove the sutures 7 to 10 days after implant surgery.
4. Instruct the patient to maintain an appropriate diet. Generally a soft diet is recommended for the first seven days. After that, the patient can gradually add more variety to his/her diet.
5. The patient should wait three months after implant surgery for mandibular implants and

six months for maxillary implant before un-covering.

Implant Uncovering Steps

1. Take panoramic or peri-apical x-rays of the implants before uncovering.
2. Use a sterile tissue punch that corresponds to the diameter of the implant and expose the cover screw. If the tissue punch is not available, a small crestal incision is a good way to expose the cover screw.
3. Remove the cover screw by using a 0.05 inch hex driver.
4. Based on the thickness of the gingival, choose a healing abutment that is 2mm taller than the thickness of the gum. Use the same 0.05 inch hex driver to screw the healing abutment over the implant.
5. Mark the location of healing abutments inside the transitional denture and use an E-cutter bur to relieve inside the denture. When the denture is seated on the ridge, there should be no contact between the healing abutments and the denture base.
6. Reline the transitional denture with tissue conditioner over the healing abutments.

Prosthetic Steps

1. If the attachment assembly design required laboratory work, 4 to 6 weeks after uncover-ing, make a pick-up impression. Otherwise, start the prosthetic phase from Step 2.
2. If the overdenture design requires a prefabri-cated stud attachment, choose an attachment with the proper transmucosal cuff height based on the gingival thickness. Otherwise, try the laboratory made attachment assembly for precision of fit by utilizing the Sheffield Test. (Refer to Chapter 7.)
3. Register the jaw relationship in the CR posi-tion, as well as the proper vertical dimension.
4. Choose proper anterior denture teeth. Se-lect posterior denture teeth that are designed for lingualized occlusion or modified regular posterior denture teeth to accommodate a lin-gualized occlusion.
5. Incorporate the attachment assembly into the denture base either by the chair-side tech-nique or the laboratory process. (Refer to the instructions that apply to the specific attach-ment being used.)
6. Check the occlusion and perform any neces-sary selective grinding to achieve a bilateral lingualized occlusion.

13
Overdenture Implants

Hamid Shafie

In recent years, a new generation of dental implants called overdenture implants have been introduced to the field of implantology. These mini implants have been designed specifically to support an implant overdenture. One of the pioneers of this concept is Dr. Victor Sendex, who conducted more than twenty years of study and documentation on Mini Dental Implants concept and design. Currently, there are several different types of these implants available on the market. The main design difference between these type of implants and traditional implants is that a part of the stud attachment, either male or female (depending on the manufacturer), has been combined with the implant body. In traditional restorative implants, the stud attachment should be screwed into the implant body as a separate component.

CLASSIFICATION OF OVERDENTURE IMPLANTS BASED ON ATTACHMENT DESIGN FEATURES

- *Implants with Male Attachment*: Maximus OS™ (Biohorizons) is a parallel sided implant and the male part of the stud attachment is part of the implant body. MDI® Implant (Imtec) is tapered.
- *Implants with Female Attachment*: ERA® implant (Sterngold) is a tapered implant and the female part of the stud attachment is part of the implant body.

These types of implants make the implant overdenture treatment more cost effective and simpler. They are narrower than most narrow-diameter traditional implants, so they can be used in cases with a deficiency in the width of the bone, avoiding a horizontal bone augmentation procedure.

TWO BASIC PURPOSES FOR OVERDENTURE IMPLANTS

Providing Immediate Stabilization for an Overdenture

Although the FDA has never approved a dental implant under 3.0mm in diameter for permanent use, overdenture implants are often used as a less expensive and simpler alternative to traditional implants for stabilizing an overdenture over a longer period of time. This technique may give the patient time to deal with the financial realities of implant dentistry or it may be a less traumatic way for the patient to get used to the idea of dental implants. In this application, it is strongly recommended to utilize advanced surface characteristics such as acid-etched or resorbable blast texturing (RBT) to enhance the implant-bone interface, as well as to expedite the osseointegration process. Placement of these implants should be limited to the anterior mandible between the two mental foramens. In fact, the greatest need for affordable implant overdentures is from patients who are unhappy with their complete lower dentures.

Acting as Transitional Implants during Initial Healing Phase

The small size of implant overdentures allows them to be placed between traditional implants, and they often fit best if placed slightly lingual to the traditional implants. If bone augmentation is part of the treatment plan, the overdenture implants provide a positive vertical stop and lateral stability to limit the force applied to the augmented area. This procedure greatly improves the success of new bone growth and limits the excess force applied to the traditional implants.

After completion of the healing period for traditional implants, the overdenture implants should be unscrewed once they have served their transitional purpose. The small bony defect usually heals with no further treatment. With this treatment scenario, it is strongly recommended to use a machined surface characteristic instead of advanced surfaces such as acid-etched or RBT, because these surfaces enhance the implant-bone interface and cause implant removal to be more difficult compared to when a machined surface is used.

The surgical procedure for overdenture implants is often composed of only a few simple steps. Many general dentists who might not perform traditional implant surgery have found placement of overdenture implants a quick, simple, and predictable procedure. Obviously, it is critical to identify important anatomical landmarks, such as the mental foramen, the mandibular nerve canal, the inferior border of the mandible, the floor of the nasal cavity, and the maxillary sinuses during treatment planning and the surgical procedure.

MAXIMUS OS OVERDENTURE IMPLANT

The Maximus OS overdenture implant is a 3.0mm diameter implant made of titanium alloy. A 2.5mm ball attachment has been added to the implant body. This implant is available with two different gingival cuff heights of 2.0mm and 4.0mm, and three different lengths of 12.0mm,

15.0mm, and 18.0mm (Figures 13.1 and 13.2).

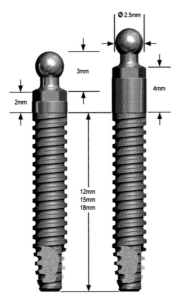

FIGURE 13.1.

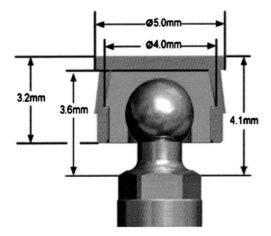

FIGURE 13.2.

Unique Features

- *Square Tread Pattern*: This tread pattern provides better force distribution and stability compared to traditional V-shaped treads.
- *RBT (Resorbable Blast Texturing) Surface Characteristic*: The surface of this implant has been blasted with an apatitic blast medium such as (tri-calcium phosphate) to create a surface roughness, and then the surface has been cleaned and passivated with acid solution.
- *Interchangeable Female Components Included with Implant Package*: The female component is available in four different retention levels from softest to firmest: Green—extra soft retention, Yellow—soft retention, Pink—medium retention, White—firm retention (Figure 13.3).
- *Parallel Body with Tapered Apical Portion*: Having a parallel body provides more surface area compared to a tapered implant with a similar length and diameter. However, its apical portion is tapered, which enhances penetration in the bone and faster stabilization.

Clinical Considerations

- Always start with the least retentive female attachment during the initial healing phase. After eight weeks, it is possible to switch to more retentive female attachments, which will minimize the chance of jeopardizing the initial stability of supporting implants. However, if the implants have been placed in D3 type bone such as a maxillary overdenture case or if the implants' primary stability is not optimum, avoid utilizing the female attachments on the day of implant placement. Instead, mark the location of the implant heads inside the denture and relieve the acrylic base in those areas. Then reline the inside of the denture with tissue conditioner for the first two weeks, replace the tissue conditioner with soft liner starting on week three, and keep the soft liner until end of week eight. Utilize the female attachments eight weeks after implant placement.
- Maximus OS implants should always be utilized with a well-fitting denture and accurate occlusion.
- Avoid utilizing the Maximus OS as a transitional implant, because its RBT surface characteristics will cause an expansive implant bone interface, which makes it very difficult to unscrew this implant without leaving a big

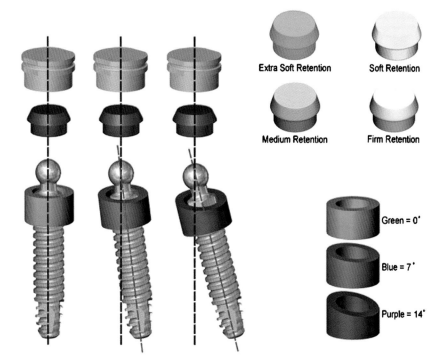

Extra Soft Retention   Soft Retention

Medium Retention   Firm Retention

Green = 0°

Blue = 7°

Purple = 14°

FIGURE 13.3.

bony defect and risking implant fracture during the unscrewing process.

- A minimum of four Maximus OS implants should be used for lower implant overdenture if the bone quality is ideal. With poor bone quality, five or six implants are recommended.
- All of the Maximus OS implants should be placed perfectly parallel to each other. Utilization of a paralleling device or an accurate surgical guide is strongly recommended. The maximum correctable discrepancy in the trajectory of each implant from the sagittal plane is 14 degrees. In this situation, a proper directional ring should be used to offset this discrepancy. There are three directional rings available with Maximus OS: 0, 7, and 14 degrees.
- The implants should be placed at least 6mm apart from center to center. However, to simplify the implant spacing, the distance between the two mental foramens can be divided into five equal columns. Then, when placing five implants, one implant can be

placed in the center of each column. When placing four implants, skip the middle column and place one implant on each side column (Figure 13.4).

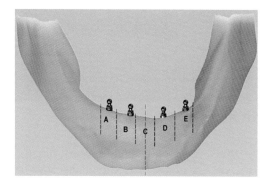

FIGURE 13.4.

Surgical Steps

1: GAINING ACCESS TO THE ALVEOLAR BONE

- *Performing a Flap Technique*: This approach provides great access and maximizes visualization of the shape and contour of the alveolar bone (Figures 13.5 and 13.6).

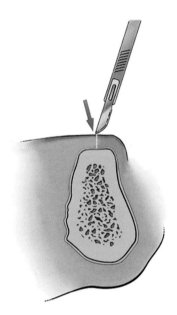

FIGURE 13.5.

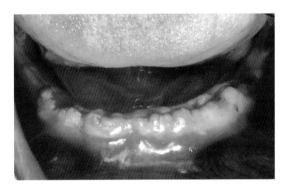

FIGURE 13.6.

When performing a flap surgery, based on the design of the surgical guide, start the drilling process before or after raising the flap. If the surgical guide has been made based on the impression of the residual ridge and sits over the gum, start the drilling process before raising the flap. Otherwise, after raising the flap, it will not be possible to insert the surgical guide in a stable manner. With this type of surgical guide, insert the guide in the

patient's mouth, mark the location of each implant by using a 2mm starter drill, and drill through the gum and alveolar bone. The drill speed should be set at 1,000rpm with constant irrigation. If the surgical guide has been made based on CT-scan data and fits over the alveolar bone, raise the flap first to make sure the guide fits perfectly over the alveolar bone, and then start the drilling process.

- *Performing a No-Flap Technique*: This approach minimizes post-operation symptoms and complications, and there is no need for suturing.

To perform a no-flap surgery, mark the location of the implants on the gum and then use the tissue punch to core-cut the gum and gain access to the alveolar bone (Figure 13.7).

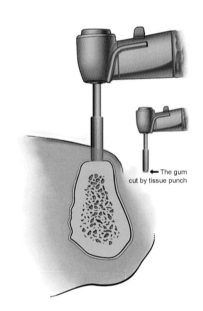

← The gum cut by tissue punch

FIGURE 13.7.

2: ALIGNING THE TRAJECTORY OF THE IMPLANT

- *Using the Alignment Drill and Guide Pins*: Use the alignment drill to initiate the first osteotomy to a depth of 5mm. After preparation of the first osteotomy, place a guide pin in that spot and start drilling the next site with a 2mm depth drill to the proper depth and exactly parallel to the guide pin. Then remove the guide pin from the first osteotomy site and place it in the second osteotomy site, and use the 2mm depth drill to drill to the proper depth. Make sure that the trajectory of the depth drill stays parallel with the guide pin. Continue preparation of the other osteotomies with the depth drill for all the implant sites (Figures 13.8–13.18).

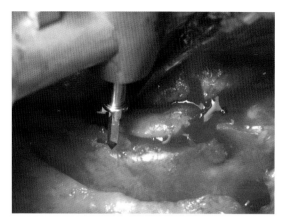

FIGURE 13.10.

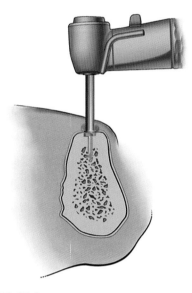

FIGURE 13.8.

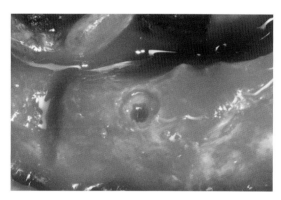

FIGURE 13.11.

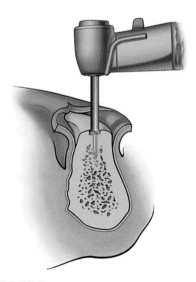

FIGURE 13.9.

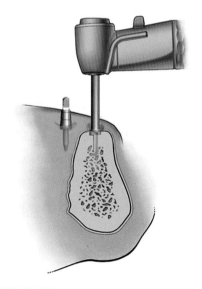

FIGURE 13.12.

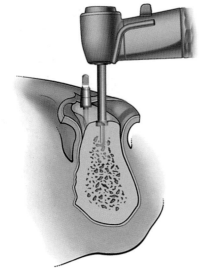

FIGURE 13.13.

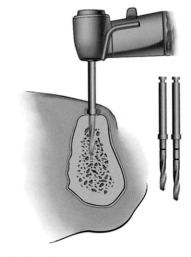

FIGURE 13.16.

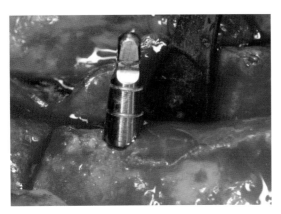

FIGURE 13.14.

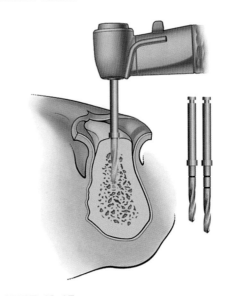

FIGURE 13.17.

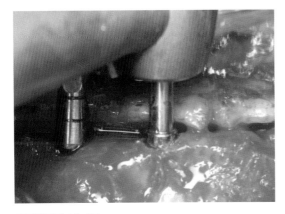

FIGURE 13.15.

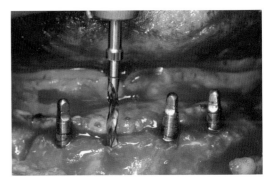

FIGURE 13.18.

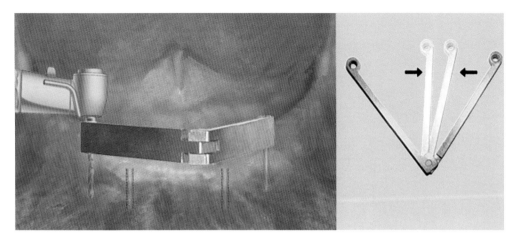

FIGURE 13.19.

- *Using Paralleling Device*: Prepare the first osteotomy with the alignment drill, and then insert the anchor pin of the paralleling device into that hole and use the 2mm depth drill to prepare the rest of the osteotomoies at the appropriate depth. Remove the anchor pin of the paralleling device from the first osteotomy site and insert it in another osteotomy, and then use the 2mm-depth drill to drill the first osteotomy site to the proper depth (Figure 13.19).

  Note: Drilling must be performed with constant irrigation and with sterile saline at a maximum of 1,000rpm rate. A pumping motion should be employed to prevent overheating of the bone. If the drill cannot advance 2mm/second in the osteotomy, it has become dull and should be replaced.

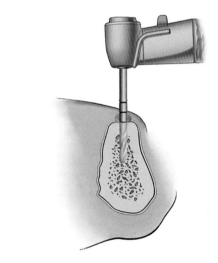

FIGURE 13.20.

3: WIDENING OF THE OSTEOTOMY
Use a 2.5mm finishing drill to widen the osteotomy at the previously established depth (Figures 13.20–13.22).

Note: The finishing drill doesn't have a cutting end, so it will automatically stop at the depth determined by the depth of the drill in Step 2. It is not recommended to use the finishing drill in poor bone quality (D3), such as in maxillary overdenture cases, because it will increase

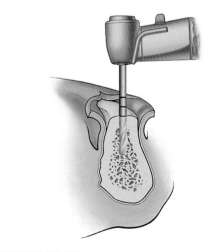

FIGURE 13.21.

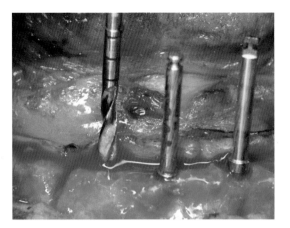

FIGURE 13.22.

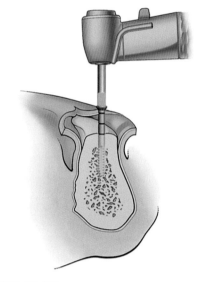

FIGURE 13.24.

the chance of over-widening the osteotomy and compromise the primary stability of the implants. Use of the bone tap is recommended if the implants are being placed in a very dense cortical bone (D1). Tap in a clockwise direction at a speed of 30rpm. Remove the tap by reversing the hand-piece's movement at the same 30rpm (Figure 13.23–13.25).

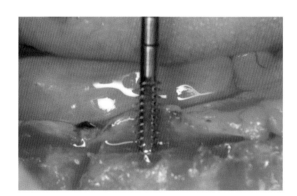

FIGURE 13.25.

4: IMPLANT PLACEMENT   Measure the thickness of the gingiva and, based on that measurement, choose a Maximus OS with a 2mm or 4mm transmucosal polished collar. Make sure that the ball attachment and its neck (total of 3mm) always stay above the gum. All of the threads and RBT surface characteristics should be completely embedded in the bone.

- *Mechanical Placement*: Insert the hand-piece adaptor into the surgical contra-angle hand-piece and then pick up the implant from its container. Place the implant in the osteotomy and drive the implant in at a rate of 30rpm (Figures 13.26–13.31).

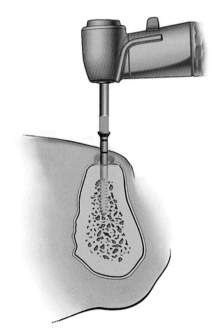

FIGURE 13.23.

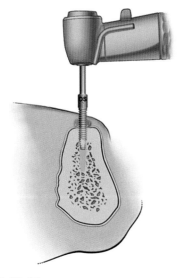

FIGURE 13.26.

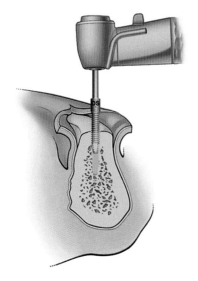

FIGURE 13.27.

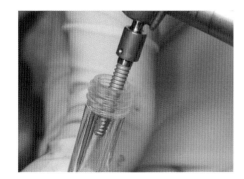

FIGURE 13.28.

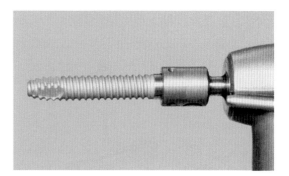

FIGURE 13.29.

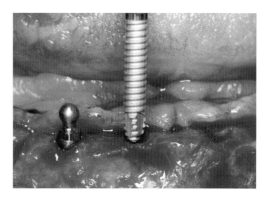

FIGURE 13.30.

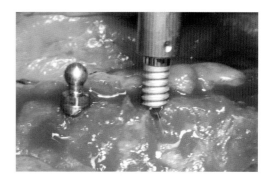

FIGURE 13.31.

- *Manual Placement*: Insert the ratchet adapter in the hand wrench and then pick up the implant from its container. Place the implant into the osteotomy and drive the implant in manually until the implant is stabilized. Then replace the hand wrench with the ratchet and complete the implant insertion (Figures 13.32 and 13.33).

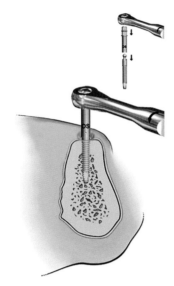

FIGURE 13.32.

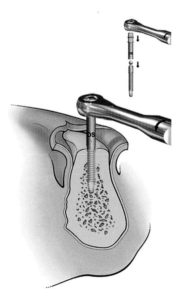

FIGURE 13.33.

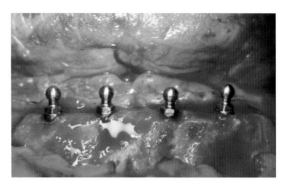

FIGURE 13.34.

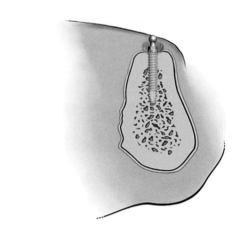

FIGURE 13.35.

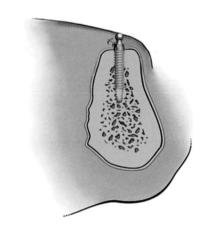

FIGURE 13.36.

Prosthetic Steps

The Maximus OS implants should be parallel in the mouth. The trajectory of the supporting implants and their relationship to each other

Note: Make sure not to over-torque the implant, as bone stripping or pressure necrosis may occur (Figures 13.34–13.36).

determine whether the 0-, 7-, or 14-degree directional ring should be used.

Chair-Side Utilization Procedure

1. Use the directional pins to determine the relation of the supporting implants with each other. Snap a 0-degree directional pin on the implant that has the best trajectory related to the ideal path of insertion for the overdenture. Use that implant as a guide to choose the appropriate directional pins, which will be parallel to the reference pin. There are three color-coded directional pins similar to the directional rings: Green—0-degree, Blue—7-degree, and Purple—14-degree.

   After achieving parallelism of all of the directional pins, the clinician can choose the appropriate directional rings based on the color of the directional pins that have been utilized.

   If none of the implants are positioned in the correct path of insertion, make a pickup impression and a master cast. Then use a surveyor to determine the discrepancy among the trajectories of the supporting implants.

2. After choosing the proper directional rings, snap a metal housing pre-loaded with a black female positioning cap onto each ball attachment.

   Note: The directional ring covers all of the undercuts. However, if a flap surgery has been performed and the tissue has been sutured, use a rubber dam to protect the sutures. Cut a small square of the rubber dam (1/2 inch by 1/2 inch) and punch a small hole in the middle of the square. The ball attachment and the hex of the implant should pass through the hole in the rubber dam. Make sure the rubber dam seats over the soft tissue and covers all of the stitches.

3. Use a large laboratory round carbide bur to cut a hole in the denture base exactly above each implant. Continue the hole toward the lingual flange and create a window. This hole should be large enough to insert a pre-loaded metal housing over the implant with no contact between the metal housing and the denture base.

4. Insert the denture and verify that no contact occurs between each attachment and the denture base. If interference is present, trim the denture base.

5. Apply self-cure acrylic around and above each metal housing as well as inside each hole in the denture base. Ensure that the external retention ridge on the outside of the metal housing is completely covered with acrylic. Insert the denture into the patient's mouth over the attachment and guide the patient into maximum intercuspation, but do not allow the patient to close firmly. Allowing the patient to close firmly could cause an improper position of the males relative to the females.

6. After the acrylic is set, remove the overdenture, fill any void with acrylic, and finish and polish the prosthesis.

7. Replace each black female nylon cap with an extra soft yellow final female. If the patient desires additional retention, replace the yellow female with a more retentive female cap six to eight weeks after the implant surgery.

   Female caps from least retentive to most retentive:
   - Green: Extra soft retention
   - Yellow: Soft retention
   - Pink: Medium retention
   - White: Firm retention

8. Verify the occlusion and perform any necessary occlusal adjustments.

ERA® OVERDENTURE IMPLANT

The ERA® Implant was developed in 1999 and introduced to the market in 2003. It is a self-tapping implant with a tapered apical portion. This implant is made of titanium alloy, and its female component is covered with a titanium nitride coating to decrease attachment wear. The aggressive thread depth of this implant helps to create a mechanical locking with the surrounding bone. Its apical end, with sharp threads all the way to the pointed tip, will cut through even dense bone. In fact, unless the bone is very dense, the apical one-third of the implant is allowed to self-tap into bone that has not been prepared.

The ERA® Implant provides hinge and vertical resiliency. The nylon male component is captured in the denture acrylic. There are six color-coded males for six levels of retention. In order from the lightest to the most retentive, they are white, orange, blue, gray, yellow, and red. An optional metal housing supports these nylon male components, and the metal housing is preloaded with a black male. The black male is slightly thicker occlusally (0.4mm) than the final males. Unlike other resilient attachments that have a separate spacer that fits between the male and female during processing, the ERA® has a spacer built into the black male. Therefore, when the black male is processed into the denture, removed using two special tools, and replaced with one of the final males, 0.4mm of empty space is left between the male and female. This procedure creates true vertical resiliency and allows a hinging function.

Design Specifications

Surface Characteristics
- Etched
- Machined

Diameter of the Threaded Part
- 2.2mm

Available Lengths
- 8.0mm
- 10.0mm
- 13.0mm
- 15.0mm

Note: Length is measured from the bottom of the female component to its apical end (Figure 13.37).

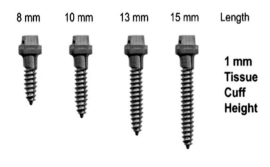

FIGURE 13.37.

Available Gingival Cuff Heights for Female Component (Figure 13.38)
- 1mm
- 2mm
- 3mm
- 4mm

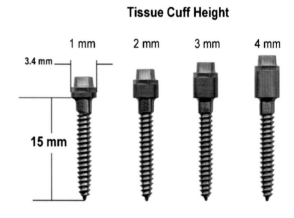

FIGURE 13.38.

Dimensions of Male Component
- *Height:* 2.0mm
- *Diameter:* 3.4mm

Surgical Steps

1: MARKING LOCATION OF THE IMPLANTS Insert the surgical guide in the mouth. Using the starter drill or the 1.6mm pilot, drill through the gum and penetrate into the bone (Figures 13.39–13.42).

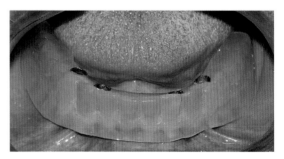

FIGURE 13.39. (Photo courtesy of Dr. Kaveh Seyedan)

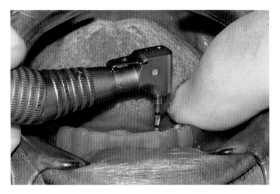

FIGURE 13.40.   (Photo courtesy of Dr. Kaveh Seyedan)

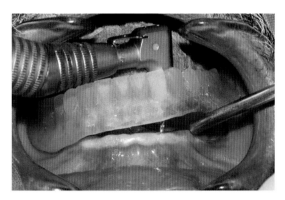

FIGURE 13.41.   (Photo courtesy of Dr. Kaveh Seyedan)

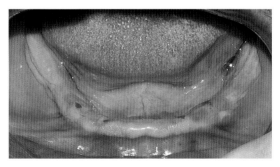

FIGURE 13.42.   (Photo courtesy of Dr. Kaveh Seyedan)

2: GAINING ACCESS TO THE ALVEOLAR BONE

- *Performing a Flap Technique*: This approach provides great access and maximizes visualization of the shape and contour of the alveolar bone (Figures 13.43–13.46).

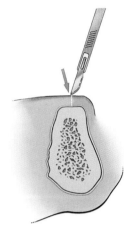

FIGURE 13.43.

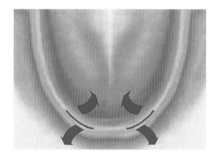

FIGURE 13.44.

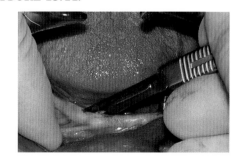

FIGURE 13.45.   (Photo courtesy of Dr. Kaveh Seyedan)

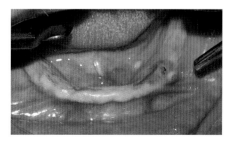

FIGURE 13.46.   (Photo courtesy of Dr. Kaveh Seyedan)

When performing a flap surgery, based on the design of the surgical guide, start the drilling process before or after raising the flap. If the surgical guide has been made based on the impression of the residual ridge and sits over the gum, start the drilling process before raising the flap. Otherwise, after raising the flap, it will not be possible to insert the surgical guide in a stable manner. With this type of surgical guide, insert the guide in the patient's mouth, mark the location of each implant by using a 2mm starter drill, and drill through the gum and the alveolar bone. The drill speed should be set at 1,000rpm with constant irrigation. If the surgical guide has been made based on CT-scan data and fits over the alveolar bone, raise the flap first to make sure the guide fits perfectly over the alveolar bone, and then start the drilling process.

- *Performing a No-Flap Technique*: This approach minimizes post-operation symptoms and complications, and there is no need for suturing.

To perform a no-flap surgery, mark the location of the implants on the gum and then use the tissue punch to core-cut the gum and gain access to the alveolar bone (Figure 13.47).

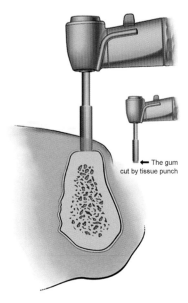

FIGURE 13.47.

3: MARKING THE BONE   Use the surgical round bur or the 1.6mm starter drill to mark the location of the implant. When using the starter drill in D2 and D3 bone quality, it is recommended to penetrate the bone 3mm shorter than the length of the designated implant. When placing the implant in D1 bone quality, prep the osteotomy at full length, which is equal to the length of the designated implant (Figures 13.48 and 13.49).

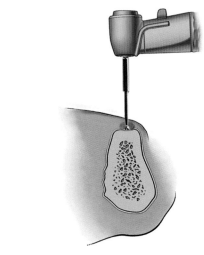

FIGURE 13.48.

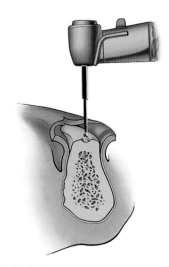

FIGURE 13.49.

4: PREPARING THE OSTEOTOMY   Use the hybrid countersink/pilot drill and finalize preparation of the osteotomy. The length of the pilot part of the hybrid drill is equal to the length of the parallel portion of the implant, which means that the tapered apical portion of the implant will self-tap in the bone. This approach maximizes the primary stability of the implant in D2 and D3 bone quality. The countersink part of the hybrid drill will create a platform on the crest of the alveolar bone that the bottom of the female component of the implant will eventually seat over. If placing the implant in D1 bone quality, after using the hybrid drill, extend the depth of the osteotomy to the full length of the implant, and use the bone tap to create the tread form in the bone (Figures 13.50–13.60).

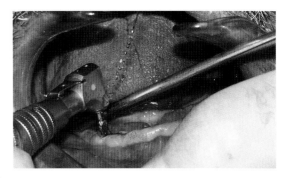

FIGURE 13.52. (Photo courtesy of Dr. Kaveh Seyedan)

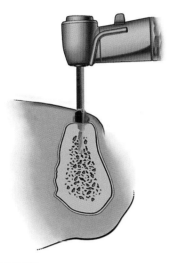

FIGURE 13.50.

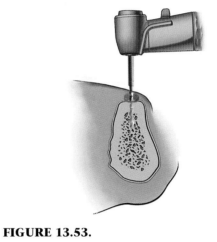

FIGURE 13.53.

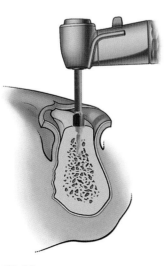

FIGURE 13.51.

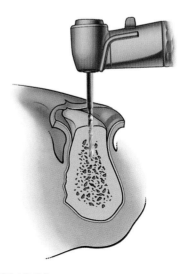

FIGURE 13.54.

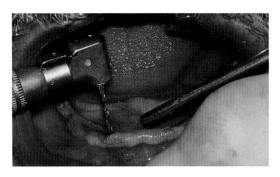

FIGURE 13.55. (Photo courtesy of Dr. Kaveh Seyedan)

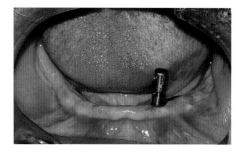

FIGURE 13.58. (Photo courtesy of Dr. Kaveh Seyedan)

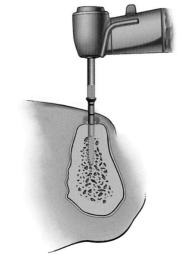

FIGURE 13.56.

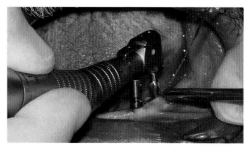

FIGURE 13.59. (Photo courtesy of Dr. Kaveh Seyedan)

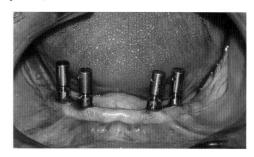

FIGURE 13.60. (Photo courtesy of Dr. Kaveh Seyedan)

5: PLACING THE IMPLANT Measure the thickness of the gingiva. Based on the measurement, choose an implant with the proper gingival cuff height. Make sure the female component of the implant always stays above the gum. All of the threads should be completely embedded in the bone.

- *Mechanical Placement*: Pick up the implant from its container using the hand wrench and begin screwing the implant into the osteotomy. Insert the hand-piece adaptor into the surgical contra-angle hand-piece and continue driving the implant into the osteotomy.

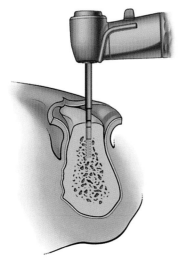

FIGURE 13.57.

Drive the implant in at 10–15rpm with irrigation (Figures 13.61–13.67).

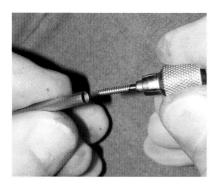

FIGURE 13.61. (Photo courtesy of Dr. Kaveh Seyedan)

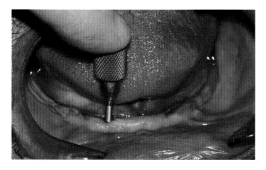

FIGURE 13.62. (Photo courtesy of Dr. Kaveh Seyedan)

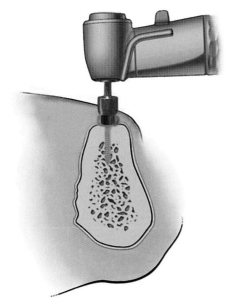

FIGURE 13.63.

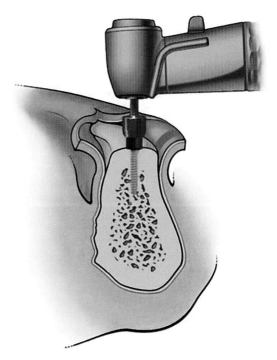

FIGURE 13.64.

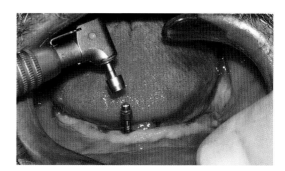

FIGURE 13.65. (Photo courtesy of Dr. Kaveh Seyedan)

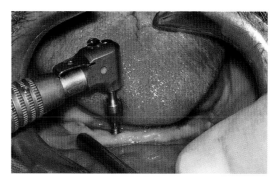

FIGURE 13.66. (Photo courtesy of Dr. Kaveh Seyedan)

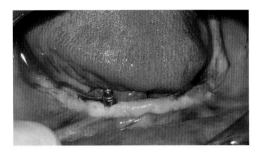

FIGURE 13.67. (Photo courtesy of Dr. Kaveh Seyedan)

- *Manual Placement*: Pick up the implant from its container with the hand wrench. Place the implant into the osteotomy and drive the implant in manually until the implant is stabilized. Next, insert the ratchet adaptor into the ratchet wrench and remove the hand wrench. Use the ratchet to drive the implant into its final position.

Note: Be sure not to over-torque the implant, as bone stripping or pressure necrosis may occur (Figures 13.68 and 13.75).

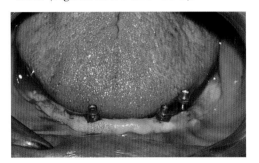

FIGURE 13.68. (Photo courtesy of Dr. Kaveh Seyedan)

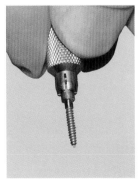

FIGURE 13.69. (Photo courtesy of Dr. Kaveh Seyedan)

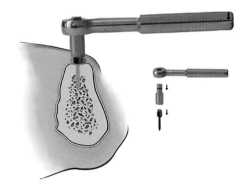

FIGURE 13.70.

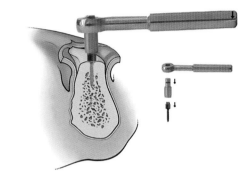

FIGURE 13.71.

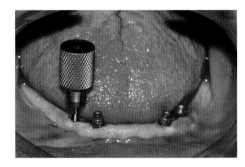

FIGURE 13.72. (Photo courtesy of Dr. Kaveh Seyedan)

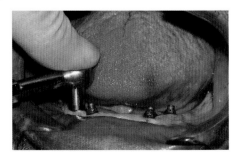

FIGURE 13.73. (Photo courtesy of Dr. Kaveh Seyedan)

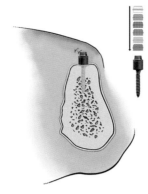

FIGURE 13.74.

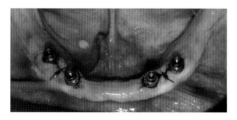

FIGURE 13.75. (Photo courtesy of Dr. Kaveh Seyedan)

Prosthetic Steps

Chair-Side Utilization Procedure

1. Use a large laboratory round carbide bur to cut a hole in the denture base exactly above each ERA implant. Continue the hole toward the lingual flange and create a window. This hole should be large enough to insert a pre-loaded metal housing over the female abutment with no contact between the metal housing and the denture base (Figures 13.76 and 13.79).

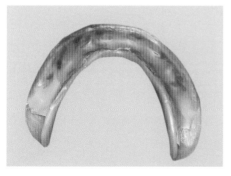

FIGURE 13.76. (Photo courtesy of Dr. Kaveh Seyedan)

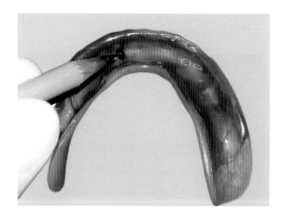

FIGURE 13.77. (Photo courtesy of Dr. Kaveh Seyedan)

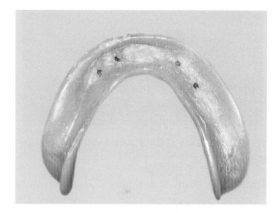

FIGURE 13.78. (Photo courtesy of Dr. Kaveh Seyedan)

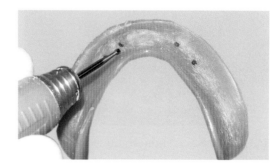

FIGURE 13.79. (Photo courtesy of Dr. Kaveh Seyedan)

2. Snap a black male, which is preloaded in a metal housing, onto each female abutment. Block out the sutures (if the flap technique has been utilized) and any remaining exposed surfaces of the female component or any

potential undercuts with small pieces of rubber dam (Figures 13.80 and 13.81).

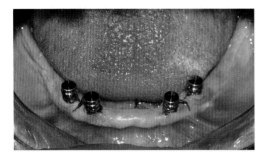

FIGURE 13.80. (Photo courtesy of Dr. Kaveh Seyedan)

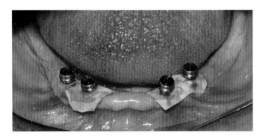

FIGURE 13.81. (Photo courtesy of Dr. Kaveh Seyedan)

3. Insert the denture and verify that there is no contact between each female component and the denture base. If interference is present, trim the denture base (Figure 13.82).

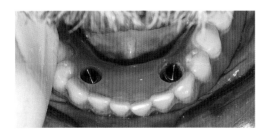

FIGURE 13.82. (Photo courtesy of Dr. Kaveh Seyedan)

4. Apply self-cure acrylic around and above each metal housing, as well as inside each hole in the denture base. Ensure that the external retention ridge on the outside of the metal housing is completely covered with acrylic. Insert the denture into the patient's mouth over the attachment assembly and guide the

patient into maximum intercuspation, but do not allow the patient to close firmly. Allowing the patient to close firmly could cause an improper position of the males to the females (Figures 13.83 and 13.84).

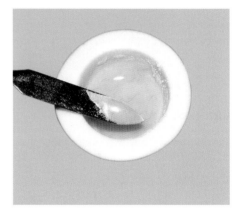

FIGURE 13.83. (Photo courtesy of Dr. Kaveh Seyedan)

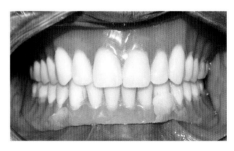

FIGURE 13.84. (Photo courtesy of Dr. Kaveh Seyedan)

5. After the acrylic is set, remove the overdenture, fill any void with acrylic, and finish and polish the prosthesis (Figures 13.85).

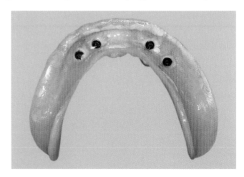

FIGURE 13.85. (Photo courtesy of Dr. Kaveh Seyedan)

6. Replace each black male nylon attachment with a white final male. Since the final male is 0.4mm shorter (inside) than the black male, it creates vertical resiliency for the prosthesis. If the patient desires additional retention, replace the white male with an orange male approximately eight weeks after the implant placement. Use the blue, gray, yellow, or red male components as necessary (Figures 13.86 and 13.89).

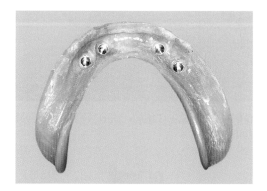

FIGURE 13.86. (Photo courtesy of Dr. Kaveh Seyedan)

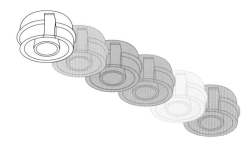

FIGURE 13.87.

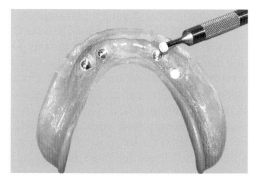

FIGURE 13.88. (Photo courtesy of Dr. Kaveh Seyedan)

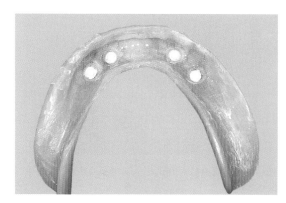

FIGURE 13.89. (Photo courtesy of Dr. Kaveh Seyedan)

7. Verify the occlusion and perform any necessary occlusal adjustments (Figure 13.90).

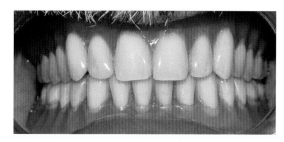

FIGURE 13.90. (Photo courtesy of Dr. Kaveh Seyedan)

Changing ERA Male Component

Note: A dentist's tool kit (core cutter and seating tool) is necessary for replacement of ERA males.

1. Use a core cutter bur and a slow speed handpiece to core the nylon male out of the metal housing at a low rpm. Use a short cutting cycle and an in-and-out motion. Push in for about one second at a time. Check to see if the core is removed. The core will remain in the core cutter and can be ejected by sliding a thin blade along the cutter's side slot (Figures 13.91 and 13.92).

2. Use a C-scaler, collapse the remaining ring into the open space created by removal of the

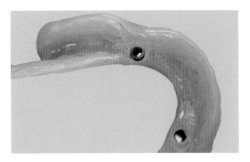

FIGURE 13.91. (Photo courtesy of Dr. Kaveh Seyedan)

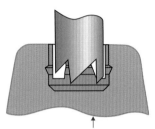

Cross section of denture base

FIGURE 13.92.

core, and then lift it out (Figures 13.93 and 13.94).

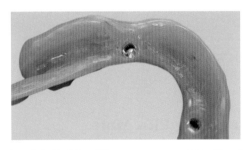

FIGURE 13.93. (Photo courtesy of Dr. Kaveh Seyedan)

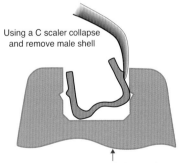

Using a C scaler collapse and remove male shell

Cross section of denture base

FIGURE 13.94.

3. Seat a new male component on the seating tool. Push the new male firmly into the metal housing until it snaps securely into place (Figures 13.95 and 13.96).

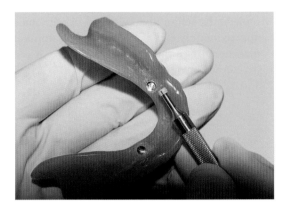

FIGURE 13.95. (Photo courtesy of Dr. Kaveh Seyedan)

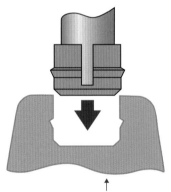

Cross section of denture base

FIGURE 13.96.

There are several different philosophies regarding how to set the fees for patients that have been treated by overdenture implants. One theme that seems to run throughout these methods is to charge about one-third the amount charged for a traditional implant. If used along with traditional implants, this additional charge should be relatively easy to justify, given the many advantages. If used alone, the lower price can be used to encourage more patients to accept this type of therapy. A significant number of those who might otherwise decide against implant dentistry based on the cost or fear of complicated surgery will accept the overdenture implant procedure. Not only will this provide a new source of income to the practice, but it will generate income from other procedures as well. Patients who are happy with the outcome of the overdenture implants are more likely to decide to proceed with more complicated implant restoration.

REFERENCES AND ADDITIONAL READING

Ahn, M. R., An, K. M., Choi, J. H., & Sohn, D. S. (2004). Immediate loading with mini dental implants in the fully edentulous mandible. *Implant Dentistry*, Dec, 13(4), 367–72.

Bulard, R. A. (2001). Mini dental implants: enhancing patient satisfaction and practice income. *Dentistry Today*. Jul, 20(7), 82–5.

Bulard, R. A. (2002). Mini implants. Part I. A solution for loose dentures. *Journal of the Oklahoma Dental Association*, 93(1), 42–6.

Glauser, R., Schupbach, P., Gottlow, J., & Hammerle, C. H. (2005). Periimplant soft tissue barrier at experimental one-piece mini-implants with different surface topography in humans: A light-microscopic overview and histometric analysis. *Clinical Implant Dentistry & Related Research*, 7 (supplement 1), S44–51.

Hubbard, L. G. (2005). Many problems, mini solutions. *Dentistry Today*, Mar, 24(3), 104, 106–7.

Kanie, T., Nagata, M., & Ban, S. (2004). Comparison of the mechanical properties of 2 prosthetic mini-implants. *Implant Dentistry*, Sep, 13(3), 251–6.

Kitai, N., Yasuda, Y., & Takada, K. (2002). A stent fabricated on a selectively colored stereolithographic model for placement of orthodontic mini-implants. *International Journal of Adult Orthodontics and Orthognathic Surgery*, 17(4), 264–6.

Mazor, Z., Steigmann M., Leshem, R., & Peleg, M. (2004). Mini-implants to reconstruct missing teeth in severe ridge deficiency and small interdental space: a 5-year case series. *Implant Dentistry*, Dec, 13(4), 336–41.

Morea, C., Dominguez, G.C., Wuo Ado V., Tortamano, A. (2005). Surgical guide for optimal positioning of mini-implants. *Journal of Clinical Orthodontics*, May, 39(5), 317–213.

Shatkin, T. E., Shatkin S., Oppenheimer, A. J., & Oppenheimer, B. D. (2003). A simplified approach to implant dentistry with mini dental implants. *Alpha Omegan*, Oct, 96(3), 7–15.

Tri mini-transitional implants the ultimate immediate loading implant for transitional or long-term use. (2003). *Journal of the Irish Dental Association*, 49(2), 75.

14
Loading Approaches for Mandibular Implant Overdentures

Dittmar May
George Romanos
Hamid Shafie

HEALING PERIOD BEFORE LOADING

Originally, the recommended waiting period between implant placement and loading was 12 weeks. Recently, however, implant manufacturers and clinicians have found it generally acceptable to practice premature loading of splinted or non-splinted implants that are being utilized for mandibular implant overdentures.

THREE CONCEPTS IN PREMATURE LOADING

Early Loading

Early loading means insertion of the prosthesis before 12 weeks—usually longer than a week but within a period of 20 to 28 days after implant placement.

Progressive Loading

Progressive loading means a gradual increase in application of the functional forces on the supporting implants, whether they are applied intentionally with the prosthesis during mastication or unintentionally via forces placed by the adjacent anatomic structure or parafunctional loading.

Immediate Loading

Immediate loading means that full occlusal and incisal loading is applied on the supporting dental implants with the overdenture the same day of implant placement or within the first few days after surgery.

CRITICAL FACTORS IN DETERMINING LOADING STRATEGIES

- Primary stability of the implant
- Bone quality
- Surgical technique
- Implant length
- Implant surface
- Implant design features

IMPORTANT INDICATING FACTORS FOR SUCCESS OF PREMATURELY LOADED IMPLANTS

- Fully functional prosthesis without any discomfort
- No changes in the patient's sensation
- No infection
- Absence or minimal marginal bone loss
- Implant stability

Premature loading can be done successfully with implants that have machined surface characteristics, but it is preferred to use implants with more advanced surface characteristics such as SLA, TiUnite, RBT, and so on. These new generations of surface characteristics provide faster bone healing and more implant-bone interface.

The concept of immediate replacement of teeth for fully edentulous patients has been in the forefront of clinical implantology research for more than 20 years. Currently, immediate loading as well as early loading of the implants placed in the fully edentulous mandible has become a very popular treatment protocol.

The most important prerequisites for successful immediate-function procedures appear to be achieving initial implant stability and controlling the immediate loading forces directed to the implant. The initial stability is achieved through biomechanical interlocking of the implant in the surrounding bone and is needed to avoid micromotion at the interface during early healing. The implant's surface properties are believed to influence the bone healing and implant stability over time. In order to optimize the initial bone healing, especially in situations with less dense bone, using an enhanced implant surface characteristic and thread design will help primary implant stability and achieve secondary stability earlier than machined surfaces through heightened bone response to more advanced surfaces.

Lederman showed in 1979 that an overdenture can be inserted over a bar attachment assembly supported by four implants in the edentulous mandible immediately after the surgery, eventually obtaining successful osseointegration as well as a fully functional implant-supported overdenture. However, making an immediate bar-supported overdenture involves considerable laboratory procedures and expenses. Furthermore, there would be a 12–24 hour delay between the surgical appointment and delivery of the overdenture.

Some implant companies have developed very sophisticated computer-milled metal substructures as well as a matching surgical guide for immediately loaded, screw-retained implant-supported overdenture. The negatives of this technique are the high cost of the overdenture, the complex surgical steps it requires, and the necessity of utilizing very sophisticated equipment and machinery to produce this type of overdenture, which requires advanced training and mastership.

ADVANTAGES OF IMMEDIATE LOADING IN IMPLANT-SUPPORTED OVERDENTURE CASES

- Reduces treatment duration and the frequency of patient visits
- Reduces chair-side time for the dentist, which reduces overhead
- Does not require second-stage surgery
- Reduces patient stress and anxiety due to the treatment process
- Benefits patient psychologically

IMPORTANT REQUIREMENTS FOR TREATMENT PROTOCOL

- Treatment protocol that is applicable for geriatric patients
- Shortened total treatment time
- High primary stability of the implants
- Immobilization of the implants immediately after surgery

- Sufficient bone quality at the implant site
- Simple clinical and laboratory steps utilizing prefabricated components as well as chair-side techniques
- Applicable with an implant system that offers multiple clinical applications
- Ease of switching treatment strategy to the conventional treatment protocol
- Good patient compliance

SYNCONE® CONCEPT

It has long been reported that full dentures can be retained with telescopic crowns. However, the high costs and labor-intensive laboratory procedures required for telescopic crowns have minimized the application of this concept. The SynCone® system is an innovative telescopic crown technique that combines technical precision with affordability. It has been developed by May and Romanos (2000) and has been used specifically for the immediate loading of oral implants in the anterior part of the mandible. For this concept, the Ankylos® implant system (Friadent, Dentsply, Mannheim, Germany) has been used.

Advantages of Telescopic Crown Techniques

- Excellent three-dimensional immobilization of the restoration
- Defined release force
- Flexibility of design
- Optimal access for oral hygiene

The treatment protocol described here is based on four implants placed between the two mandibular foramens and utilization of 4-degree taper SynCone® abutments. No reliable long-term clinical data are available on the use of higher or lower numbers of implants and SynCone® abutments in the maxilla. Deviation from the following protocol is not advisable when the implants will be loaded immediately after their placement.

Patient Selection

Selecting patients who are generally good health and good compliance is important. The candidate for this treatment option should have at least 12–14mm of bone height in the anterior mandible. The width of the alveolar ridge and the bone quality are of great importance in order to get high primary stability.

Pre-Surgical Steps

1. Fabricate an ideal denture with perfect tissue adaptation. However, avoid overextension of the flanges, because this can prevent the overdenture from fitting properly over the telescopic attachment assembly.
2. Fabricate a precise surgical guide by duplicating the fabricated final denture.
3. Insert titanium guide tubes in the surgical guide. These tubes must be parallel with each other to ensure parallelism in the trajectory of the supporting implants.

Surgical Steps

1. After administration of the peripheral infiltration anesthetic, make two crestal incisions 3mm distal to the midline. The untouched soft tissue bridge in the middle will reduce the risk of dehiscence (Figures 14.1 and 14.2).

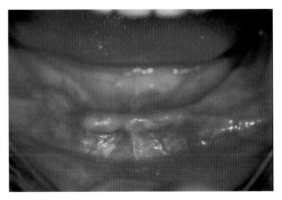

FIGURE 14.1.

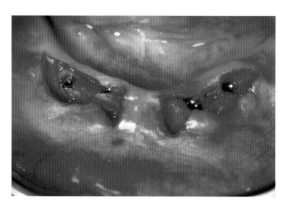

FIGURE 14.2.

2. Release the flap and observe the crest of the alveolar ridge. If necessary, use a surgical round bur and perform alveoloplasty to level the ridge (Figure 14.3).

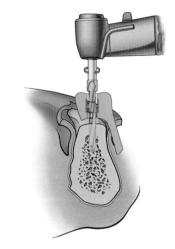

FIGURE 14.4.

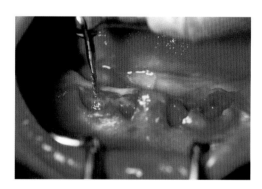

FIGURE 14.5.

allow the implant to be placed slightly below the crest of the ridge (Figure 14.6).

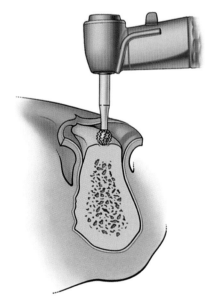

FIGURE 14.3.

3. Use the surgical guide and matching twist drill to establish the trajectory of the supporting implants (Figures 14.4 and 14.5).
4. Continue with the next drill to widen the osteotomy. The depth of the osteotomy should

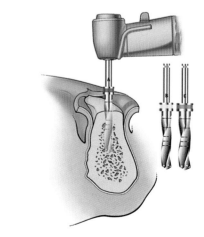

FIGURE 14.6.

5. Choose the matching tapered bone reamer for the Ankylos® implant. Mount the bone reamer on the hand ratchet and start reaming the osteotomy. The reamer doesn't have a cutting end. Therefore, it will not change the depth of osteotomy, but will shape the osteotomy to a taper. The reaming process should be done with slight pressure to avoid pressure necrosis (Figure 14.7).

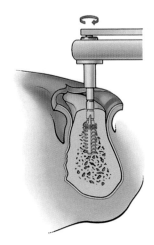

FIGURE 14.8.

the osteotomy with saline, and tap the site again (Figures 14.9 and 14.10).

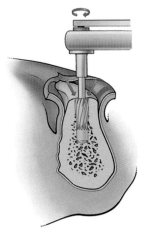

FIGURE 14.7.

6. After widening the osteotomy, the upper edge of the reamer must be approximately 0.5mm below the crest of the ridge. If the reamer doesn't go below the crest of the ridge, the osteotomy should be deepened with the last pilot drill. After deepening the osteotomy, perform the remaining steps.

7. Choose the proper tapping drill according to the Ankylos® implant. Mount the tap drill on the hand ratchet and start tapping the osteotomy. As soon as the tap drill reaches the bottom of the osteotomy, stop ratcheting. Otherwise, all of the formed threads will be stripped (Figure 14.8).

8. Use the hand wrench to drive the implant into the prepared osteotomy. The minimum length of the implant should be 11–14mm. Drive the implant into the osteotomy until the lower edge of the polished collar contacts the bone. If the driving of the implant into the osteotomy becomes difficult and stops before the polished collar reaches the crestal bone, turn the implant back up, rinse

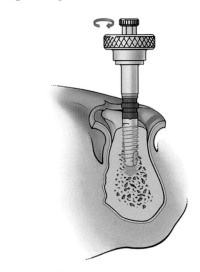

FIGURE 14.9.

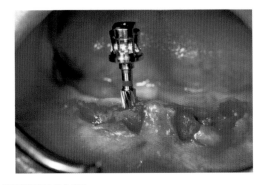

FIGURE 14.10.

9. Remove the hand wrench and drive the implant into its final position using the ratchet (Figures 14.11 and 14.12).

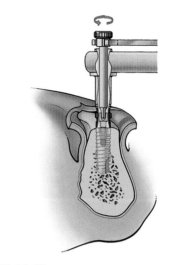

FIGURE 14.13.

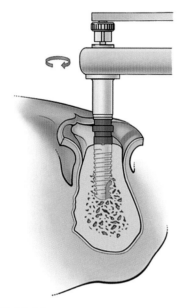

FIGURE 14.11.

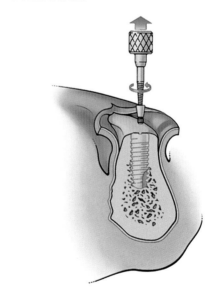

FIGURE 14.14.

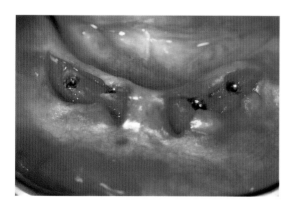

FIGURE 14.12.

Note: In D1 type bone quality, drive the implant slowly to eliminate the possibility of overheating and pressure necrosis.

10. Remove the mount and the cover screw (Figures 14.13–14.15).

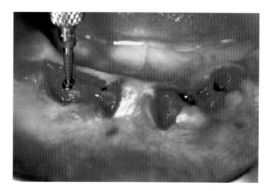

FIGURE 14.15.

Note: If the implant rotates in the osteotomy during removal of the cover screw, the implant should not be loaded immediately and should be submerged for a delayed approach.

Prosthetic Steps

1. Choose the proper prefabricated 4-degree SynCone® abutment. The SynCone® abutment comes in three different cuff heights: 1.5mm, 3mm, and 4.5mm. Based on the thickness of the gingiva, choose the abutment with the proper cuff height. The abutment should be tightened to 15Ncm using a torque wrench. Before inserting the abutment, make sure that the inner cone of the implant is carefully rinsed with saline and then dried (Figure 14.16–14.18).

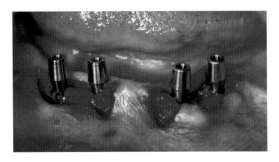

FIGURE 14.18.

Note: If there is a discrepancy between the trajectories of the supporting implants, use a SynCone® 15-degree abutment to make sure all of the abutments are as parallel as possible. To find the correct abutment position, place alignment tools with extensions on the abutments. These extensions help to visualize the orientation of the abutment. One of the advantages of implants that have a conical tapered abutment connection, such as Ankylos® implant, is the unlimited possibilities of changing the orientation of the abutment. In implant systems with different implant-abutment connections, such as hexagon or octagon, Camlog and Camtube, the number of flat surfaces or guiding planes dictate the number of abutment orientation possibilities (Figures 14.19 and 14.20).

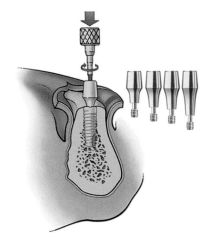

FIGURE 14.16.

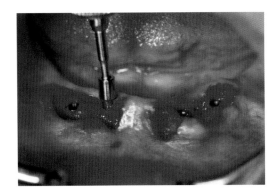

FIGURE 14.17.

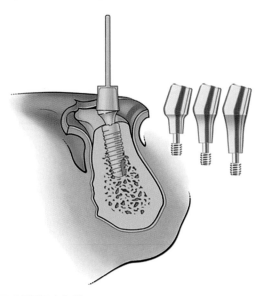

FIGURE 14.19.

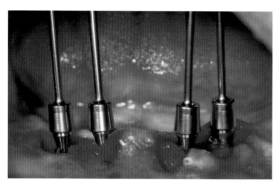

FIGURE 14.20.

2. Suture the soft tissue around the SynCone®
   abutments. The convergent transmucosal
   portion of the abutment allows the gum to
   form a tight seal around the implant (Figures
   14.21 and 14.22).

3. Insert a SynCone® cap over each abutment.
   SynCone® caps should be kept in cold, sterile
   solution before insertion over the abutments.
   These caps engage the height of the contour
   of the tapered abutment and prevent penetration of the self-cure acrylic into the undercut
   area. However, to eliminate any possibility of
   interlocking of the acrylic into the undercut
   area, place a small square of the rubber dam
   over each abutment (Figures 14.23–14.25).

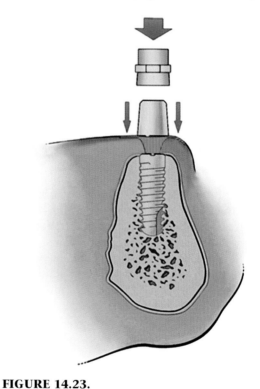

FIGURE 14.23.

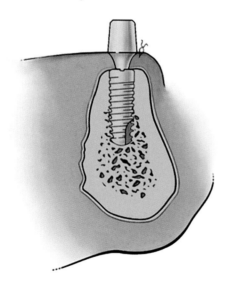

FIGURE 14.21.

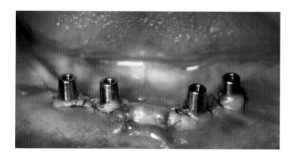

FIGURE 14.22.

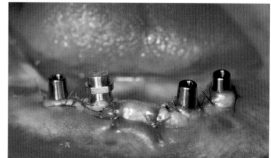

FIGURE 14.24.

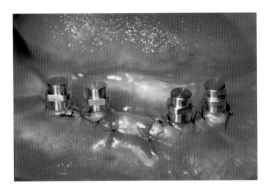

FIGURE 14.25.

Note: Ensure that no sutures are trapped between the cap and the abutment.

4. Start preparing the denture by cutting a large window or windows in the lingual flange of the denture. The window should be large enough to allow no contact between the SynCone® caps and the denture base. However, to prevent excessive polymerization shrinkage of the self-cure acrylic, be very cautious and conservative in cutting the denture base. The denture must have functioned properly prior to placing the implants. An ill-fitting denture will not fit accurately over the abutments and will not make a stable implant overdenture. Reduce the flanges all around (Figure 14.26 and 14.27).

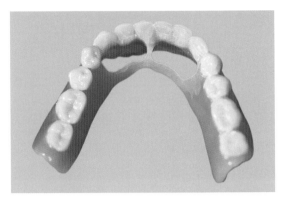

FIGURE 14.27.

5. Apply self-cure acrylic around the caps as well as inside the denture base. It is important that the entire surface of the SynCone® caps is embedded in the acrylic. Then guide the patient into the centric occlusion and ask the patient to keep the upper and lower teeth in this position with a light pressure until the acrylic is completely polymerized and hardened (Figures 14.28–14.30).

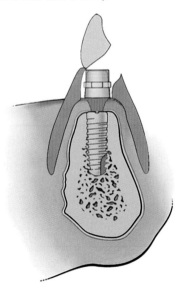

FIGURE 14.26.

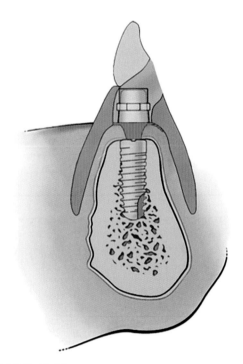

FIGURE 14.28.

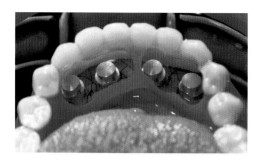

FIGURE 14.29.

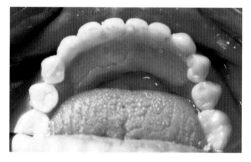

FIGURE 14.30.

Note: If the patient applies excessive pressure during this step, the denture base will displace the supporting tissues. After completion of the polymerization and after the patient releases pressure, the soft tissue will rebound and push the denture base up, which will disengage the SynCone® caps from the abutments.

6. Remove the denture from the patient's mouth after completion of the polymerization, and then finish and polish the area around the SynCone® caps. Trim back the acrylic 1mm away from the margins of the SynCone® caps (Figures 14.31–14.33).

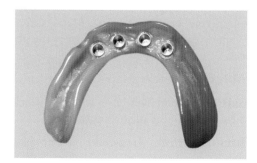

FIGURE 14.31.

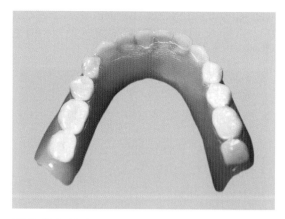

FIGURE 14.32.

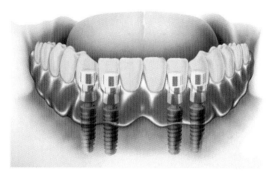

FIGURE 14.33.

7. Check the occlusion in the centric and lateral excursion.
8. Prescribe an antibiotic for one week.

Postoperative Instructions for Patient

- Do not remove the overdenture for one week.
- Eat soft foods for the next 14 days.
- Take the prescribed antibiotic for one week.
- Rinse mouth twice a day with chlorhexidine mouthwash.
- Return seven days after surgery to have sutures removed.

One week following removal of the sutures, the denture is removed from the mouth for the first time and the patient should wear it again for two consecutive three-day periods. At the end of these two weeks, the patient is instructed fully on how to maintain good oral hygiene as well as maintaining the overdenture. After this period, there are no further restrictions on eating (Figures 14.34 and 14.35).

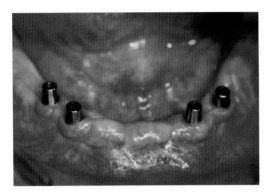

FIGURE 14.34.

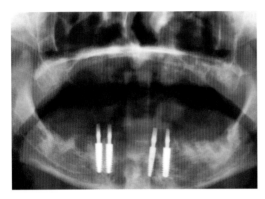

FIGURE 14.35.

The patient should be seen every six months. During the recall visit, evaluate the patient for possible changes in the supporting bone, the attachment assembly, and the fit of the denture base. If necessary, reline the denture base.

Based on the above protocol, 51 patients (age: 65.60 +/− 8.84 years; 204 Ankylos® implants) were treated. After a mean loading period of 17.7 months, the investigative team showed a cumulative success rate of 97.54 percent. All implants were clinically stable and surrounded by a healthy and non-irritated peri-implant mucosa.

A recent study with 54 patients (66.4 +/− 9.6 years old) and 189 implants using the SynCone® concept in the anterior interforaminal part of the mandible showed only two failures after a loading period of 24.6 +/− 14 months. The high

success rate (98.95 percent) of this surgical and prosthetic technique is probably related to the implant system design as well as the four conical prefabricated abutments (SynCone®), which allow a stable and positive seating of the denture (via secondary caps). This method has a high predictability because it provides stability, function, and aesthetic results.

Furthermore, it is possible to connect the implants with the remaining teeth using the SynCone® telescopic abutments, allowing the general practitioner a high number of clinical applications. This has positive psychological effects for the patient. This technique is not well evaluated; more clinical studies are necessary in order to use this concept in daily practice.

Delayed Loading Protocol with SynCone® Concept

The SynCone® concept can be used to retain osseointegrated implants. This technique can be used chair-side or as an indirect laboratory technique. With the indirect approach, fabrication of a metal framework to reinforce the denture base is strongly recommended.

When the chair-side technique is utilized, the SynCone® caps are picked up with self-cure acrylic.

TROUBLESHOOTING

Problem: Insufficient retention.

Possible Cause: The caps are not fully engaged with abutments.

Solutions: During the pick-up process, the patient should be in centric occlusion but without applying heavy pressure. Make sure the SynCone® caps are fully seated over the abutments.

Problem: Excessive retention of overdenture.

Possible Cause: Self-cure acrylic is stocked in the undercut area of the abutment.

Solutions: Block undercuts with plastic sleeves or small pieces of rubber dam. Self-cure acrylic should not have runny consistency.

SYNCONE® ABUTMENTS AND FRAMEWORK-REINFORCED OVERDENTURE

In general, conventional techniques to fabricate telescopic restorations are difficult, expensive, and time-consuming. Because of these drawbacks, telescopic restorations are not very popular among dentists and lab technicians. The use of a prefabricated telescopic abutment (SynCone®) eliminates the need for the waxing, casting, and milling steps in the lab. SynCone® is a very retentive attachment assembly.

PROCEDURAL SEQUENCES

1. The trajectory of the implant analogs in the master cast is a guide for the lab technician to choose the proper SynCone® abutment. The angulations of the abutments should be determined and corrected by using alignment tools (Figure 14.36).

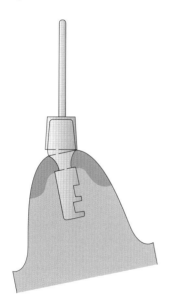

FIGURE 14.36.

2. After choosing the abutments, the metal framework should be fabricated on the master cast.

3. Insert the abutments in the patient's mouth by utilizing a custom-made positioning jig and then tighten the retaining screws.
4. Place the prefabricated external conical copings (matrices) over the abutments. The matrices will be picked up and connected to the metal framework by utilizing self-cure acrylic or self-cure composite cement (Nimetic-Cem®, Espe, Seefeld, Germany) intra-orally for an accurate fit (Figures 14.37 and 14.38).

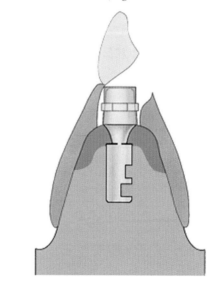

FIGURE 14.37.

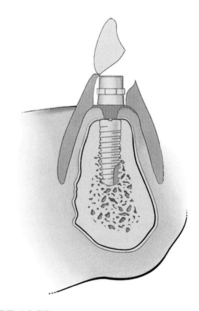

FIGURE 14.38.

5. Use the metal framework to register an accurate jaw relationship record.
6. Make a pick-up impression of this framework to reproduce and finalize the base of the overdenture.

In conclusion, the innovative SynCone® abutment provides a simple, reproducible, and cost-effective option in modern oral implantology.

REFERENCES AND ADDITIONAL READING

Academy of Prosthodontics. (1999). The Glossary of prosthodontic terms (7th edition). *Journal of Prosthetic Dentistry*, 81, 41–110.

Albrektsson, T., Zarb, G. A. (1998). Determinants of correct clinical reporting, *International Journal of Prosthodontics*, 11, 517–521.

Carr, A. B. (1998). Successful long-term treatment outcomes in the field of osseointegrated implants: Prosthodontic determinants. *International Journal of Prosthodontics*, 11, 502–512.

Cochran, D. L. (1999). A comparison of endosseous dental implant surfaces. *Journal of Periodontology*, 70, 1523–1539.

Cochran, D. L. (2001). The scientific basis for and clinical experiences with Straumann implants including the ITI Dental Implant System: A consensus report. *Clinical Oral Implants Research*, 11(supplement 1), 33–58.

Ericsson, I., Randow, K., Nilner, K., & Peterson, A. (2000). Early functional loading of Branemark implants. 5-year clinical follow up study. *Clinical Implant Dentistry and Related Research*, 2, 70–77.

Espositio, M., Coulthard, P., Worthington, H. V., & Jokstad, A. (2000). Quality assessment of randomized controlled trials of oral implants. *International Journal of Oral & Maxillofacial Implants*, 16, 783–792.

Fourmousis, I. & Bragger, U. (1999). "Radiographic interpretation of peri-implant structures." In *Proceedings of the 3rd European Workshop on Periodontology-Implant Dentistry*, ed. Lang, N. P., Karring, T., & Lindhe, J. Chicago: Quintessence Publishing, 228–241.

Friberg, B., Sennerby, L., Linden, B., Grondahl, U. K., & Lekholm, U. (1999). Stability measurements of one-stage Branemark implants during healing in mandibles. A clinical resonance frequency analysis study. *International Journal of Oral & Maxillofacial Surgery*, 28, 266–272.

Jemt, T., Chai, J., Harnett, J., et al. (1996). A 5-year prospective multicenter follow-up report on overdentures supported by osseointegrated implants. *International Journal of Oral & Maxillofacial Implants*, 11, 291–298.

Lekholm, U. & Zarb, G. A. (1985). "Patient selection and preparation." In *Tissue Integrated Prostheses: Osseointegration in Clinical Dentistry*, ed. Branemark, P. I., Zarb, G. A., & Albrektsson, T. Chicago: Quintessence Publishing, 199–210.

Mericske-Stern, R. (1998). Treatment outcomes with implant-supported overdentures: Clinical considerations. *Journal of Prosthetic Dentistry*, 79, 66–73.

Naert, I., Gizani, S., Vuylskeke, M., & van Steenberghe, D. (1999). A 5-year prospective randomized clinical trial on the influence of splinted and unsplinted oral implants retaining a mandibular overdenture: Prosthetic aspects and patient satisfaction. *Journal of Oral Rehabilitation*, 26, 195–202.

Payne, A. G. T., Solomons, Y. F., & Lownie, J. F. (1999). Standardization of radiographs for mandibular implant-supported overdentures: Review and innovation. *Clinical Oral Implants Research*, 10, 307–319.

Payne, A. G. T., Solomons, Y. F., Lownie, J. F., & Tawse-Smith, A. (2001). Inter-abutment and peri-abutment mucosal enlargement with mandibular implant overdentures. *Clinical Oral Implants Research*, 13, 179–187.

Payne, A. G. T., Tawse-Smith, A., Duncan, W. J., & Kumara, R. (2002). Conventional and early loading of unsplinted ITI implants supporting mandibular ovedentures: Two-year results of a prospective randomized clinical trial. *Clinical Oral Implants Research*, 13, 603–609.

Payne, A. G. T., Tawse-Smith, A., Kumara, R., & Thomson, W. M. (2001). One-year prospective evaluation of the early loading of unsplinted conical Branemark fixtures with mandibular overdentures: A preliminary report. *Clinical Implant Dentistry & Related Research*, 3, 9–18.

Schmitt, A. & Zarb, G. A. (1998). The notion of implant-supported overdentures. *Journal of Prosthetic Dentistry*, 79, 60–65.

Sul, Y. T., Johansson, C. B., Jeong, Y., Wennerberg, A., & Albrektsson, T. (2002). Resonance frequency and removal torque analysis of implants with turned and anodized surface oxides. *Clinical Oral Implants Research*, 13, 252–259.

Szmukler-Moncler, S., Piattellie, A., Favero G. A., & Dubruille J. H. (2000). Considerations preliminary to the application of early and immediate loading protocols in dental implantology. *Clinical Oral Implant Research*, 11, 12–25.

Tawse-Smith, A., Duncan, W., Payne, A. G. T., Thomson, W. M., Wennstrom, J. L. (2002). Effectiveness of electric toothbrushes in peri-implant maintenance of mandibular implant overdentures. *Journal of Clinical Periodontology*, 29, 275–280.

Tawse-Smith, A., Payne, A. G. T., Kumara, R., & Thomson, W. M. (2001). A one-stage operative procedure using 2 different implant systems: A prospective study on implant overdentures in the edentulous mandible. *Clinical Implant Dentistry & Related Research*, 3, 185–193.

Tawse-Smith, A., Payne, A. G. T., Kumara, R., & Thomson, W. M. (2002). Early loading of un-splinted implants supporting mandibular overdentures using a one-stage operative procedure with two different implant systems: A 2-year report. *Clinical Implant Dentistry & Related Research*, 4, 33–42.

Watson, G., Payne, A. G. T., Purton, D. G., & Thomson W. G. (2002). Mandibular implant overdentures: Comparative evaluation of the prosthodontic maintenance during the first year of service using three different systems. *International Journal of Prosthodontics*, 15, 259–266.

Wismeijer, D., van Waas, M. A. J., Mulder, J., Vermeeren, J. I. J. F., & Kalk, W. (1999). Clinical and radiological results of patients treated with three treatment modalities for overdentures on implants of the ITI Dental Implant System. *Clinical Oral Implants Research*, 10, 297–306.

Zarb, G. A. (1983). The edentulous milieu. *Journal of Prosthetic Dentistry*, 49, 825–831.

15
Clinical Applications for the Measurement of Implant Stability Using Osstell™ Mentor

Neil Meredith
Hamid Shafie

Osstell™ Mentor is the latest generation of clinical diagnostic instrumentation designed to measure the stability of a dental implant using resonance frequency analysis. This technique was developed approximately ten years ago by Professors Neil Meredith and Peter Cawley at Imperial College, London. It has evolved from an academic and research concept into a clinical diagnostic instrument benefiting everyday clinical practice (Figure 15.1).

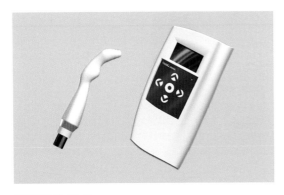

FIGURE 15.1.

The technique works by stimulating a small transducer similar to an electronic tuning fork that is attached to an implant fixture or abutment. However, the implant itself is not vibrated directly. It is the change in stiffness of the implant and surrounding tissues and its height in the surrounding bone that enables a measurement of stability to be derived from the resonance frequency of this transducer (Figure 15.2).

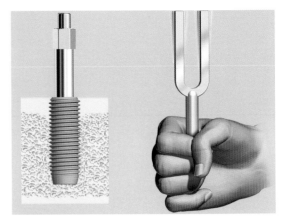

FIGURE 15.2.

In its latest form, Osstell™ Mentor presents an extremely ergonomic clinical instrument. The transducer is a small precision-made pin containing a high-quality and high-powered rare earth magnetic. The new transducer is called Smart Peg and may be screwed into the implant fixture or into an implant abutment. The Osstell™ Mentor Analyzer is a small handheld instrument with a probe that is held close to the Smart Peg (Figures 15.3 and 15.4).

The Mentor instrument senses the presence of the magnetic field from the Smart Peg and stimulates it, measuring the resonance frequency a number of times and in a number of directions. The reading is given as an Implant Stability Quotient (ISQ), derived from the resonance frequency measurements via a simple arithmetic algorithm. The ISQ is scaled 0–100 for easy clinical measurements. A typical measurement is between 40–80, where 40 represents a failed or failing implant and 80 represents an implant with the highest stabilitya (Figure 15.5).

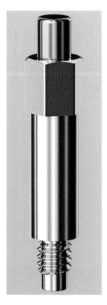

FIGURE 15.3.

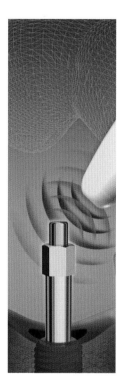

FIGURE 15.5.

Unlike its predecessors, Osstell™ Mentor measures stability in a number of directions simultaneously, rather than giving a single measurement of ISQ, if there is a clear difference in the stability of the implant in different directions due to fenestrations, dehiscence, or variations in the local anatomy. The instrument will present two ISQ values, both of which are clinically valuable and should be recorded. It often may be clinically obvious that there is such an abnormality.

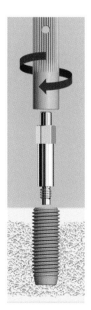

FIGURE 15.4.

CLINICAL STAGES WHEN ISQ MEASUREMENT CAN BE RECORDED

- At the time of implant placement for immediately loaded implant overdenture cases
- For one-stage implants, at the time of implant placement and/or during various clinical periods thereafter, as the implant is exposed in the oral environment
- In a two stage surgical procedure for implant overdenture cases, a second measurement can be made at the time of uncovering and attachment connection

The ISQ measurement is valuable because it makes it possible to determine if osseointegration has taken place. Generally in the mandible there should be a relatively small change in the ISQ between placement and attachment connection. The reason for this small change is that bone density is commonly much higher in the mandible than in the maxilla during the healing process. There is remodeling rather than new bone formation and a small early change. There may also be a decrease in stability over a period of a few days, but over a period of 8–10 weeks the implant stability will increase and slightly exceed that of the original stability of placement. This is an indication of a sound and healthy osseointegrated implant.

In the maxilla, it is quite different. For example, there should be lower ISQ values at implant placement than in the mandible. However, with time there is an increase in new bone formation, which has been supported by histological and radiographic studies. This new bone formation leads to a greater increase in implant stability from the initial measurements. Therefore, over a period of time in a single-stage or two-stage procedure, there should be a significant increase in the original ISQ values. Over a period of 10–20 months, the changes in stability in the mandible and the maxilla move together to create a zone of symmetrical osseointegration where the maxillary and mandibular measurements of stability will overlap.

It is thus possible to obtain valuable and useful information regarding the suitability of implants for immediate loading. Since implants are not generally immediately loaded, there are clinical conditions that affect the optimum osseointegration after implant placement in immediately loaded overdentures.

CLINICAL CONDITIONS AFFECTING THE OUTCOME OF IMMEDIATELY LOADED IMPLANTS

- Bruxism
- Heavy occlusal function
- Location of the implants
- The number of supporting implants
- Force distribution of loading conditions of the overdenture
- Bone quality and quantity

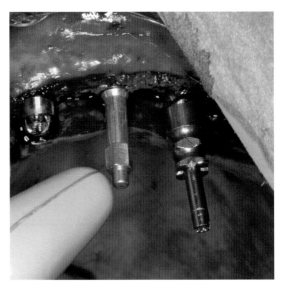

FIGURE 15.6.

ISQ measurements, however, can be an invaluable aid to the real-time measurement of clinical implant stability. This not only gives valuable information as to the placement stability of an implant at the time of insertion, but also as to how that stability is changing. For example, in the case of single-stage, immediately loaded implant supported overdentures, it is possible to monitor the stability with time, and this is strongly recommended at two, four, six, and eight weeks. In the cases of Bruxism and para-function, there are indications and reported cases that this may lead to a decrease in stability and potential failure of such implants.

Before clinical or radiographic signs are apparent, there will be a significant decrease in the ISQ measurement (e.g., from 60 down to 50). A decrease of 5 or 10 points in the ISQ at a measurement period is a sign of a noticeable decrease in stability, and corrective clinical treatment is strongly indicated. In an immediately loaded overdenture case, if after two or three weeks of loading, there is a significant decrease in ISQ, it is recommended to remove the overdenture or perform an occlusal adjustment to provide either a complete load relief to the supporting implants or eliminate overloading of the implants.

Case reports have indicated that it is possible to recover the stability and maintain the success of implants under such conditions. ISQ measurements are straightforward and simple to make. However, on occasions, if the asymmetry of the implant and the bone condition is extreme, then a double peak may occur in the implant measurement. This problem is not as much of an issue with the new Osstell™ Mentor instrumentation, but there has been a traditional point of uncertainty.

This problem occurs typically if the implant has been placed in the bone at an unusual angle or in the lower canine region. In such cases, it is recommended that the transducer be rotated until a single, clear peak measurement can be achieved. Trapping soft tissue between the implant and the bone (common if no-flap surgery has been performed) or between the implant and the Smart Peg will cause a false reading that is easily observed.

RFA measurements with Osstell™ Mentor have been designed to measure with great sensitivity the range of stiffness and stability of an implant from placement to restoration. In clinical function, the stiffness of a failed implant is considerably less; therefore, the measurements recorded by a failed implant are likely to be false and of little value.

Osstell™ Mentor can be used to measure the majority of implant systems, and information about the corresponding Smart Peg can be obtained from integration technology.

16
Follow Up and Maintenance of the Implant Overdenture

Valerie Sternberg Smith
Roy Eskow

Success of implant-supported overdentures is related both to a correct biomechanical design and maintaining a healthy oral environment. The focus in implant dentistry, all too often, is successful placement of the implant, establishing osseointegration, and building the restoration. The real driving force must be to maintain a steady state of bone around the implant for the patient's lifetime. This success will only be achieved by proper biomechanics and healthy gingival tissues with adequate dimensions and contours that will allow for ideal maintenance.

The forces generated by the overdentures in function and the constant accumulation of plaque place the success of the overdenture at risk. The nature of the soft tissue surrounding the implant component as it enters the oral cavity can influence the patient's ability to control plaque. Non-keratinized peri-implant tissues can be easily traumatized and therefore uncomfortable for the patient to perform oral hygiene. Also the shape of the soft tissue, which can be a result of the underlying residual ridge, can interfere with the proper plaque control. The tissue contours as well as the attachment assembly design must allow for easy and thorough maintenance.

CHARACTERISTICS OF IDEAL PERI-IMPLANT TISSUES

- Pink
- Firm/adherent
- Keratinized tissue circumferentially around the implant

CONSEQUENCES FOR FAILURE TO ACHIEVE CLEANSABLE ATTACHMENT DESIGN

- *Peri-Implant Mucocitis:* Inflammation limited to soft tissue
- *Peri-Implantitis:* Resorption of the bone around the implant (Figure 16.1)

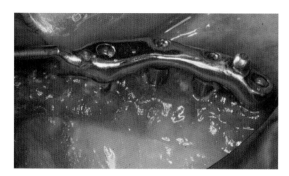

FIGURE 16.1.

- *Recession:* Exposure of the implant surface
- *Tissue Overgrowth*
- *Calculus Formation and Retention*

All attachment assemblies in the oral environment provide surfaces for bacterial growth. The plaque biofilm in proximity to the peri-implant soft tissue can result in the following peri-implant diseases:

- *Peri-Implant Mucositis:* Inflammation limited to the soft tissue
- *Peri-Implantitis:* Bone resorption around the implant

Both the patient and the clinician have a defined responsibility to care for the implant-soft tissue interface of the attachment assembly. Effective daily plaque removal prevents not only the initiation of peri-implant disease, but also the development of calculus, which can interfere with the function of the attachment assembly components.

The clinician contributes to the preventive regimen by discriminating between the presence of health and disease and by evaluating the status of the attachment assembly. The soft tissue, through which the implants enter the oral cavity, and the mucosal surfaces covered by the overdenture should be evaluated for evidence of inflammation. In addition, the examination should include palpation of the peri-implant tissues to detect bleeding or suppuration.

HOME CARE IMPLEMENTS

There are many plaque-control implements from which to choose. Those recommended should be simple and effective for the patient to use. Often patients who require implant-supported overdentures have limited anatomical access due to the extent of previous alveolar ridge resorption as well as the structural complexity of attachment assembly.

Toothbrushes

Toothbrushes should be selected based on the type of attachment assembly and the limited access to the surface intended to be cleaned.

END-TUFTED TOOTHBRUSHES   End-tufted toothbrushes may be used where the oral anatomy may limit the use of a full-headed toothbrush. These are ideal for site-specific plaque removal around stud attachments.

ACCESS BRUSH   The Access brush (Imtec Implant Company) is designed to clean the buccal and lingual surfaces of the abutment and the bar simultaneously (Figure 16.2).

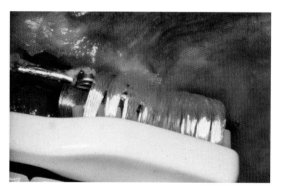

FIGURE 16.2.

INTERDENTAL BRUSHES   Interdental brushes can be used on the proximal aspect of abutments that support the bar, provided that sufficient clearance exists between the abutment, bar, and soft tissue. All interdental brushes should have a nylon or plastic coating over the center wire so the abutment is not deformed or scratched in the cleaning process.

PROXY TIP   Proxy Tip (Advanced Implant Technologies) is an all-plastic type of interdental brush that can be used as an alternative.

Flossing Cords

Floss can be used circumferentially around the abutment to clean the peri-implant crevice.

THORNTON BRIDGE AND IMPLANT CLEANER   Thornton bridge and implant cleaner is a floss with stiff threaders on both ends with a yarn-like portion in the middle. It can be an effective cleaning approach for the bar attachment assemblies. The threader allows the patient to thread the floss around the abutments and bar (Figure 16.3).

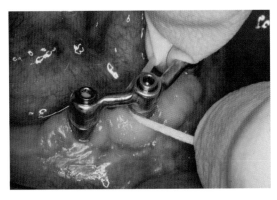

FIGURE 16.3.

POSTCARE   Postcare (Sunstar Butler) is a nylon-woven flossing cord that is abrasive enough to remove calculus. It has a pre-formed end similar to a hook, enabling the patient to thread it circumferentially around the abutment and the bar. This is a good item for patients who tend to form heavy calculus (Figures 16.4 and 16.5).

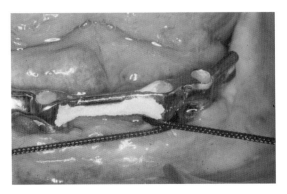

FIGURE 16.4.

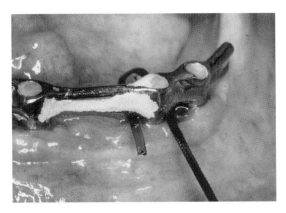

FIGURE 16.5.

Denture Brushes

Denture brushes can be used for the removable prosthesis. The patient should be directed to manually brush the underside (tissue side) of the overdenture where the attachment assembly is located. Denture tablets alone are not enough to clean the denture, and brushes must be used. Patients who are fully edentulous should be warned not to use the denture brush intraorally.

Antimicrobials

Chlorhexidine (0.12 %) should be considered if the patient demonstrates peri-implant disease. Long-term rinsing, however, can affect the patient's taste sensations. Furthermore local application can lead to stain and a more pronounced calculus accumulation. The clinician needs to weigh the benefit-to-risk quotient.

RECOMMENDED ROUTINES AT RECALL VISITS

Radiographic Examination

An essential part of assessing the peri-implant tissues is the radiograph. A baseline film should be taken at the time that the prosthesis is placed, another at six months post loading, another 12 months later, and every 2 years thereafter. The radiograph records the crestal bone level, the bone-to-implant interface, and the integrity of the implant restorative component connection.

Removal of Accretions

REMOVAL OF SOFT ACCRETIONS The clinician can use any homecare item mentioned above for removal of plaque both supra- and sub-gingival. A prophy cup with a fine prophy paste or flour of pumice can be used on the abutments and the attachment assembly.

REMOVAL OF HARD ACCRETIONS The procedure for removing hard accretions is determined by the location and tenacity of the calculus. Access to the lingual surfaces in some of these cases can be difficult to achieve with traditional instrumentation. Plastic reinforced scalers designed like a hoe or back-action chisel are ideal for these restorations.

These instruments are excellent for removal of heavy calculus on the direct lingual or facial of the abutment and attachment assembly surfaces (Figures 16.6 and 16.7).

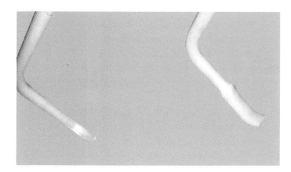

FIGURE 16.6.

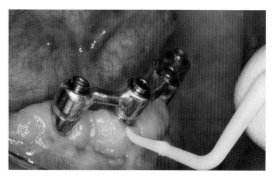

FIGURE 16.7.

RECOMMENDED INSTRUMENTS FOR HARD AND HEAVY CALCULUS

- Implant facial scaler (Premier)
- Back-action chisel (Surgical Innovations)
- Implant ultrasonic scaler (Tony Riso Co)
- Graphite piezoelectric tips (Satelec)
- Profin with plastic insert (Dentatus)

RECOMMENDED INSTRUMENTS FOR LIGHT CALCULUS THAT IS READILY ACCESSIBLE

- Implacare (Hu-Friedy)
- Prophy + scaler (Advanced Implant Technologies)
- Implant curette (Premier)
- Curette (Surgical Innovations)

Cleaning the Prosthesis

During office visits the overdenture should be placed in an ultrasonic bath with a chemical tarter-and-stain-remover solution. The clinician should then brush it with a denture brush to make certain all accretions are removed.

Evaluation of the Attachment Assembly Components

Attachment assembly components should be evaluated to ensure that retaining screws which connect the attachment to supporting implants are completely tight and secure. Furthermore the attachments components, such as clips/riders, should be evaluated to ensure proper functioning; any broken or worn-out component should be replaced (Figure 16.8).

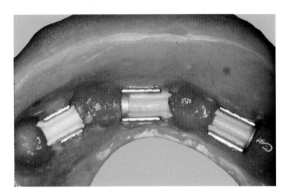

FIGURE 16.8.

In summary, preventive care consists of responsibilities of the patient and the clinician. The patient must be trained and supervised in the use of plaque-control implements.

The clinician should evaluate the peri-implant tissues, implant, and prosthetic components. In addition, debridement is performed at the appropriate intervals to remove soft and hard accretions.

REFERENCES AND ADDITIONAL READING

American Academy of Periodontology. Position paper: maintenance and treatment of dental implants, April 1995.

Baily, G., Gardner, J., Day, M., Kovanda, B. (1998). Implant surface alternations from a nonmetallic ultrasonic tip. *Journal of the Western Society Periodontology/Periodontol Abstracts*, 46(3), 69.

Briner, W. W., et al. (1986). Effect of chlorhexidine gluconate mouth rinse on plaque bacteria. *Journal of Periodontal Research*, 16, 44.

Brough, W. A., et al. (1988). The dental hygienist's role in the maintenance of osseointegrated dental implants. *Journal of Dental Hygiene*, 62(9), 448.

Callan, D., O'Mahony, B., & Cobb, C. (1998). Loss of crestal bone around dental implants: a retrospective study, *Implant Dentistry* 7, 258.

Daniels, A. (1993). The importance of accurate charting for maintaining dental implants. *Journal of Practical Hygiene*, 9 Sep/Oct.

English, C. (1995). Hygiene, maintenance, and prosthodontic concerns for the infirm patient: clinical report and discussion. *Implant Dentistry*, 4, 166.

Felo, A., et al. (1997). Effects of chlorhexidine irrigation on peri-implant maintenance. *American Journal of Dentistry*, 10, 107.

Gantes, B. & Nilveus, R. (1991). The effects of different hygiene instruments on titanium implant surface modifications: SEM observation. *International Journal of Periodontics and Restorative Dentistry*, 11(3), 225.

Ganz S. (1993). Communication: an essential building block for a successful implant practice—the hygienist's role. *Journal of Practical Hygiene*, 2(5), 27.

Garber, D. A. (1991). Implants—the name of the game is still maintenance. *Compendium* 12(12), 876.

Garg, A., Duarte, F., & Funari, K. (1997). Hygienic maintenance of dental implants: the key to long term success. *Journal of Practical Hygiene*, 6(2), 13.

Garg, A. *Practical Implant Dentistry*. Dallas: Taylor Publishing, 1997.

Gould, T. R. L., Brunette, D. M., & Westbury, L. (1981). The attachment mechanisms of epithelial cells to titanium in vitro. *Journal of Periodontal Research*, 16, 611.

Grondahl, K. & Lekholm, U. (1997). The predictive value of radiographic diagnosis of implant instability. *International Journal of Oral & Maxillofacial Implants*, 12, 59.

Hallmon, W., Waldrop, T., Meffert, R., & Wade, B. A comparative study of the effects of metallic, nonmetallic, and sonic instrumentation on titanium abutment surfaces. *International Journal of Oral & Maxillofacial Implants*, 11, 96, 1996.

Karayiannia, A., Lang, N. P., Joss, A., & Nyman, S. (1992). Bleeding on probing as it relates to probing pressure and gingival health in patients with a reduced but healthy periodontium. A clinical study. *Journal of Clinical Periodontology*, 19, 471.

Koutsonikos, A., Fednco, J., & Yunka, R. (1996). Implant maintainance. *Journal of Practical Hygiene*, 5(2), 11.

Kracher, C. M. & Smith, W. S. (1998). Oral health maintenance of dental implants: a literature review. *Dental Assistant*, 67(5), 2.

Lang, N. P., Adler, R., Joss, A., & Nyman, S. (1990). Absence of bleeding on probing: an indicator of periodontal stability. *Journal of Clinical Periodontology*, 17, 714.

LeBeau, J. (1997). Maintaining the long-term health of the dental implant and the implant bone restoration. *Compendium of Continuing Education in Oral Hygiene*, 3(3), 3.

Matarasso, S., et al. (1996). Maintenance of implants: an in vitro study of titanium implant surface characteristics of titanium implant surface modifications subsequent to the application of different prophylaxis procedures. *Clinical Oral Implants Research*, 7, 64.

Meffert, R. (1995). Implantology and the dental hygienist's role. *Journal of Practical Hygiene*, 4(5), 12.

Meschenmoser, A., et al. (1996). Effects of various hygiene procedures on the surface characteristics of titanium abutments. *Journal of Periodontology*, 67, 229–235.

Minichetti, J. & Colplanis, N. (1997). Considerations in the maintenance of the dental implant patient. *Journal of Practical Hygiene*, 2(5), 15.

Mobelli, A., van Oosten, M. A. C., Schurch, E., & Lang, N. P. (1987). The microbiota associated with successful or failing osseointegrated titanium implants. *Oral Microbial Immunology*, 2, 145.

Papaioannou, W., Quirynen, M., & van Steenberghe, D. (1996). The influence of periodontics on the subgingival flora around implants in partially edentulous patients. *Clinical Oral Implants Research*, 7, 405.

Probster, L. & Lin, W. (1992). Effects of fluoride prophylactic agents on titanium surfaces. *International Journal of Oral & Maxillofacial Implants*, 2(7), 390.

Shuman, E. Early crestal bone loss. Why? *Journal of Practical Hygiene*, 42, May/Jun 1997.

Siegrist, A. E., et al. (1986). Efficiency of nursing with chlorhexidine digluconate in comparison of phenolic and plant alkaloid compounds. *International Journal of Periodontal Research*, 21(16), 60.

Silverstein, L., et al. (1994). The microbiota of the peri-implant region in health and disease. *Implant Dentistry*, 3, 170.

Steele, D. & Orton, G. (1992). Dental implants: clinical procedures and homecare considerations. *Journal of Practical Hygiene*, 4, 9.

Strong, S. (1995). The dental implant maintenance visit. *Journal of Practical Hygiene*, 4(5), 29.

Technique for implant polishing. *Journal of Practical Hygiene*, 35, Mar/Apr 1997.

Tillmanns, H., et al. (1997). Evaluation of three different dental implants in ligature-induced peri-implantitis in the beagle dog. Part II. Clinical evaluation. *International Journal of Oral & Maxillofacial Implants*, 12(5), 6–11.

Tillmanns, H., et al. (1998). Evaluation of three different dental implants in ligature-induced peri-implantitis in the beagle dog. Part II. Histology and microbiology. *International Journal of Oral & Maxillofacial Implants*, 13, 59.

Wilken, E. *Clinical Practice of the Dental Hygienist* (7th edition). Pennsylvania: Williams & Wilkins, 1994.

Yukna, R. (1993). Optimizing clinical success with implant: maintenance and care. *Compendium of Continuing Education in Dentistry*, 15, 554.

17

Core Principles of the Successful Implant Practice

Sean Crabtree

In coaching peak dental practices all across North America for nearly a decade, I have found the principles of success to be the same regardless of the clinician's area of focus. However, the specifics of creating the peak performing implant practice of your dreams require that implementation of these principles be combined with a strong business model perhaps in the most traditional sense. For some this can be a stretch, as most dental schools have no significant curriculum focus on business.

While the success of any business is certainly beyond the scope of a few pages, my intent is to share, principally from a business standpoint, that which I have found to be at the core of any successful implant practice. This core model can then become the foundation on which all areas of the practice rest. A similar outcome of the following pages is to provoke thought that may challenge current beliefs that can sabotage your success.

VISION, TEAM, SYSTEMS, SALES, MARKETING

Core Belief: My Practice Is an Entrepreneurial Business.

My first challenge to you is to see your practice as not a practice at all. Instead see it as I see it—an entrepreneurial business. As such, it can become an asset that can be invested in, bought, sold, and even transitioned to new ownership. As you'll see, this view serves your patients, your team, and your bottom-line profitability.

With that in mind, consider that an overall picture of your business might look much like a spinning saucer. The business is divided into four segments that spin around a central point—your vision. Your vision gives direction, meaning, purpose and clarity to each of the four segments (Figure 17.1).

Center Point VISION

Defining and communicating your identity.

In his book *The 21 Indispensable Qualities of a Leader*, John Maxwell titles one of the chapters,

216

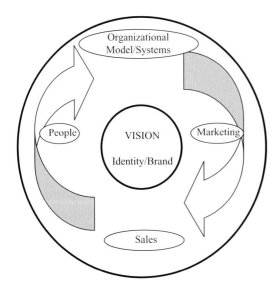

FIGURE 17.1.

"VISION: You Can Seize Only What You Can See." The word "vision" has become a buzzword in referring to business and desired outcomes, perhaps causing it to lose some of its original meaning. However, your vision of exactly who it is, how it is, and what it is that you and your team want to be for yourselves, each other, and your patients must be at the heart of your business. It must incorporate your beliefs, values, and attitude about business and indeed life in general. Once clearly defined, it must be at the very center of everything that you do, everything you are, and how your patients perceive you. Any and all decisions must be filtered through this vision so that it becomes your identity and creates the culture of your practice. Great questions to get you started include:

- How much do I want to earn in the next twelve months?
- How many days am I willing to work to earn it?
- How many patients am I willing to see to earn it?
- How do I want my practice to look?
- How do I want my team to look?
- How do I want my patients to look?

Once answering these questions with your team, you'll then begin to shape a single paragraph that will become your identity and indeed the culture of your practice. It must be the higher purpose that motivates everyone on your team. This identity you've created will become the brand that separates you from others in the marketplace and will be communicated in all forms of marketing.

Organizational Model/Systems

- People VISION Marketing
- Identity/brand
- Sales
- Organization and systems
- Creating a better mousetrap!

For your entrepreneurial business to be a solid asset, two components must be in place. First, it must have a model that allows it to be self sustaining. That is, while the people you have in place can bring their own strengths to support the systems within the model, the model itself drives success and must be the continual focus. Secondly, with this focus in mind, every single person, including the doctor, must be replaceable. In other words, if decision-making and progress lie at the feet of any one person, the saucer slows its spin and that person becomes the bottleneck. Similarly, when that person is no longer there, the business can cease to exist. So the model, by design, must bring success, and this will be accomplished in part by empowering the people inside it to make decisions.

Without a successful model in place, the owner of a small business must be the human resources manager, the sales manager, the manufacturing supervisor, the collection manager, the president of marketing and even the bookkeeper. In addition to these roles, the owner of an implant practice is the only one in the office who can actually perform the production. Again, add all this to the fact that most dental schools spend little or no time on business management, and the whole thing can begin to seem overwhelming. The organizational model that follows is what I call the *front line management* concept. It directly addresses this and the previously mentioned components, when applied with key system strategies (Figure 17.2).

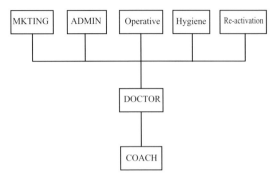

FIGURE 17.2.

Based loosely on what I learned as an undergraduate in the school of business and with my own additions and twists, this model allows for the doctor to make a staff person directly responsible and accountable for a respective front line area. This is not to divide duties, as you'll see in the system layout. Instead it is to have a person responsible for game plans in a particular area and accountable for the results in that area. In the example, a typical implant practice could be divided into five departments: marketing, administration, operative, hygiene, and reactivation. The front line reports directly to the doctor, and both report to the coach. From the bottom up the coach supports the doctor in a leadership role and supports the team to ensure that these areas are getting results. The doctor supports the team from an informational and emotional standpoint. The model is customized depending on the circumstances of the practice. If, for example, a doctor had a full-time, in-house lab that made dentures, there would be a sixth front line box labeled "lab" added to the mix.

This model supports the doctor by freeing him to produce implant dentistry as well as focus on long-term directional business issues. The staff is then enabled to take on more of a partnership role by being empowered to create and implement game plans. In order to support them, decision-making criteria must be in place. Four possible questions for decision-making criteria include:

1. Is it good for our patients?
   No. Create another game plan.
   Yes. How? Go to question 2.
2. Is it good for our referral sources?
   No. Create another game plan.
   Yes. How? Go to question 3.
3. Is it good for our team?
   No. Create another game plan.
   Yes. How? Go to question 4.
4. Is it good for our bottom line?
   No. Create another game plan.
   Yes. How? Implement the game plan.

The final piece of this model is the system layout that supports it. It is based on five questions that front line staff will use to manage each area. The intent is to ensure constant growth by being proactive rather than reactive in your management style. Weekly use of this system at staff meetings will support this focus.

Front Line Accountability System
1. What opportunities exist for improvement in this area?
2. What is a game plan that would possibly enable us to meet this challenge?
3. Which part of this plan will I do, and what do I need support to do?
4. How will I measure the results of this game plan?
5. How will I coach and report on this game plan to my team?

In his book *Leadership*, Rudolph Giuliani explains how, by using a model of accountability and a system he dubbed *Compstat*, he reduced crime by 70 percent in New York in just a few years. Similarly, I see amazing boosts in production and collection in practices that implement the above model and system.

People

Creating your best asset!

As mentioned earlier, all four of these segments will be driven by and filtered through your vision. When it comes to the people who will eventually make up your team, it is most important to use your vision as a hiring tool. My belief is that choosing the right people on the front end is paramount to a successful implant practice.

A few things to consider when assembling a team:

- Make sure they will fit with who it is, how it is, and what it is (your vision) that you want your business to be.

  It may sound like a given, but it is a big challenge that I see throughout the profession. People are chosen without giving thought to the broader vision. You have incorporated your beliefs, attitude, and values into your vision. It is imperative that this person fits with those fundamentals. Otherwise, he or she will be at odds with everything your team and your business represents. How do you find out what this person's beliefs, attitude, and values are? One way is simply to ask, keeping two things in mind. First, make sure you are within the boundaries of labor law and fair hiring practices for your state and country. Second, if interviewing is part of your process, remember that this person will display their best "game face" in answering questions. Another way is to share your beliefs and values and how that fits into your business. Then gauge their responses.
- When talking to a prospective team member, picture the person talking about you to a patient.

  When this person communicates, what are they saying to you outside of the words? Studies show that human beings communicate with tonality and physiology much more than with words. When you picture this person communicating with a prospective patient or a prospective referral source about you, do you see that as a fit for your vision?
- Is this someone you can see yourself spending time with outside the office?

  This does not mean that you will. However, what better way to gauge whether or not this person is a good fit? My assertion is that any staff member you have that you would not spend time with outside the office is probably not currently "fitting in." That person may do a wonderful "job." You and your team, however, need more than that.
- When it's time to add a team member, let the team decide who that person will be.

When this is handled properly, it will not only result in a great team member, but it will also promote unity and cohesion with the others, which, in turn, will save you much grief later. Have the team conduct the search through interviews and other processes, and then narrow the list to three people they really like and think will be a great fit. The doctor will then conduct his or her own interviews of the three and make the final choice. If none of the prospects seems to work for the doctor, the team continues the search.

- Hire for the right reason.

  The most significant mistake I see consistently is basing the decision to hire on experience only. Training is certainly an issue, and training will be required regardless of the level of experience. Instead, place more emphasis on beliefs, attitude, and values. Experience can be acquired, especially if these principles are in place. In the long run, it will serve your patients, your team, and your bottom line to hire based on these principles rather than experience.
- Analyze your strengths and weaknesses and those of your team.

  In finding the best person for the job, make sure the strengths they bring to the table not only support the position, but that they complement the weaknesses that exist, as well. This will require a serious look at yourself and your team. The team will perform best when each member brings different strengths and contributions to support the overall outcome.
- Have the courage to remove staff members who are not a good fit with your beliefs, attitude, and values.

  This seems to be common sense, yet I see different teams encounter this challenge on a continuing basis. Let's face it. There is no easy way to ask a team member to leave. However, it is possible to look at the situation in an empowering way. It is not a personal attack on the person's character or work ethic. It is simply a question of proper fit. If this is the case, then the employee is probably also not happy with the situation. I remember a particular instance with a periodontist who had a team member who needed to go. He and I brainstormed all the strengths and weaknesses he saw in her and then he spoke with colleagues who he knew that needed staff members. He found a general dentist who was looking for someone with her strengths and qualifications. The colleague called her the next day for an interview. She left and has been there four years. She never missed a paycheck. While I am not suggesting this will work for everyone, or even that you try it, the principle of making sure it is not personal and is sincerely helping your staff, even if it means helping them be somewhere else, will serve all involved. As the old saying goes, a bad apple will ruin the bunch.

Hiring good people is only part of the process. Once the "right people" are on board, you must take several steps to keep them. While the list is long and varied as to what it takes to keep good people, following are a few key points:

- Give your team members something to work towards beyond a paycheck.

  Most studies show that money is not a sole motivator for anyone in the long term. However, bonuses are great incentives to exceed set goals. Take care to ensure the goals are set high enough so the bonuses do not become expected. Expected bonuses can be perceived as paychecks and lose their value as incentives. Bonuses can also take the form of trips or gift certificates, for example. In addition, make the team a part of your "grand scheme." In other words, put the vision out in front; it's this higher purpose that they are there for, not just the paycheck.

- Invest in their growth and consistently acknowledge it.

  Ray Crock said that when we are green, we grow, when we are ripe, we rot. Most people may justify, even to themselves, that they leave a position for better hours and pay. Studies show that people leave because of lack of acknowledgements and/or because they felt as though they were going nowhere. Make continuing education a part of who you are and take staff along consistently. Then find reasons to acknowledge them. Some business owners are naturally gifted at

acknowledging team members. If you are not, start a good habit by beginning each day with ten quarters in your left pocket and challenge yourself to have them in your right pocket by the end of the day by moving one at a time when you give a heartfelt acknowledgement.

- Become a leader.

Leadership can be learned. While this subject is beyond the scope of these pages, it is one of the most important aspects of keeping great people. Read and learn all you can about becoming an effective leader. John Maxwell has written many books on the subject, as have many others. My belief is that leadership begins with the way you think and the first step is always to see things as better than they are. Additionally:

- Make motivation a part of who you are.
- Never see things as worse than they actually are.
- Become a great influencer.
- Acknowledge, acknowledge, acknowledge.
- Do what you say, when you say.
- Begin all corrections with what is working.
- Acknowledge, acknowledge, acknowledge.

While strong clinical skills lay the foundation for your trade, the success of your business depends on how well you master the relationships with your team, referral sources, and patients.

Sales

Embrace the concept.

Use the word "sales" in a roomful of healthcare practitioners, and you can observe all variations of facial contortions. Many equate negative connotations to the word and think in terms of used car salesmen, or vacuum cleaner salesmen. While there are certainly professionals in both these areas, they don't immediately come to mind for some. I have addressed this issue from coast to coast for nearly 10 years and continue to do so. Consider the following:

Fiction: I am healthcare professional, sales is beneath me.
Fact: You are the healthcare professional; it is your responsibility to influence your patients' decision-making to help them choose

the treatment plan that will give them what they want.

Fiction: You cannot sell healthcare, you can only offer solutions to the patient's problems. It is up to the patient to do whatever she or he think, is best.

Fact: Again, you are the healthcare professional; you know all the benefits of the treatment you provide. You owe it to your patients to find out not only what is happening clinically, but indeed to find out what they want. Then, show them how what you have to offer will get them what they want.

Fiction: I am competing with other general and implant dentists for market share.

Fact: Your competition is the professional salesperson who sells the big screen plasma TVs, the vacation travel packages, the home audio components, new cars, or anything else that goes after the same discretionary dollars you are. Patients see what you offer as a luxury item; therefore, you are offering a product and service in the same category as the things just mentioned. The only solution is to embrace the idea of becoming a professional salesperson to compete.

Fiction: Salespeople are pushy and I would have to become that to be good at sales.

Fact: Some salespeople in the world give sales a bad name, just as some dentists, specialists, and attorneys give their respective careers a bad name. The truth is that sales is a respected profession and those who master it are paid very well. If your intent is to have a successful implant practice, it is imperative that you make a conscious decision to embrace sales and master it.

Very simply put, sales is the art of making friends. It is finding out what people want and giving it to them. If you do not master this concept, you are destined to hear one inevitable sentence from each patient, "How much does it cost?" My challenge to you is that from this point forward, any time you hear that question, see these words in your mind's eye:

THE PATIENT SEES NO VALUE.

Hygienists see this concept in action nearly daily. They can show a patient how to floss, talk about what flossing accomplishes, put the mirror in the patient's hand so they see flossing, and in general spend lots of time "educating" patients on flossing. This is a free service to the patients and yet many will simply never do it because even though they were educated, they weren't sold. So they did not see the value.

The doctor sees it when he has a patient in the chair, perhaps someone he knows, who obviously has money. He talks of how many implants are needed, spends time educating the patient on how the procedure will go, the time involved, and all the care that will go into making sure the patient is taken care of, but when the patient learns the price, she says she just can't afford that. On the way out the door, she changes her hygiene appointment because of a month-long vacation in Australia and then gets in her Lexus and drives away.

The vast majority of my lectures and training are based strictly in this area. Professionally trained salespeople will tell you that no one has ever or will ever buy anything based on price. We all buy things based on the value we perceive them to have, as they relate to how they will benefit us. Therefore the focus must be on creating value. Doing this is as easy as finding out what patients want and then showing them how they can have what they want by purchasing what you have to offer. It is best remembered by the acronym PLAST:

- Probe by asking open-ended questions.
- Listen for emotional values.
- Amplify the pain.
- Save them from pain with benefits.
- Trial close.

PROBE BY ASKING OPEN-ENDED QUESTIONS There is no better question than a direct one. The doctor examines the patient and knows exactly what prosthesis he is going to recommend. However before making the recommendation he asks, "What are the most important things to you about your teeth?"

LISTEN FOR EMOTIONAL VALUES The doctor then listens for emotional responses. It is important to continue to ask these questions until the patient provides an emotional response. Write down the response and continue to probe until you get three emotional responses in total. Writing down the responses tells the patient that you're listening and that it is important. Following is a sample question/response dialog:

Question: "What is most important to you about having teeth?"
Non-Emotional Response: "That I am able to chew properly."
Question: "What is important to you about chewing properly?"
Emotional Response: "I know this sounds crazy, but my most favorite thing in the world is a T-bone steak, and right now these dentures just flop around in my mouth and I'm not able to chew. I am tired of trying to make them work with that sticky glue."
Question: "What else is most important to you about having teeth?"
Non-Emotional Response: "That they not look like dentures."
Question: "What is most important to you about the way they look?"
Emotional Response: "My grandson told me the other day that I had horse teeth. Tears just came to my eyes. I want something that is part of me, not something I put in a glass."

It is interesting to note that an actual patient told a doctor this in an office I coach, just after we had role-played these steps. Remember that it is not the dentistry that is important—no one wants dentistry. It is the emotional benefit that the patient is after.

AMPLIFY THE PAIN   Remember, all of us buy based on emotions. So here I am speaking of the emotional pain. This is the transitional point. It is here that the patient takes ownership of the problem. Without this step in place, you as the healthcare provider own the problem, and the patient's response will again be, "How much does it cost?" To amplify pain, ask a question that does the work for you. Questions that amplify pain might be:

- How long have you felt this way?
- How does it feel now?

- How will it feel in the future if you continue in this way?

Using the last emotional response, the dialog might sound like the following:

Question: "When your grandson told you that, how did that make you feel?"
Response: "I was embarrassed and ashamed. I really want to get this fixed."

SAVE THEM FROM PAIN WITH BENEFITS   While the patient is in pain mode, you now get to be the hero and save them with the benefits of the services you provide. This is a key distinction. You cannot save them with the treatment plan you provide; instead, you must save them with the *benefits* of this treatment plan. Now is the time to recommend treatment and bridge the gap between what the patient wants and what you have to offer. Use verbiage such as "what that means to you is." In the same scenario, it might sound like the following:

"After getting a good look at your x-rays and what is going on in your mouth and now knowing what is most important to you, I would recommend *this kind of implant supported overdenture*. What that means to you is that you'll be able to enjoy that T-bone steak, you'll no longer have to use that sticky glue, and your grandson will be proud of his grandmother's smile."

TRIAL CLOSE   Trial close. If you have done everything properly up to this point, you'll have no trouble closing. If there is still some value yet to be discovered, simply reiterate the things the patient said were important, and then start from the top again.

A major area of opportunity that has come along in the past few years is in the area of patient financing. Never before in the history of dentistry has it been easier to afford major dental work. There are at least nine financing companies that I consistently recommend. From 90-days, no-interest to the patient and no fees to the doctor, to as much as 60-months for nominal fees.

As with anything, the key is in the orchestration. Unfortunately, so many offices get so far with the patient and then lose the big cases in the financing. Make sure that your administrative accountability person is orchestrating the verbiage properly. As an example, I was in an office recently when the patient asked if the office would allow her to pay them "a little at a time." The administrative person said, "No. We don't do financing, but we'll set you up with a third party to finance it."

While there is no reason for any dental office to ever do in-house financing, this is not the way to handle this question. If a patient ever asks if you can finance it say sure, we partner with *xyz*, just have a seat here and we'll get it started. Role-playing verbiage like this in every scenario is important to do consistently. The scary part is that most big cases are lost in bad verbiage over the phone before you even get a chance to see the patient.

Marketing

You are only limited by your own imagination!

While a whole book could be dedicated to marketing for the implant practice, there are several focuses and factors to keep in mind. As with each segment, your vision must be the center point. By properly communicating your vision to your team, your patients, and the general public, it will become your brand. Your brand is how people can identify with you. It is what separates you from others who do what you do. The environment in your practice should live around this brand. It should become the culture of who you are—your identity. Everything discussed up to this point is what makes up this identity. This is where marketing starts.

- Internal marketing is the most effective and least expensive form.

    Since the beginning of time it seems, word-of-mouth referral was the best source of marketing. Even with the advent of the Internet, the same is true today. The key is to devise a plan that orchestrates it comfortably for your team and maintains the focus for the life of your practice. There are many great books on the subject; get one or several and become a student of marketing. If room permitted, I would share what my offices do to get results in this area. Again, role-playing with video is a tool I often use for referral marketing.

- Target your marketing to your vision.

    When marketing an implant practice, it is extremely important to let your vision dictate how you will define yourself in the marketplace. In other words, if what excites you about implants is smile re-creation, your marketing will be much different than if you are interested mainly in prosthetic applications. Your marketing must be targeted to the proper patient.

    To target your marketing, find out as much as you can about the demographics in your area. The chamber of commerce is a good start. Your dental supply company can get you very specific information by area. Again, obtain as much information as possible—age, marital status, income, career, commute time, hobbies, shopping, and so on. The Internet is a great source, as well. Then begin to paint as specific a picture as possible of your ideal patient from this information. Male or female, age, kids, where they shop, their leisure activities, whether they have a long morning commute or a short drive, and so on. Then, begin to think of how you might interface with this person.

- Consistency is key to market penetration.

    By some accounts, the average consumer is bombarded by nearly three thousand advertisements a day. Because of that, we have become numb, and it takes seeing, watching, or hearing the ad many times to digest what the ad is saying, what it is offering, and what action is required. By keeping your marketing message consistent and changing only the offer and action, that time frame can be reduced.

- Referral sources are key, but they are not do or die.

    A challenge I often see is that a doctor will see his referrals from other doctors as the only real source of marketing. The truth of the matter is that there are many more, sometimes better, alternatives. One great way is to market directly to patients through seminars. A seminar is a great way to hold yourself out as the expert. From a marketing standpoint, it is one of the few ways to ensure that your dollars are going right to a specific target— everyone in the room is there because they are interested in implant-supported overdentures.

- Create alliances.

  Find other companies who are outside dentistry and going after the same target market and then partner with them. This could be as simple as customizing offers for their clients about your services, or as formal as an exclusive reciprocal marketing relationship.

- Always reward referrals.

  The fact that most offices do not reward their referrals makes your rewards even more valuable—people will notice. Now you have someone accountable to make sure there is a consistent game plan and constant implementation. Similarly you'll be tracking results daily.

My final advice is to get a coach to support you in everything discussed up to this point. Even if you have been trained in this arena, someone who is far enough outside the game to keep an eye on the ball, no matter where it is on the field, is invaluable. There are many great coaches available; find one with a proven track record who can relate to you like a best friend. Your return will be triple-fold.

WHY MAKING IMPLANT OVERDENTURES CAN MAKE YOUR RESTORATIVE PRACTICE CLICK

Paul Homoly, DDS

Dr. Tom was having trouble with dentures. Not his dentures—Tom has a full set of fine teeth. No, he was having trouble with his patients' dentures. Or, more specifically, the lack thereof.

"I just don't see many patients who need implant overdentures," Tom was telling me following one of my workshops. "I can't make them if they don't walk in the door."

Tom is about 30 years old with a busy general practice. He does a lot of cosmetic dentistry and traditional fixed prosthetics, restoring one to three teeth at a time. He wants to expand his practice into rehabilitative care but seems to be stuck doing smaller cases.

"How many overdentures did you make last year," I asked.

"Very few, probably less than five."

"Your problem is that you have too many patients with teeth in your practice," I told him. "Too many teeth can interfere with practice growth." Tom laughed, but stopped after he realized I wasn't kidding.

"I suspect most of your patients are plus or minus five years of your age. Your circle of influence—friends, family, acquaintances—is predominately under forty years old. How many people in your circle of influence wear dentures?"

"None of my friends do. A few of my relatives do, but they're not patients in my practice," he replied.

"Tom, if you want to do more overdenture cases, you must do two things: First, you need to age your patient base by one or two decades. Next, you need to attract the partially and fully edentulous patient to your practice. It's like we're in the car repair business. Would we do more work by focusing on new cars or old cars? Old cars. Tom, you need more 'old cars' in your practice," I said.

Like many dentists, Tom is caught in the generation gap—the gap between himself and the patients he wants to treat. Tom's generation and that of most of his patients is too young to support a rehabilitative implant dentistry practice.

Attracting Older Patients

A predictable way to attract patients who are at least fifty years old and need complex restorative care is to market to the full-denture patients. There are some solid reasons why marketing to full-denture patients is great for your restorative practice.

First, when you market to the fully edentulous patient, they respond well to your messages.

The deepest and most devastating disability in dentistry for most patients is total edentulism. Unlike a thirty-year-old with a missing first molar, the older totally edentulous patient is more profoundly affected by her dental condition. It affects her health, appearance, and self-confidence. The full-denture patient is aware of the problem every moment. Because of this awareness of their profound disability, they respond well to your marketing messages.

Second, marketing to full-denture patients will attract patients with a wide variety of dentistry needs—implant surgery, hard- and soft-tissue engineering procedures, oral surgery, extensive prosthetic treatment—people who want to look better, feel better, and speak better. I marketed to the fully edentulous patient for 20 years. My primary purpose was to treat dental implant patients. In the process of attracting the fully edentulous patient, I also attracted patients who needed cosmetic care and crown and bridge work, which kept my full-time associate very busy and happy.

Third, older patients are willing to spend on their dental health. There is an unmistakable passage we all experience when we realize we're growing older. A full denture is the icon of old age. Many older patients have the money and are willing to spend what it takes to postpone the emotional tolls of the aging process.

The first rule when marketing implant overdentures is appealing to the emotions of the target market, and the emotions of the target market have two components: Things they want more of, and things they want less of. They are pulled toward things that they want more of and pushed away from things they want less of. Smart marketing of implant overdentures does both—it pulls patients toward what they want and pushes them away from what they don't.

The leading pull for most women is aesthetics and for most men it's function. Women are pulled toward better face and lip support, whiter teeth, more natural-looking denture base shades, and more display of teeth when talking and smiling. Men are pulled toward being able to chew steak, eat corn on the cob, hold a pipe between their teeth, and speak more clearly.

The push, what removable denture patients want less of, is the opposite of the pull. For women the push is looking old; having short, dull teeth; having cheap-looking teeth, and suffering from facial creases. A phenomenally strong push for women is being seen without their dentures. The push for men is soft diets, inconvenience, and slurred speech.

Case Acceptance for Complete Dentistry

Just knowing what Tom needs in his practice to increase his implant overdenture practice is not enough. For most dentists, performing sophisticated dental care is easier than convincing the patient to accept these kind of treatment modalities. The limits to which we treat our patients are usually not determined by our clinical skills. The limits are set by our relationship skills.

Adapted from my book *Dentists: An Endangered Species*, the following sections describe some guidelines for case acceptance.

INCREASE THE IMPACT OF YOUR LANGUAGE   Increase the impact of your language by injecting energy in your voice and having an engaging attitude with your patients. Give people your full attention. Don't look at their record or a radiograph as you speak. Hold eye contact as you listen and speak. Most of my clients break eye contact half the time during a conversation. Let patients know you beyond your role as a dentist; let them know you as a parent, spouse, athlete, and so on. This disclosure of your other side expands the patient's associations with dentistry, relates with you on a personal level, and establishes a sense of trust.

DO NOT RELY ON PATIENT EDUCATION   The older patient has heard it all before. The last thing they need is to hear another lecture about plaque and floss, or watch another video on home care. Traditionally in dentistry we believe that patient education raises the patient's dental IQ, thereby leading to case acceptance. I disagree. I believe the leading criteria for case acceptance is patient readiness.

When patients are ready, they'll act. Readiness comes from other areas of the their life—divorce, promotion, death in the family, sudden poor health, and so on. We don't make patients ready through the process of patient education.

Instead, focus on finding patients who are ready. This is the function of marketing—to attract people who are compelled to have fine dentistry. Case acceptance is linked to marketing to people who are ready but don't know who or where you are. Marketing is the invitation. Spend less time trying to make patients ready and more time on identifying those who are.

KNOW YOUR PATIENT'S BUDGET BEFORE YOU RECOMMEND REHABILITATIVE CARE   The big fear in case acceptance is not the fear of hearing "No." It's the fear of hearing "Hell no!" and watching the patient streak out the front door, requesting that their records be sent down the street! A great way to avoid the anger and embarrassment many patients experience after they hear the fees is to know their budget before you recommend care. This is done at the end of the examination appointment just before they schedule for the consultation. Suggest to them that they think about their budget. Here's a phrase that has worked for hundreds of my clients: "I'm really good about staying within a budget if I know I need to. Have you thought about your budget?" Don't push for a dollar value. Just plant the seeds that at the next appointment you'll discuss money. "Next time we'll discuss your care, and I guarantee you I'm good at staying within my patients' budgets."

Usually the patient is the first to talk about money. That's a mistake with rehabilitative care. You should be the first one bringing up the issue of money. Tell them you'll stay within their budget. Then if they object to your fee, tell them that's why you asked about the budget. With fee objections, suggest that you do their case over time, staying within their budget. By being budget-oriented, you'll end up doing many cases for $5,000, instead of no cases for $10,000.

In closing our conversation, I gave Tom some action steps to follow in order to increase his practice.

Step One: Upgrade his implant overdenture denture clinical techniques.

Step Two: Direct-mail his patients who are over 45 years of age, highlighting his new and/or improved implant-overdenture denture services.

Step Three: Speak to civic and church groups about the miracle of modern dentistry.

Step Four: Host public seminars about implant overdentures.

Step Five: Team up with colleagues who share his vision and cooperatively advertise to attract the older patient.

In a year's time, Tom will be on the road to a more lucrative implant practice. And you can be, too.

BRANDING OF AN IMPLANT PRACTICE

Andreas Charalambous, AIA

In every profession, and more so in organizations such as dental practices that deal with the public, creating a strong *identity* and *branding* of your practice can make the difference between success and failure.

Because potential patients are unable, in most instances, to immediately quantify the quality of the care provided by the doctor, they rely on other clues to tell them that they are in good hands: The quality and attention to detail in the built environment (the office space itself, the updated and modern equipment, the lighting of the space, how comfortable the patient feels while waiting for treatment, as well as how comfortable they feel while being treated,) are as important as the quality of the treatment they get from the doctor and staff.

Identity Ambassadors

Just as important as the quality of the built environment and other sensory experiences (how the patients are greeted when they arrive, the kind of music they hear while they are on hold on the phone, and so forth) are the visual materials that the practice uses to introduce and represent itself to the public. These materials, starting with the practice logo, begin to create a strong brand for your practice that sets it apart from your competition. The understanding of the brand value early on can make the difference between doing well and doing great.

Everything that is being sent out to, or being seen by, the public matters. They become the ambassadors of your practice at any given moment.

Followings are some examples of identity ambassadors for the practice:

- Business cards
- Letterhead and envelopes that the practice uses for written communication
- Announcements sent to the public on various occasions (relocation announcement, holiday wishes, personal cards, advertising, banners or posters in fundraiser or other events that promote the name and good aura that the practice builds, and so on)
- The practice website; as a general rule the site should have a simple and clever design. This allows a potential new or existing patient to easily navigate through it to find information.

It is important that all these materials are well coordinated and send a consistent message to the public. The branding of the implant practice needs to be smart and appropriate to the field of implant dentistry and appealing to the prospective patients' demographic.

Another element that is important, especially in an implant practice, is introducing the personal factor of who the doctor is and his/her level of expertise in the field of implant dentistry. The common concept of seeing the neighborhood dentist for routine dental care usually doesn't apply to the field of implant dentistry. People understand that there is more complexity in implant dentistry than regular dental care, so they do extensive research to find the best doctor with the most experience for this kind of treatment modality. If the branding of your practice as the place to go for implant treatment is weak, potential patients may bypass your practice and go to another office which has done a better job of identifying itself as capable of offering the services they are looking for. You might lose the patient to another better-branded company, even if you are a better implantologist. All these elements need to be incorporated in the mix while the branding of the practice is being created.

The following sections discuss the initial steps you may want to consider to begin your branding process.

External Marketing Objectives

- Distinguish yourself from other dentists in your area.
- Increase implant IQ of targeted demographic.
- Build momentum by creating consistency in your messages.
- Create an image for yourself as an implantologist.

Marketing Research

- What are the demographics in your area?
  US Census Bureau: www.census.gov
  US Department of Commerce, Bureau of Economics Analysis: www.bea.doc.gov
- Who are your competitors and what type of marketing are they doing?
- What types of patients are your primary focus?

Create a Brand Name for Your Practice

- Avoid individual or long names.
- Give an identity to your practice.
- Choose a name with an acceptable abbreviation.
- Make sure the domain name for your brand is available.

Website

- Secure an implant-related domain name.
- Avoid using your name as domain name.
- Have a comprehensive FAQ.
- Have clinical images of each implant treatment modality.

- Register your site with different search engines.
- Write a complete list of key words so search engines can find you easily.

DESIGN CRITERIA FOR AN IMPLANT PRACTICE

Peter Warkentin
Kornelius Warkentin

Innovation, technology, and architecture are crucial design elements for a successful implant practice! Proper elements can improve overall efficiency, increase productivity, and create an atmosphere worthy of patient return. The use of a simple mental tool can teach you element basics. With it, you will understand why they are crucial and how to apply them. You will see how new trends will influence design, and you will understand new requirements like HIPAA. Whether you are designing an implant practice from scratch, want to add something new, or simply want to be better informed, this tool is your basic approach to design.

The design process should start by dividing the practice into its various core components. A typical implant practice should have following the components:

- Reception area
- Waiting room
- Consultation room
- Surgical operatory
- Prosthetic operatory
- Hygiene and recall operatory
- Sterilization area
- Staff lounge

Once the practice is divided, you will need to draft a mental map as a tool for how the implant practice is broken down and also how to address the flow issues. Upon analysis, you will find patients, practitioners, technicians, and receptionists all performing different functions in various areas and having different needs. The map becomes more detailed as you gain more knowledge of the needs from each individual.

You should keep this in mind or even draw a picture if necessary.

It's important to understand why the elements of innovation, technology, and architecture are considered crucial. First, patient satisfaction is imperative to the operation of your practice. To maintain patient comfort, individuals, including staff and practitioner, must meet the needs of the patient. For this to happen, their own needs must be met. Collectively, all individuals have different needs, and this map describes these needs. A more detailed map shows greater differences. This creates an obstacle to patient satisfaction. If you meet the needs of all individuals, whether separate or at the same time, in each area, you have essentially created a successful practice with people able to work for the common goal of patient happiness.

Innovation, technology, and architecture have proven their ability to meet individual needs inside a practice at all times. Therefore, they are considered crucial. This is true because a patient's need to restore what was lost or damaged has not really changed. However, the elements have changed to better assist the goal to restore. Keeping up with the elements takes time and effort. Hence, it is necessary that you keep up with them.

The success of your practice depends on your knowledge of available elements and how you use them to assist in the common goal of patient fulfillment.

The rest of this section is devoted to providing application examples of the elements. To do this, create a mental map of a typical implant practice consisting of the following areas:

- Reception area
- Waiting room
- Consultation room
- Surgical operatory
- Prosthetic operatory
- Hygiene and recall operatory
- Sterilization area
- Staff lounge

Walk through each area and consider the needs of each individual. The more you know the needs, the more detailed your map becomes with greater potential to use crucial elements to meet them.

Reception Area

A reception area is, of course, the first experience of your potential or returning patient. It is also where you deliver your first impression and introduction to the patient. Nevertheless, it is easy to see why an area alone can make a difference without ever speaking to a person. Recall some of your very own medical office experiences as a first-time patient. Do you remember struggling to get yourself physically to the reception because of an overcrowded waiting area? Did you decide to wait a little longer until you noticed another obstacle of concern—the glass window separating you from a reception clerk? Were you beginning to feel that even if you made it to the reception area, the glass window conveyed the message that there was more wrong with you than needing a cavity filled? All these are common complaints by many patients.

Ask yourself what really was needed to make the experience a more pleasant one. How could the elements have been applied? What could have made your experience more enjoyable?

The common needs of patients in reception are accessibility and privacy. Innovation, architecture, and possibly new material technology can accomplish this. First, reception areas should not be places of congestion. Congestion creates an uncomfortable and frustrating experience. The goal should be to place the reception area such that it does not create a standing line of guests. The last message you want to deliver is one of being herded through a process. Second, the reception counter should provide an open and welcome feeling to the patient while still enabling privacy. Patients should feel valued and free to communicate privately with reception staff. A way to create an open sense is by building a wall with materials capable of dampening or blocking sounds not intended for others. You also want to leave glass dividers a material of the past.

Since patient privacy is a necessity in the reception area, it is a good time to explain how HIPAA works with your map. HIPAA is a mandated need to protect patient privacy. Since your mental map shows individuals and their needs in various areas, HIPAA fits in quite well. It acts like any other individual with needs. However, failing to meet its need can result in large penalties and even the closure of your practice! Everywhere patient information goes, this individual will follow. There will be hundreds of these in your practice. Sometimes they will be grouped together and sometimes lounging around.

Waiting Room

Your waiting areas should be a place of comfort because this is the heaviest need in the mind of a patient. However, to increase comfort, you'll need to lower anxiety, as this is a feeling expected by the patient receiving a procedure or a potential patient receiving consultation. To combat anxiety, use elements that are soothing in nature. This may come in the form of custom furniture, artwork, soft music, special lighting, and proper interior color choices.

When selecting furniture, custom European furniture functions well, because it can be crafted to provide comfort in a variety of styles, woods, and colors. Its timeless nature differentiates it from other furniture that becomes outdated over time and with changing trends. It further can deliver a message that the practice is on top of current technologies. It should be noted that furniture is essentially art, and art adds flavor to good architecture.

Artwork can add or detract from a feeling of comfort. Artworks containing minimal colors, that are impressionistic in style, or that present scenic views calm an anxious mind and are the best choices.

Employ technical elements like audio and video to provide additional comfort. Music is a great sedative in all areas of a practice. It can lower anxiety not just for patients but also for practitioners and assistants. It is always best to err on a softer side in both style and volume.

Video is another great tool to lower anxiety, because it gives your patient something else to think about while waiting. However, video messages should not contribute to anxiety or stress. Too often, practices contain televisions with news channels broadcasting disaster and negativity. This can only add to the anxiety your patient already had on the way to the appointment. Consider using an informational video containing patient success stories or soothing videos of nature. Instead of a standard TV set, consider a flat-panel display that functions as another piece of artwork while saving space.

Your waiting area is great place to incorporate newer lighting technologies that increase comfort. Full-spectrum lighting simulates natural sunlight by using all the colors found in the color spectrum. When installed and distributed properly, it has proven to display a better sense of individual well being, lowers depression, and lessens feelings of lethargy. Science has proven that fluorescent lighting for extended periods contributes to depression and lowers a person's energy level. Full-spectrum lighting should be implemented throughout your practice so a patient's mood remains stable and your staff can enjoy its benefits as well. Even your existing practices can be fitted with full-spectrum lighting to add additional comfort anywhere in your practice. Full-spectrum lighting has other benefits that are explained later in this chapter.

Consultation Room

Although a waiting area may do well to lower patient anxiety and increase comfort, more is needed to gain trust, and a well-designed consultation room can help. Your consultation room is really an extension of your waiting area. A patient's move from one environment to another may change mood, increase fear, and cause rash decision-making. If your need is for the patient to remain comfortable, you need to provide a smooth transition. Your goal should be to minimize a change in the environment for your prospective patient. Attend to all elements that will accomplish this goal.

Surgical Operatory

In the past, practitioners would often consult prospective patients in their office or even right in an operatory. Although an office environment is more comforting than an operatory chair, the elements inside could be intimidating, private to the practitioner, or may even violate HIPAA requirements, as other patient information may be contained within. An operatory area is a strong change of environment for your patient. Moreover, they could feel as though a surgery is about to take place while they are considering a procedure. An alternate approach is to use a video message, implying that an implant procedure "isn't as bad" as it might seem. It could also free your time, as a practitioner, to perform other tasks while your patient is "entertained" to the idea of a procedure. The improper use or lack of the elements could mean the loss of a patient.

Prosthetic Operatory

Surgical or prosthetic operatories must meet the needs of patients and implant practitioners while having enough space for everyone to work simultaneously. This area is where your patients' fear and anxiety can surge. To lower anxiety, implement the same elements you use in the waiting area, including soothing music and soft colors. Because different practitioners, such as a prosthodontist, may use this area, it must be customized. The needs of all individuals will be heavy and diverse. Consider their movement, access to instruments, and resources required. The area requires customized sink and cabinetry for surgery, organized drawer structure, and efficient tool access, and it must match the flow of dirty-to-clean sterilization procedures. Access to a single microscope by two professionals without disrupting the flow of personnel is a possible scenario. A new technology in carpet fiber can change the floor to something comfortable while the correct color choice can help personnel locate items that are dropped. Just as HIPAA acts on your map as an individual with specific needs, OSHA will influence the design of this area, ensuring that its standards are met. The technical element of video can be used to record surgeries for later discussion and training. Because successful surgery depends on the level of sterilization, make sure you meet the need with elements of material technology. Corian®, aluminum, and glass are great sterile material choices that can be cut, shaped, and placed ergonomically while conforming to OSHA standards.

Knowing the needs of all individuals is highly required before choosing what elements fit this area because of its complexity. It's important to communicate the needs of everyone to anyone involved in the actual design and creation of this area. For the most part, designers have experience and suggestions to share.

Hygiene and Recall Operatory

Your hygiene and recall operatory will need to reacquaint your patient with comfort. After all, waking up in a foreign place after surgery can be awkward. Use elements that provide comfort as in the waiting area. Although the surgery was performed, its verification takes time with follow-up visits. Follow-up visits by the patient will require sterilization. In the meantime, meet the need of sterilization with materials used in other operatories.

Sterilization Area

The sterilization area should uphold the highest sterilization principles that will safeguard your patient and your implant practice. This is crucial for the long-term success of an implant practice. Careful sterilization guidelines should become routine, and the ergonomics of the facility need to assist in this process. No patients should have access to this area, and proper materials will assist in meeting sterilization standards.

Staff Lounge

Kitchen and staff areas are other great places to continue with proper lighting and materials used elsewhere. They can contain similar elements used in a waiting area but convey more of a relaxing message than a comforting one.

Furthermore, a practitioner's office introduces further security requirements from HIPAA but can remain friendly in appearance. The practitioner's office and access to patient information are of heavy concern to HIPAA individuals on your map. This is because practitioners generally have higher access to patient information. Therefore, it is extremely important that you remain up to date on HIPAA requirements. It may come in the form of a custom-designed desk with a locking keyboard drawer. X-ray viewers can often be placed in improper locations and viewing angles. Consider the need to customize their location and lighting control.

After you have performed a mental walkthrough for each area of your practice and applied the elements, you must consider traffic flow as a whole. Congestion can make staff and personnel very frustrated when they find themselves bumping into each other. Staff may find themselves willing to go around areas they would normally pass through to be more productive and efficient. Combat this problem by combining ergonomic furniture with a well thought-out architectural layout. Ergonomics provides a better flow for both patients and practitioner.

Proper element utilization will lead to an efficient, safe practice and more return patients. In conclusion, innovation, technology, and architecture combined are crucial design elements that when used properly will lead to a successful implant practice.

Index

Abscess around cover screw, 147
Abutment
    inability to perfectly connect, to implant, 147
    SynCone, 194, 198–199, 203–204
Access brush, implant overdentures and, 211
Accretions, removal of, implant overdentures
        and, 213
Acid-etched surface, 154, 169
Acrylic denture base, clinical and laboratory
    procedures for VKS-OC rs attachment, 45, 49
    embedded in, 45
Alignment, 37, 172
    of stud attachments, 37
    of trajectory of implant, Maximus OS,
        overdenture implant and, 168–171
Alignment drill aligning trajectory of implant
        and, 172, 175
Allogeneic bone, bone grafting and, 141
Allograft, bone grafting and, 140–141
Alloplast, bone grafting and, 140–141
Alveolar bone, access to, 33, 144, 171–172,
        181–183
    ERA Overdenture Implant and, 171–172,
        181–183
    Maximus OS overdenture implant and, 169
Alveolar ridge
    sagittal relationship of bar to, 66
    vertical relationship of bar to, 66

Ambassadors, successful implant practice and,
        227
Anchors, retentive. *See* Retentive anchors
Anesthesia, 147
Angle correction gauge kit, ERA, 39–40
Ankylos implant system, 90
Anterior crestal incision with or without
        vestibular release, 133–134
Anterior interferences, elimination of, 124,
        127–129
Anterior mandible, lingual swelling after
        implant placement in, 146
Anterior-posterior distance rule, bar
        attachments and, 68
Antimicrobials, 212
Apical portion, tapered, parallel body with,
        170
Artwork, selection of, in waiting room,
        229–230
Aspirin, effect of, on coagulation process,
        132
Astra ball abutment, 57
Astra implant, 57–58
Attachment assemblies
    evaluation of components of, 213–214
    factors influencing diagnosis and resiliency
        level of, 33
    for Straumann implants, 155

Attachment design
    classification of overdenture implants based
        on features of, 168–169
    cleansable, failure to achieve, 210–211
Attachments
    bar. *See* Bar attachments
    Clix, 57–60
    combination resilient, 32
    ERA, 37
    hinge resilient, 32, 81
    resiliency of, 76
    restricted vertical resilient, 32
    rigid non-resilient, 25, 32, 107
    rotary resilient, 32
    stud. *See* Stud attachments
    universal resilient, 32
Attachment selection
    biomechanical considerations and, 33
    biomechanics of maxillary overdenture and,
        33
    criteria for, 32–33
    different attachment assemblies and, 33
    distal extension to bar and, 33
    factors influencing design and resiliency level
        of attachment assembly and, 33
    load distribution of stud *vs.* bar attachments
        and, 33
    principles of, 31–33
    types of attachments based on resiliency and,
        32
Autograft, bone grafting and, 140–141
Available bone quantity in diagnosis and
    treatment planning, 15

Balanced occlusion, set-up procedure for,
    utilizing Vita Physiodens teeth, 113
Balancing excursion, eccentric jaw movements
    and, 129
Balancing side, eccentric balance and, 127
Ball bearings (BBs), 12–13
Bar
    distal extension to, 33
    Dolder. *See* Dolder bar
    flexibility of, 64
    Hader. *See* Hader bar
    parallel, 78–79
    passive seat of, 82
    sagittal relationship of
    to alveolar ridge, 66–67

    to hinge axis, 67
    vertical relationship of, to alveolar ridge, 66
Bar arrangement, 64
Bar assembly, incorporation of, into denture, 82
Bar attachments, 33, 63–81
    bar materials and, 63
    based on cross-sectional shapes, 63
    based on nature of their resiliency, 64
    Dolder bar and, 72–75
    fundamentals of bar arrangement and, 64
    Hader bar and, 63, 69–73
    load distribution of, 33
    Vario Soft Bar Pattern VSP and, 76
Bar clips, 63
Bar joint, 32, 64, 72–73, 75–76
Bar materials, 63
Bar riders, 63, 69–73, 213
Bar unit, 64, 72, 75
BBs. *See* Ball bearings (BBs)
Betamethasone, 132
Bio-Gide, 143
Biomechanics
    attachment selection and, 31–33
    lingualized teeth and, 122–123
    of maxillary overdenture, 33
    risk factors for lower implant overdentures
        and, 106
    risk factors for upper implant overdentures
        and, 105
BioMend, 142
BioMend Extend, 143
BIOS. *See* Breda Implant Overdenture Study
    (BIOS)
Blood pressure of surgical patient, 132–133
Bone
    allogeneic, 141
    alveolar. *See* Alveolar bone
    cancellous, 17–18, 144
    compact, 17–18
    ERA Overdenture Implant and, 179–180
    height of, 11–15
    length of, 15
    porous, 18
    shape of, 15
    thick, 17–18
    thin, 17–18
    width of, 15
    xenogeneic, 141
Bone grafting, 15, 17, 104, 140–141, 144, 163

Bone quantity
   available, in diagnosis and treatment
      planning, 11–19
   classification of edentulous ridges based on,
      17
Bone-spreading sequence, split-control system
   and, 144
Bone supported surgical guides, 26
Branding of implant practice, 226–227
Brand name, successful implant practice and,
   227
Brealloy F 400, 80
Breda Implant Overdenture Study (BIOS), 5
Bredent PiKuPlast HP36, 79
Bredent "Thixo Rock," 78
Bredent Vario Soft Bar Pattern, 76
Bredent VSP bar, 81
Brush
   access, 211
   denture, 212
   interdental, 211
Buccal corridor, 117
Buccal cusp interferences, maxillary,
      elimination of, 124, 126
Buccal incision, mandibular surgery and, 136
Buccolingual position, mandibular teeth and,
   124
Budget, patient's, successful implant practice
   and, 226
Burs, careful handling of, disinfection and, 140

Calculus, instruments for, 213
Camlog, 198
Camtube, 198
Cancellous bone, classification of edentulous
   ridges based on, 17–18
Cap, healing, difficulty inserting, 147
Case acceptance, successful implant practice
   and, 225–226
Castable bar, plastic, advantages of, 77
Castable ERA attachment, mandibular
   implant-supported overdenture utilizing
      Hader bar and, 72
Castable Hader bar attachment with gold alloy
   clips/riders, fabrication procedures for,
      70–71
Castable Hader bar attachment with plastic
   clips/riders, fabrication procedures for,
      70–71

Cawley, Peter, 206
Center point vision, successful implant practice
   and, 216–217
Centric occlusion contacts, reestablishing,
   128
Centric relation, 5, 11, 48, 52, 78, 81, 90, 93,
   120, 129
Centric stops, mandibular, equilibration and,
   128
Chair-side utilization procedures
   of Astra implant, 57
   of Clix attachment, 57
   ERA attachments and, 39
   ERAOverdenture Implant and, 179
   Maximus OS overdenture implant and,
      169–170
   prosthetic steps and, 167, 178, 187, 198
   of retentive anchor abutment and elliptical
      matrix, 55–56
Chlorhexidine, 133, 147, 166, 201, 212
Chrome cobalt framework, clinical and
   laboratory procedures for VKS-OC rs, 49
   attachment cast within, 49
Cleansable attachment design, failure to
      achieve, 210–211
Clips
   bar, 104
   gold alloy, 71–73
   Hader, placement of, 82
   metal. See Metal clips
   metal, vs. plastic Hader, 63, 72
   parallel-sided, for rectangular bar, 77
   plastic, castable Hader bar attachment with,
      fabrication procedures for, 70–71
   snap-on, 77–78
      with no extension, 78
      with parallel-sided extension, 77
   VKS-OC rs stud attachment and, 44–45
Clix attachment, 57–60
   design specifications of female component of,
      57, 59, 170
Clix inserts, replacing, 57–58
Clopidogrel (Plavix), effect of, on coagulation
      process, 132
Cobalt framework, chrome, clinical and
   laboratory procedures for VKS-OC rs,
   49
   attachment cast within, 49
CO-Comfort GC, 166

Coe-Comfort, 139

Collar, polished, Straumann Implant System and, 153, 155, 157, 159

Combination resilient attachments, 32

Compact bone, classification of edentulous ridges based on, 17–18

Compstat, 218

Computed tomography (CT scan) , 12, 14–15, 26-28, 147, 172, 182

Consultation room, successful implant practice and, 228, 230

Continuous sutures, 138–139

Conventional suture *vs.* implant overdenture, 3

Cords, flossing, implant overdentures and, 212

Core principles of successful implant practice. *See* Implant practice, successful, core principles of

Coumadin. *See* Warfarin (Coumadin)

Cover screw, 134, 147, 165–167
    abscess around, 147
    exposed, 147

Crestal incision, 133–134, 136, 167, 194
    anterior, with or without vestibular release, 133–134
    extended, mandibular surgery and, 134
    full arch extended, 134
    mandibular surgery and, 134
    maxillary surgery and, 136
    with vestibular releasing incisions, 134
    without releasing incisions, 134

Crock, Ray, 220

CT scan. *See* Computed tomography (CT scan)

Curve
    of Spee, 125
    of Wilson, 125

Curved occlusal plane, mandibular teeth and, 122

Cusps, maxillary lingual, equilibration and, 122–123

Delayed loading protocol with SynCone concept, 202

Dentists: An Endangered Species, 225

Denture
    conventional, *vs.* implant overdenture, 3
    incorporation of bar assembly into, 82

Denture base, acrylic, clinical and laboratory procedures for VKS-OC rs attachment, 45 embedded in, 45

Denture base extensions, bar attachments and, 68–69

Denture brushes, 212

Denture teeth, occlusal schemes formed by, 112–113

Dexamethasone, effect of, on patient's ability to heal after surgery, 132

Diabetes, effect of surgery on patient with, 132

Diagnosis and treatment planning, 11–23
    anatomical considerations during diagnosis and treatment planning process and, 15
    benefits of diagnostic mounting and, 11
    diagnostic workup for implant overdentureand, 11
    joint treatment planning and, 15
    radiographic evaluation and, 12

Diagnostic mounting, benefits of, 11–12

Diagnostic stent, surgical guide and. *See* Surgical guides and diagnostic stent

Diagnostic workup for implant overdentures, 11

DICOM-3-format, 27

Disinfection
    of hands, 133
    of instruments, 133

Distal extension to bar, attachment selection and, 33

Dolder, Eugen, 72

Dolder bar, 5, 32, 63, 72–73, 75–76
    contraindications for, 73
    dimensional specifications of, 73
    fabrication procedure for, 75
    indications for, 72–73

Dolder bar joint, 32, 75–76
    fabrication procedure for, 75

Dolder bar joint attachment assembly, relining an overdenture with, 76

Dolder bar unit attachment assembly, relining overdenture with, 75

Draping of patient for surgery, 133

Drilling, hemorrhaging during, 146

Drilling sequence for standard implants, 156
    Straumann Implant System and, 153–159

Drills
    alignment, aligning trajectory of implant and, 137, 156, 163, 172–173
    careful handling of, disinfection and, 140

Early loading, mandibular implant, 192
  overdentures and, 192–203
Eccentric balance, implant-supported, 127
  overdenture and, 127
Eccentric jaw movements, implant-supported,
    129
  overdenture and, 129
Edentulous ridges, classification of, based on
  bone quantity, 15–17
Education, patient. *See* Patient education
Elliptical matrix, retentive anchors and,
    53–56
Emotional pain, 146
  in patient's decision to have treatment,
    222
  successful implant practice and, 222
Emotional values, listening for, successful,
    implant practice and, 221
Endopore dental implant system, 17,
    161–167
  advantages of, 162
  implant uncovering steps for, 167
  post surgical instructions for, 166–167
  prosthetic steps for, 167
  short, mechanical rationale for, 162–163
  surgical steps for, 163
Endosseous diameters, Straumann Implant
    System and, 154–155
End-tufted toothbrushes, implant overdentures
    and, 211
Epinephrine, anesthesia and, 133
Epoxy, 92
ePTFE. *See* Polytetrafluoroethylene (ePTFE)
Equilibration
  after processing, 128
  completion of, by adjusting incline planes of
    mandibular posterior teeth, 129
  sequence of, after processing, 128
Equipment. *See* Instruments
ERA angle correction gauge kit, 39–40
ERA attachment, 37, 72
  castable, mandibular implant-supported,
    72
  overdenture utilizing Hader bar and, 72
ERA implant, 187
ERA male component, changing, 43,
    189
ERA Overdenture Implant, 179–180
  changing male component of, 168

design specifications of, 168, 180
  surgical steps and, 171–172
ERA plastic handle gauges, 39
Erosion, spark. *See* Spark erosion
Error, magnification, of panoramic x-rays,
    determining, 11–14
Excessive retention of overdenture, SynCone
    concept and, 202–203
Expectations, patient. *See* Patient preferences
  and expectations
Exposed cover screw, 147
Exposed implant threads, 146
Extended crestal incision, full arch, 134
Extended crestal incision, mandibular surgery
    and, 134–135
External marketing objectives, successful,
    implant practice and, 227, 228

Fabrication procedures, 70–75
  for castable Hader bar attachment, 70
  with gold alloy clips/riders, 71
  with plastic clips/riders, 72
  for Dolder bar joint, 72
  of hinge resilient overdenture using Bredent
    VSP bar, 81
  of rigid fully implant-borne overdenture,
    using parallel bar, 78
Failure to achieve cleansable attachment design,
    210–211
Female attachments
  implants with, 170
  interchangeable, 170
First lower premolar, setting up, for balanced
    occlusion, 114, 116
First upper premolar, setting up, for balanced
    occlusion, 113
Fishtailing, attachment selection and, 31–32
Fixed implant-supported prosthesis *vs.* implant
    overdenture, 3–4
Flap designs
  basic, 133
  incisions and, 133
Flaps, mini, 134
Flap technique, gaining access to alveolar bone
    and, 171–172, 181, 187
Flexibility of bar, bar attachments and, 64
Flossing cords, implant overdentures and,
    212
Fluorescent lighting, effect of, on mood, 230

Follow up and maintenance of implant
        overdentures, 210–213
    characteristics of ideal peri-implant tissues
        and, 210
    consequences for failure to achieve
        cleansable, attachment design and, 210
    home care implements and, 211
    recommended routines at recall visits and,
        213
"Forgiving" intercuspation, 120–121
Framework-reinforced overdenture, SynCone
        abutments and, 202–203
Front line management concept, 217–218
Full arch extended crestal incision, 134
Full implant-supported implant overdenture,
        4–5, 68–69
Full-spectrum lighting, effect of, on mood,
        230
Fully edentulous ridges, classification of, based
        on bone quantity, 15–16
Fully implant-supported overdentures, 4–5, 69,
        85
Furniture, selection of, in waiting room,
        229

George Schick Dental Company, 29
Gingival cuff heights of Astra ball abutment,
        38, 57
Gingiva supported surgical guides, 26
Giuliani, Rudolph, 218
Gloves, sterile, 133
Glucose metabolism, diabetes and, 132
Gold alloy clips/riders, castable Hader bar
        attachment with, fabrication procedures
        for, 69–71
Gold screw, difficulty inserting, 147
GORE-TEX, 142
Grafting, bone, 140–141, 163
Granulation tissue around implant head, 147
Guide pins, aligning trajectory of implant and,
        46, 49
Gysi, 123

Hader, Helmut, 69
Hader bar, 32, 63, 69–72
    Castable, 70
        with gold alloy clips/riders, fabrication,
            procedures for, 71, 72

        with plastic clips/riders, fabrication,
            procedures for, 70, 72
    mandibular implant-supported overdenture,
        utilizing, 72
    metal clips and, 72
Hader bar attachment assembly
        troubleshooting for, 72–73
Hader clip placement, 71–72
Hader Vertical, 69
Hard accretions, removal of, implant
        overdentures and, 213
Healing cap, difficulty inserting, 147
Healing period
    before loading, mandibular implant
        overdentures and, 192
    for Straumann implants with SLA surface,
        160
Healing phase, initial, overdenture implants
        acting as transitional implants during,
        169
Height of bone in diagnosis and treatment
        planning, 11–17
Hemoglobin A1C in assessment of glucose
        control, 132
Hemorrhaging during drilling, 146
Hinge axis, sagittal relationship of bar to, 67
Hinge movement, attachment selection and,
        32–33
Hinge resilient attachments, 32
Hinge resilient overdenture, fabrication,
        procedures of, using Bredent VSP bar, 81
HIPAA, 228–231
Home care, VKS-OC rs stud attachment and,
        44–45
Homecare implements, plaque-control, 211
Hygiene and recall operatory, successful
        implant practice and, 228, 231
Hypertension, effect of surgery on patient with,
        132–133

Ibuprofen, 133
Immediate loading, mandibular implant
        overdentures and, 192
Immediately loaded implants, clinical
        conditions affecting outcome of, Osstell
        Mentor and, 208
Immediate stabilization for overdenture as
        purpose of overdenture implants, 169

Implant. *See also* Implant overdentures; Overdenture implants; Overdentures;
    alignment of trajectory of, Maximus OS overdenture implant and, 169–171, 176
    Astra, 57
    body of, rough surface on, Straumann Implant System and, 154, 160
    Endopore. *See* Endopore dental implant System
    with female attachments, 168
    fracture of, during insertion in osteotomy, 147
    immediately loaded, clinical conditions affecting outcome of, Osstell Mentor and, 208
    inability to perfectly connect abutment to, 147
    with male attachments, 168
    marking location of, ERA Overdenture Implant and, 180
    mobile, 147
    painful, 147
    placement of
        ERA Overdenture Implant and, 179–180
        Maximus OS overdenture implant and, 169–170
        sensitive but immobile, 147
        Straumann. *See* Straumann Implant System
        successful integration of, with surrounding tissue, 140
        supporting, loading of, effect of shape of mandible on, 107
    transitional, during healing phase, overdenture implants acting as, 162, 169
Implant bed, preparation of, Straumann Implant System and, 155
Implant 3D software, 28
Implant head, granulation tissue around, 147
Implant insertion, Straumann Implant System and, 156–157
Implant mobility after placement, 146
Implant overdentures, 168–191. *See also* Implant Overdenture implants; Overdentures
    bar attachments, 75
    clinical applications for measurement of implant stability using Osstell Mentor, 206
    comparison of treatment strategies for, 4
    core principles of successful implant practice, 216–231
    diagnosis and treatment planning, 11–19
    Endopore Dental Implant System, 161–167
    follow up and maintenance of. *See* Follow up and maintenance of implant overdentures
    fully implant-supported, 4–5, 69
    indications for, 4
    mainly tissue-supported, 4–5
    mandibular, loading approaches for. *See* Mandibular implant overdentures, loading approaches for
    occlusion and implant-supported overdentures, 112–130
    overdenture implants, 168–191
    patient preferences and expectations, 3–5
    principles of attachment selection, 31–33
    spark erosion, 85–100
    Straumann Implant System, 153–159
    stud attachments, 37–59, 105, 211
    surgical considerations for. *See* Surgical considerations for implant overdentures
    surgical guide and diagnostic stent, 24–29
    tissue-implant-supported, 4, 79
    treatment success with overdentures, 104–107
Implant placement, osteotomy and, 137–138
Implant practice, 216–231
    branding of, 226–227
    criteria for, 228
    successful, core principles of, 216–231
        branding of implant practice and, 226–227
        design criteria for implant practice and, 228
        marketing and, 216–227
        restorative practice and, 224
        sales and, 220–221
        systems and, 217–218
        team and, 216–226
        vision and, 216–230
Implant site, tapping of, Straumann Implant System and, 156
Implant stability, clinical applications for measurement of, using Osstell Mentor, 193, 206–209
Implant Stability Quotient (ISQ), 207

Implant-supported overdentures
common mistakes in contruction of, 6
mandibular, utilizing Hader bar and castable ERA attachment, 72
occlusion and. *See* Occlusion and implant-supported overdentures
Implant-supported prosthesis, fixed, *vs.* implant overdenture, 3–4
Implant survival, 104
Implant threads, exposed, 146
Incisions
anterior crestal, with or without vestibular release, 133–134
buccal, mandibular surgery and, 134
crestal. *See* Crestal incision
extended crestal, mandibular surgery and, 134
flap design and, 133–134
full arch extended crestal, 134
palatal, mandibular surgery and, 134
releasing, crestal incision without, 134
vestibular, 133–135
Incline planes of mandibular posterior teeth, completing equilibration by adjustment of, 129
Inhalation anesthesia, 133
INR. *See* International Nornalized Ratio (INR)
Instructions, postoperative. *See* Patient Education
Instruments, 133
for calculus, 213
disinfection of, 133
treatment room preparation and utilization protocol and, 133
Insufficient retention, SynCone concept and, 73, 202
Insulin in assessment of glucose control, 132
Interchangeable female components, 170
Intercuspation, "forgiving," 120–121
Interdental brushes, implant overdentures and, 211–212
International Nornalized Ratio (INR), 132
I shape of VSP bar, 77
ISQ. *See* Implant Stability Quotient (ISQ)
Ivoclar, 28, 123, 126
Ivoclar ortholingual teeth, set-up procedure for, 123
lingualized occlusion utilizing, 123

Jaw movements, eccentric, implant-supported overdenture and, 129
Joint treatment planning, 15
Language, successful implant practice and, 225
Leadership, 218, 220
Leadership, 218, 220
Length of bone in diagnosis and treatment planning, 15
Lighting, effect of, on mood, 229–231
Lingual contact occlusion, 122–123
Lingual cusps, maxillary, equilibration and, 122–123, 125, 129
Lingualized occlusal scheme, 122–123
Lingualized occlusion, 81, 122, 123
history of, 123
utilizing Ivoclar ortholingual teeth, set-up procedure for, 123
Lingualized teeth, 133–134
Lingual swelling after implant placement in anterior mandible, 146
Lip, lower, postoperative sensory disturbance of, 147
Load distribution of stud *vs.* bar attachments, 33
Loading
early, 192
healing period before, 192
immediate, 192
premature, 192
progressive, 192
of supporting implants, effect of shape of mandible on, 107
Loading approaches for mandibular implant overdentures. *See* Mandibular implant overdentures, loading approaches for
Locking sutures, 139
Loose bone, classification of edentulous ridges based on, 17
Loosely structured cancellous bone, 17–18
classification of edentulous ridges based on, 17
Lower first molar, 118
occlusal contacts of, 114–120
setting up, 116
Lower first premolars, occlusal contacts, 113
between upper first premolars and, 113–114
Lower implant overdentures, biomechanical risk factors for, 105

Lower lip, postoperative sensory disturbance of, 147
Lower second molar, 117, 122
    occlusal contacts of, 114-120
    setting up, 116
Lower second premolars, 116
    occlusal contacts of, 116
    setting up, 113

Magnetic attachments, 32–33
Magnification error of panoramic x-rays, determining, 11–14
Male attachments, implants with, 168
Mandible
    anterior, lingual swelling after implant placement in, 146
    shape of, effect of, on loading of supporting implants, 107–108
Mandibular centric stops, equilibration and, 129–130
Mandibular implant overdentures, loading approaches for, 192
    advantages of immediate loading in implant-supported overdenture cases and, 193
    determining loading strategies and, 192
    healing period before loading and, 192
    premature loading and, 192
    procedural sequences and, 203
    success of premature loaded implants and, 193
    SynCone abutments and framework-reinforced overdenture and, 203
    SynCone concept and, 194
    treatment protocol requirements and, 193
    troubleshooting and, 202
Mandibular implant-supported overdenture utilizing Hader bar and castable ERA attachment, 72
Mandibular posterior teeth, incline planes of, completing
equilibration by adjustment of, 129
Mandibular surgery, 134
Mandibular teeth, position of, 124
Marketing, successful implant practice and, 216, 223
Matrices
    elliptical, retentive anchors and, 53–54

parallel-sided, for rectangular bar, 77–78
    snap-on, with no extension, 78
    snap-on, with parallel-sided extension, 77–78
    VKS-OC rs stud attachment and, 44
Mattress, horizontal, 139
Maxillary buccal cusp interferences, elimination of, 126
Maxillary lingual cusps, equilibration and, 129
Maxillary overdenture, biomechanics of, 33
Maxillary surgery, 136–146
Maxillary teeth, position of, 125
Maximus OS implant, 170–171, 178
Maxwell, John, 216, 220
MDI Implant, 168
med3D technology, components and advantages of, 27
Meredith, Neil, 206
Metal clips, 63, 71–72
    advantages of, 72
    disadvantages of, 72
    vs. plastic Hader, 72
Microsaws, surgical, 143
Mini dental implants, 168
Mini flaps, 134
Modified posterior setup, 123
Molars, setting up, 116
Mounting, diagnostic, benefits of, 11–12
Mouth, patient's, preparation of, for surgery, 144
Mucocitis, peri-implant, 210
Mucosa, compression of, by bar, 66
Music, relaxation and, 229–230

Neomem, 143
Nimetic-Cem, 203
No-flap technique, gaining access to alveolar bone and, 172, 182
Non-anatomic teeth, 120, 121
Noncurved occlusal plane, mandibular teeth and, 124–125
Non-locking sutures, 138
Non-resobable membranes, bone grafting and, 140, 142
Non-resorbable materials for suturing techniques, 142–143

Occlusal adjustment, 43, 57, 78, 113, 120, 123, 128

Occlusal contacts
   of lower first molar, 114
   of lower second molar, 114
   of lower second premolar, 115
   between upper and lower first premolars,
      114
   of upper first molar, 117
   of upper second molar, 119
   of upper second premolars, 114
Occlusal plane, height of, mandibular teeth
      and, 124–125
Occlusal radiographs, 147
Occlusal scheme
   formed by denture teeth, 112
   lingualized, 122
Occlusion
   balanced, set-up procedure for, utilizing Vita
      Physiodens teeth, 113
   central, reestablishing, 128
   and implant-supported overdentures, 112
   eccentric jaw movements and, 129
   equilibration after processing and, 128
   history of lingual contact and, 123
   history of lingualized occlusion and, 120
   occlusal adjustment and, 120
   occlusal schemes formed by denture teethand,
      112
   set-up procedure for balanced occlusion
      utilizing Vita Physiodens teeth and,
      113
   set-up procedure for lingualized occlusion
      utilizing Ivoclar ortholingual teeth and,
      123
   lingual contact, 123
   lingualized. See Lingualized occlusion
Older patients, attracting, successful implant
      practice and, 224–225
Open-ended questions, successful implant
      practice and, 221
Operatory
   prosthetic, 230
   recall, 231
   surgical, 230
Organizational model/systems, successful
      implant practice and, 217
Ortholingual teeth, 123
   Ivoclar, set-up procedure for lingualized
      occlusion utilizing, 123
OSHA, 230–231

Osstell Mentor, clinical applications for
   measurement of implant stability using,
      206–208
   clinical conditions affecting outcome of
      immediately loaded implants and,
      208
clinical stages when ISQ measurement can be
      recorded and, 208
Osteoporosis, edentulous ridges and, 15–17
Osteotomy
   fraction of implant during insertion in,
      147
   and implant placement, 137
   preparation of, ERA Overdenture Implant
      and, 179–180
   widening of, Maximus OS overdenture
      implant and, 169
Overdenture implants, 168–191 See also
      Implant; Implant overdentures
Overdentures
   basic purposes for, 169
   classification of, based on attachment design
      features, 168
   ERA, 179
   Maximus OS, 169
Overdentures, 168–191. See also Implant;
      Implant overdentures; Overdenture
      implants
   excessive retention of, SynCone concept and,
      202
   framework-reinforced, SynCone abutments
      and, 203
   hinge resilient, fabrication procedures of,
      using Bredent VSP bar, 81
   immediate stabilization for, as purpose of
      overdenture implants, 169
   implant. See Implant; Implant overdentures;
      Overdenture implants
   implant-supported, occlusion and. See
      Occlusion and implant-supported
      Overdentures
   lower implant, biomechanical risk factors for,
      106
   mandibular implant-supported, utilizing
      Hader bar and castable ERA attachment,
      72
   maxillary, biomechanics of, 33–34
   relining. See Relining an overdenture site
      preparation for

treatment success with. *See* treatment success
    with overdentures
upper implant, biomechanical risk factors for,
    105
Ownership of problem in patient's decision to
    have treatment, 222

Pain
    emotional. *See* Emotional pain postoperative
Palatal incision, maxillary surgery and, 136
Panoramic landmarks, 13
Panoramic radiograph, 12
Panoramic x-rays, magnification error of,
    determining, 12–13
Parallel bar, fabrication procedures of rigid fully
    implant-borne overdenture using, 78
Parallel body with tapered apical portion, 170
Parallel-sided matrices/clips for rectangular bar,
    77–78
Parelling device aligning trajectory of implant
    and, 172–173
Passive seat of bar, verification of, 82
Patient education, 225–226
    postoperative, SynCone concept and, 201
    presurgical, 132
    successful implant practice and, 216–223
Patient preferences and expectations, 3–5, 32
    Breda Implant Overdenture Study and, 5–6
    common mistakes in constructing,
        implant-supported overdentures and, 6
    comparison of treatment strategies for
        implant overdentures and, 4–5
    implant overdenture *vs.* convention denture
        and, 3
    implant overdenture *vs.* fixed, 4
    implant-supported prosthesis and, 4
    indications for implant overdenture and, 4
    overdenture treatment strategies and, 6
    successful implant-supported overdenture
        and, 6
Patients
    budget of, successful implant practice and,
        226
    older, attracting, successful implant practice
        and, 224–225
    selection of, SynCone concept and, 194
    successful implant practice and, 216–223
    treatment room preparation and utilization
        protocol and, 133

treatment success with overdentures and,
    104–107
Peri-implantitis, 210–211
Peri-implant mucocitis, 210–211
Peri-implant tissues, ideal, characteristics of,
    210
Personnel. *See* Team
Plaque-control implements, home-care, 211,
    214
Plastic castable bar, advantages of, 77
Plastic clips/riders, castable Hader bar
        attachment with, fabrication procedures
        for, 70
Plastic Hader *vs.* metal clips, 72
Plastic handle gauges, ERA, 39–40, 165
Plavix. *See* Clopidogrel (Plavix)
Polished collar, Straumann Implant System and,
    153
Polytetrafluoroethylene (ePTFE), bone grafting
    and, 139, 142
Porcelain, spark erosion and, 88
Porous bone, classification of edentulous ridges
    based on, 17–18
Positioning device X1, 29
Posterior teeth, mandibular, incline planes of,
    completing equilibration by adjustment
    of, 129
Post-healing criteria for successful integration
    of implant with surrounding tissue, 140
Postoperative care, 201
    implant overdentures and, 201
Postoperative instructions. *See* Patient
    education
Postoperative pain, 146
Pound's Triangular, 124
Prednisone, effect of, on patient's ability to heal
    after surgery, 132
Prefabricated titanium bar, advantages of, 77
Preferences, patient. *See* Patient preferences and
    Expectations
Premature loading, mandibular implant
    overdentures and, 192
Premolars, setting up, for balanced occlusion,
    113
Presurgical instructions. *See* Patient education
Presurgical steps, SynCone concept and, 194
Procedural sequences, SynCone concept and,
    203
Processing, equilibration after, 128

Progressive loading, mandibular implant, overdentures and, 192

Prosthesis
  cleaning of, 213
  fixed implant-supported, *vs.* implant overdenture, 4

Prosthetic operatory, successful implant practice and, 230

Prosthetic steps, 167, 178, 187, 198
  ERA Overdenture Implant and, 179
  Maximus OS overdenture implant and, 169
  SynCone concept and, 194–203

Prosthetic success, 104

Protrusion, eccentric balance and, 128

Protrusive contacts, eccentric jaw movements and, 128

Proxy Tip, implant overdentures and, 212

Questions, open-ended, successful implant practice and, 242

Radiographic examination, 213
  implant overdentures and, 213
  occlusal, 13
  panoramic, 12

RBT. *See* Resorbable blast texturing (RBT)

Recall visits, recommended routines at, implant overdentures and, 213

Reception area, successful implant practice and, 229

Recommended routines at recall visits, implant overdentures and, 213

Rectangular bar, parallel-sided matrices/clips for, 77-78

Rectangular shape of VSP bar, 77

Releasing incisions, 134
  crestal incision without, 134
  vestibular, crestal incision with, 134

Relining an overdenture, 140
  with Dolder bar joint attachment assembly, 75
  with Dolder bar unit attachment assembly, 75

Research, marketing, successful implant practice and, 227

Resiliency
  of attachments, 31–33
  classification of bar attachments based on, 32

Resilient attachments
  combination, 32

hinge, 32
  restricted vertical, 32
  rotary, 32
  universal, 32

Resilient Dolder bar, 72

Resorbable blast texturing (RBT), 169–170

Resorbable materials, 139
  bone grafting and, 140
  for suturing techniques, 138

Resorbable membranes, bone grafting and, 139

Restorative practice, successful implant practice and, 224

Restricted vertical resilient attachments, 32

Retention
  excessive, of overdenture, SynCone concept and, 202
  insufficient, SynCone concept and, 73, 202

Retentive anchors, 52–56
  adjusting retention of female component of, 54–55
  chair-side utilization of, 55–56
  contraindications for, 58–59, 60, 61
  design specifications of, 53
  elliptical matrix of, 53
  Straumann, 52

RH-BMP2, bone grafting and, 140–141

Riders
  bar, 63
  gold alloy, castable Hader bar attachment with, fabrication procedures for, 71–72
  plastic, castable Hader bar attachment with, fabrication procedures for, 70

Rigid Dolder bar, 72–73

Rigid non-resilient attachments, 32

Robot, stationary, 29

Rotary resilient attachments, 32

Rotation movement, attachment selection and, 32, 33

Rough surface on implant body, Straumann, Implant System and, 153

Rübeling, Günter, 102

SAE Secotec Spark Erosion technique, 88

Sagittal relationship
  of bar to alveolar ridge, 66–67
  of bar to hinge axis, 67

Sales, successful implant practice and, 216, 220

Screw
  cover, abscess around, 147

cover, exposed, 147
   gold, difficulty inserting, 147
   transfer, difficulty inserting, 159
Secotec-System impression copings, 97
Semi-anatomic teeth, 120–121
Sendex, Victor, 168
Sensory disturbance, postoperative, of lower
   lip, 147
Shape of bone in diagnosis and treatment
   planning, 15
Sheffield test, 85
   spark erosion and, 85–86
Site preparation for overdentures, 140
SLA surface, 160
   Straumann implants with, healing period for,
   160
Smart Peg, 207, 209
Snap-on matrices/clips
   with no extension, 77–78
   with parallel-sided extension, 77–78
Soft accretions, removal of, implant
   overdentures and, 213
Software, implant 3D planning, 27–29
Spark erosion, 85–101
   common reasons for ill fit and, 88
   process of, 88
   Sheffield test and, 85
Spee, curve of, 125
Spinniing, attachment selection and,
   31–32
Split-control system, 144
Spreaders, split-control system, 144
Square tread pattern, Maximum OS implant
   and, 170
Stability, implant, clinical applications for
   measurement of, using Osstell Mentor,
   206-208
Stabilization, immediate, for overdenture, as
   purpose of overdenture implants, 169
Staff lounge, successful implant practice and,
   231
Standard Plus implants, 153
Stationary robot, 29
Stent, diagnostic, surgical guide and. *See*
   Surgical guides and diagnostic stent
Sterilization area, successful implant practice
   and, 26
Steroids, effect of, on patient's ability to heal
   after surgery, 132

Straumann Implant System, 153–159
   endosseous diameters and, 154
   healing period for Straumann implants with
      SLA surface and, 160
   recommended attachment assemblies for, 155
   regular neck implants and, 155
   surgical steps for standard implants, 155
   wound closure and, 159
Straumann Retentive Anchor and Abutment,
   52–53
Straumann Standard implants, 153
Stud attachments, 37
   alignment of, 37
   Astra Implant and, 57
   Clix attachment assembly and, 57
   ERA attachment and, 37
   height of, 37
   load distribution of, 33
   relationship of, with each other, 37
   relationship of, with path of insertion, 37
   Straumann Retentive Anchor Abutment and,
      52–53, 55
   VKS-OC rs Stud Attachment and, 44
Success, treatment, with overdentures. *See*
   Treatment sucess with overdentures
Successful implant practice. *See* Implant
   practice, successful, core principles of
Successful implant-supported overdentures, 6
Surgical considerations for implant
   overdentures, 132–147
   incisions and flap design and, 133
   mandibular surgery and, 134
   maxillary surgery and, 136
   osteotomy and implant placement and, 137
   post-surgical care and, 139
   presurgical instructions and, 132
   procedural considerations during, 137
   procedural considerations during surgery
      and, 137
   site preparation for overdentures and, 140
   split-control system and, 144
   surgical-related problems and, 146
   suturing techniques used for implant
      overdenture surgeries and, 139
Surgical guides
   classification of, 26
   and diagnostic stent, 26–27
      components and advantages of med3D
      technology and, 27

Surgical hand disinfection, 133

Surgical microsaws, 143–144

Surgical operatory, successful implant practice and, 230

Surgical related problems, 146

Surgical steps, 163, 171, 180, 194

  ERA Overdenture Implant and, 179

  Maximus OS overdenture implant and, 169

  for standard implants, Straumann Implant System and, 155

  SynCone concept and, 194–203

Suture material, 139, 160

Suturing techniques, 149–150

  continuous, 138

  horizontal mattress, 150

  locking, 139

  most commonly used, 139

  non-locking, 138

  non-resorbable material for, 139

  resorbable material for, 139

SynCone abutment, 203

  and framework-reinforced overdenture, 203

SynCone cap, 199–201

SynCone concept, 194–203

Systems, successful implant practice and, 216

Tapered apical portion, parallel body with, 170, 179

Tapered Effect implants, 153

Tapping of implant site, Straumann Implant System and, 156

Team

  members of, addition of, team decision on, 240

  successful implant practice and, 237–245

Teeth

  denture, occlusal schemes formed by, 112

  Ivoclar ortholingual, set-up procedure for lingualized occlusion utilizing, 123

  lingualized, 122

  mandibular, position of, 124

  mandibular posterior, incline planes of, completing equilibration by adjustment of, 129

  maxillary, position of, 125–126

  non-anatomic, 120

  semi-anatomic, 120

  Vita Physiodens, set-up procedure for balanced occlusion utilizing, 113

Telescopic crown techniques, advantages of, 194

Telescopic riggings, 33

The 21 Indispensable Qualities of a Leader, 216–217

Thick bone, classification of edentulous ridges based on, 17–18

Thin bone, classification of edentulous ridges based on, 18

Thornton bridge and implant cleaner, implant overdentures and, 212

Threads, exposed, 146

3D planning software, implant, 27

Ti6Al4V alloy, Endopore Dental Implant System and, 161

Tissue

  granulation, around implant head, 147

  peri-implant, ideal, characteristics of, 210

  surrounding, successful integration of implant with, 140

Tissue-implant-supported implant overdenture, 4, 69

Tissue punch technique, maxillary surgery and, 136

Tissue-supported implant overdenture, 4, 69

Titanium bar, prefabricated, advantages of, 77

Titanium plasma spray (TPS), 153

Toothbrushes, implant overdentures and, 211

TPS. See Titanium plasma spray (TPS)

Trabecular core, bone with, classification of edentulous ridges based on, 17–18

Trajectory of implant, alignment of, Maximus OS overdenture implant and, 169

Transfer screw, difficulty inserting, 147

Transitional implants during healing phase, overdenture implants acting as, 169

Translation, attachment selection and, 31

Treatment

  comparisons of, for implant overdentures, 104–107

  planning of, diagnosis and. See Diagnosis and treatment planning, 11

Treatment room preparation and utilization protocol, 133

Treatment success with overdentures, 104–107

  biomechanical risk factors for lower implant overdentures and, 105

  biomechanical risk factors for upper implant overdentures and, 105

implant survival and, 104
  patient related factors and, 105
  prosthetic success and, 104
  shape of mandible and its effect on loading of
    supporting implants and, 107
Trial close, successful implant practice and,
    221–222
Tri-calcium phosphate, resorbable blast
    texturing and, 170
21 Indispensable Qualities of a Leader,
    216–217

Universal resilient attachments, 32
Upper first molar
  occlusal contacts of, 119
  setting up, 119
Upper first premolars, occlusal contacts
    between lower first premolars and, 114
Upper implant overdentures, biomechanical
    risk factors for, 105
Upper second molar
  occlusal contacts of
  setting up, 114
Upper second premolars
  occlusal contacts of, 115
  setting up, 115
Utilization procedures, chair-side. *See*
    Chair-side utilization procedures

Vario Ball-Snap-OC, 44
Vario Soft Bar Pattern VSP, 76–77
  clips of, shapes of, 76
  shapes of, 76
Verification of passive seat of bar, 82
Vertical movement, attachment selection and,
    31
Vertical relationship of bar to alveolar ridge,
    bar attachments and, 66

Vertical resilient attachments, restricted, 32
Vestibular incision, 135
Vestibular incisions, mandibular surgery and,
    134
Vestibular release, anterior crestal incision with
    or without, 133–134
Vestibular releasing incisions, crestal incision
    with, 133–134
Video, lessening of anxiety and, 223, 229–230
Vision, successful implant practice and, 216
Vita Physiodens teeth, set-up procedure for
    balanced occlusion utilizing, 113–114
VKS-OC rs stud attachment, 44

Waiting room, successful implant practice and,
    229
Warfarin (Coumadin), effect of, on coagulation
    process, 132
Website, successful implant practice and, 227
Widening of osteotomy, Maximus OS
    overdenture implant and, 137
Width of bone in diagnosis and treatment
    planning, 15
Wieland Dental-Technik Germany, 92
Wilson, curve of, 125
Working excursion, eccentric jaw movements
    and, 127
Working side, eccentric balance and, 127
Workup, diagnostic, for implant overdentures,
    11
Wound closure, Straumann Implant System
    and, 159–160

X1, positioning device, 29
Xanax, 133
Xenogeneic bone, bone grafting and, 141
X-rays, panoramic, magnification error of,
    determining, 11–12